Naked to the Bone

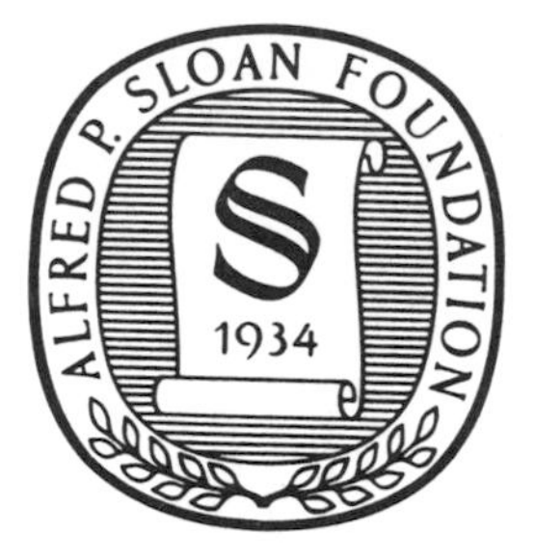

The Sloan Technology Series

Dark Sun: The Making of the Hydrogen Bomb by Richard Rhodes

Dream Reaper: The Story of an Old-Fashioned Inventor in the High-Tech, High-Stakes World of Modern Agriculture by Craig Canine

Turbulent Skies: The History of Commercial Aviation by Thomas A. Heppenheimer

Tube: The Invention of Television by David E. Fisher and Marshall Jon Fisher

The Invention That Changed the World: How a Small Group of Radar Pioneers Won the Second World War and Launched a Technological Revolution by Robert Buderi

Computer: A History of the Information Machine by Martin Campbell-Kelly and William Aspray

Naked to the Bone: Medical Imaging in the Twentieth Century by Bettyann Holtzmann Kevles

A Commotion in the Blood: A Century of Using the Immune System to Battle Cancer and Other Diseases by Stephen S. Hall

Beyond Engineering: A New Way of Thinking about Technology by Robert Pool

The One Best Way: Frederick Winslow Taylor and the Enigma of Efficiency by Robert Kanigel

Crystal Fire: The Birth of the Information Age by Michael Riordan and Lillian Hoddeson

Naked to the Bone

Medical Imaging in the Twentieth Century

Bettyann Holtzmann Kevles

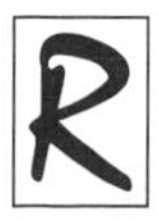

Rutgers University Press
New Brunswick, New Jersey

Library of Congress Cataloging-in-Publication Data

Kevles, Bettyann Holtzmann.
Naked to the bone : medical imaging in the twentieth century / Bettyann Holtzmann Kevles.
p. cm. — (Sloan technology series)
Includes bibliographical references and index.
ISBN 0-8135-2358-3 (cloth : alk. paper)
1. Diagnostic imaging—History. 2. Radiography, Medical—History. I. Title. II. Series.
RC78.7.D53K48 1997
616.07'54'0904—dc20 96-2844
CIP

British Cataloging-in-Publication information available

Manufactured in the United States of America
Published by Rutgers University Press, New Brunswick, New Jersey

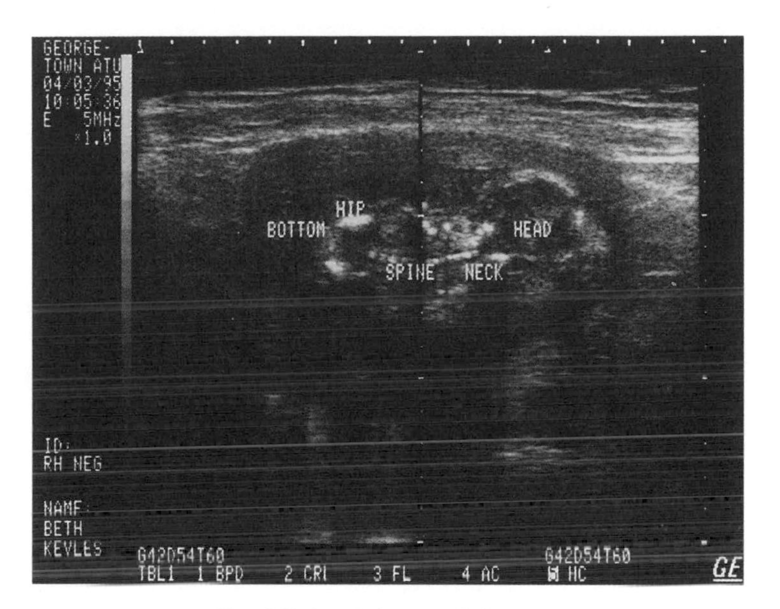

For Michael Aaron Salzman,
born September 23, 1995

Contents

List of Illustrations ix
Preface to the Sloan Technology Series xiii

Introduction 1

Part I The X-Ray Years

One The Discovery of X-Rays: Seeing Is Believing 9
Two Medical Applications: The Living Body beneath the Skin 33
Three Technological Innovation 1897–1918: Building a Better Mousetrap 54
Four Medical Politics between the Wars: Setting Standards 77
Five Technological Innovation 1918–1940: Sharper, Clearer, Deeper 97
Six X-Rays in the Imagination: The Avant-Garde through Surrealism 116

Part II Beyond the X-Ray

Seven The Perfect Slice: The Story of CT Scanning 145
Eight A Subtler Slice: Magnetic Resonance Imaging 173
Nine From the Inside Out: PET (Positron Emission Tomography) in Nuclear Medicine 201

Ten Looking through Women: The Development of Ultrasound and Mammography *228*

Eleven The Transparent Body in Late Twentieth-Century Culture *261*

Epilogue *297*

Timeline *303*
Acknowledgments *319*
Notes *323*
Bibliography *345*
Index *365*

List of Illustrations

1. Alexander Graham Bell with President Garfield 11
2. Bullet in President Garfield's spine 12
3. Wilhelm Conrad Roentgen 18
4. Frau Roentgen's hand, 1895 21
5. "The Wondrous X-rays" 25
6. "Naked Truth" R. V. Wagner & Sons advertisement 29
7. Tolman Cunnings being X-rayed at McGill 31
8. Painting showing fluoroscopic examination of a woman 34
9. Radiograph by Michael Pupin of Prescott Butler's hand 35
10. Edison examines a hand through his fluoroscope 37
11. Mihran K. Kassabian 50
12. Friedlander X-ray protective suit 56
13. Radiograph of a face with and without the Bucky grid 65
14. Picture of the spine using Potter improvement of the Bucky grid 66
15. Marie Curie driving a "petit curie" during World War I 72
16. Marie Curie with seventeen-year-old Irène 73
17. En route to the X-ray room, World War I 75
18. Chest X-rays, 1902 78
19. Air in the brain, 1913 98
20. The first encephalograph, 1919 101

21. Pablo Picasso, *Les Demoiselles d'Avignon* *125*
22. Marcel Duchamp, *Nude Descending a Staircase* *128*
23. Francis Picabia, *Mechanical Expression as seen through our own Mechanical Expression* *129*
24. Pablo Picasso, *Girl Before a Mirror* *133*
25. Frida Kahlo, *The Broken Column* *135*
26. John Heartfield, *Hitler Swallows Gold and Spouts Junk* *138*
27. John Heartfield, *Das ist das Heil, das sie bringen!* *139*
28. Oldendorf's model CT scanning machine *150*
29. First transmission section scan of a living human thorax, 1965 *154*
30. First clinical prototype EMI brain scanner, 1972 *159*
31. First clinical CT image *160*
32. Five CT brain scans, 1974–1980 *164*
33. MRI of normal spine *174*
34. Fetal mice in the living womb *190*
35. Surgery performed in an open MRI machine *192*
36. MRI of brain with multiple sclerosis *195*
37. MRI of brain with pituitary macroadenoma *196*
38. MRI of ruptured silicone breast implant *197*
39. MRI of human molar *200*
40. Whole body PET/FDG study *212*
41. Serial PET study of glucose metabolism *213*
42. Serial PET studies in patients with high-grade brain tumors *214*
43. Pre- and posthemispherectomy PET scan of child *218*
44. PET/FDG-glucose study of local cerebral metabolic rates in normal human infant and adult *219*
45. A comparison of CT, MRI, and PET brain images *222*
46. Diagram of a fetus from X-rays, 1917 *231*
47. A hyperphonogram *233*
48. A "patient" demonstrating early ultrasound *237*
49. Cross-section of the neck with ultrasound *238*
50. Demonstration of Wild's breast scanner *239*
51. B-mode water-bath scanner *240*
52. A 1964 ultrasound scan of the fetal head *242*
53. Ultrasound image taken through the mother's abdomen *248*
54. Georges Chicotot, self-portrait with breast cancer patient *251*
55. Mammography of R. Leborgne *252*
56. First xeroradiograph of the breast *255*
57. Steve Miller, *Portrait of Veronique Maxe* *259*
58. Francis Bacon, *Head Surrounded by Sides of Beef* *270*

59. Robert Rauschenberg, *Booster* 272
60. Laura Ferguson, *Rib Cage with Spine* 274
61. Tori Ellison, *X-Dress* 276
62. Ted Meyer, *Structural Abnormalities* 277
63. Agnes Denes, *Introspection III—Aesthetics (X-rays of the Masters)* 279
64. Sheila Pinkel, *Instinct Extinct?* 280
65. Sheila Pinkel, *Kachina Transform* 281
66. David Teplica, *Birth of Man with Homage to Michelangelo* 282
67. Pavel Tchelitchew, *Hide-and-Seek* 284
68. Alex Grey, *Pregnancy* 285
69. Andy Warhol, *Philip's Skull (CAT Scan)* 288
70. Steve Miller, *L'Origine du Monde* 290
71. May H. Lesser, *Sagittal Series 1/10* 291
72. Joyce Cutler Shaw, *The Anatomy Lesson: Memory Picture with CT* 293
73. Nina Sobell, *Interactive Electroencephalographic Brainwave Drawing* 294
74. Annie Liebovitz, *Laurie Anderson MRI* 295

Preface to the Sloan Technology Series

Technology is the application of science, engineering, and industrial organization to create a human-built world. It has led, in developed nations, to a standard of living inconceivable a hundred years ago. The process, however, is not free of stress: by its very nature, technology brings change in society and undermines convention. It affects virtually every aspect of human endeavor: private and public institutions, economic systems, communications networks, political structures, international affiliations, the organization of societies, and the condition of human lives. The effects are not one-way; just as technology changes society, so too do societal structures, attitudes, and mores affect technology. But perhaps because technology is so rapidly and completely assimilated, the profound interplay of technology and other social endeavors in modern history has not been sufficiently recognized.

The Sloan Foundation has a long-standing interest in deepening public understanding about modern technology, its origins, and its impact on our lives. The Sloan Technology Series, of which the present volume is a part, seeks to present to the general reader the story of the development of critical twentieth-century technologies. The aim of the series is to convey both the technical and human dimensions of the subject: the invention and effort entailed in devising the technologies and the comforts and stresses they have introduced into contemporary life. As the century draws to an end, it is hoped that the series will disclose a past that might provide perspective on the present and inform the future.

The Foundation has been guided in its development of the Sloan Technology Series by a distinguished advisory committee. We express deep gratitude to

John Armstrong, Simon Michael Bessie, Samuel Y. Gibbon, Thomas P. Hughes, Victor McElheny, Robert K. Merton, Elting E. Morison (deceased), and Richard Rhodes. The foundation has been represented on the committee by Ralph E. Gomory, Arthur L. Singer, Jr., Hirsch G. Cohen, A. Frank Mayadas, and Doron Weber.

Alfred P. Sloan Foundation

Naked to the Bone

Introduction

On a warm summer afternoon in 1996, six middle-aged people sat around a conference table. It had been a long day and the men's ties lay limp on the backs of chairs while one of the women, her high-heeled shoes discarded nearby, wriggled her toes to restore circulation.

"That reminds me of Berlin in 1936," a man observed. "My mother used to take me to a shoe store where I put my feet under a fluoroscope to watch my bones." The group sat up, revived by nostalgia. They were all children again, recalling the same experience in Indianapolis, Bakersfield, Manhattan, Wellington, and Shanghai. The memory triggered grins at first, and moments later, the barefoot woman was the first to shudder. She was trying to estimate the quantity of radiation she had unwittingly absorbed.

For each the shoe store was a first encounter with a technology that allowed them to see into their own bodies. Since then the six had also sampled all the daughter technologies of X-rays—computerized tomography, magnetic resonance imaging, positron emission tomography, and ultrasound. They had benefited from the revolution that transformed diagnostic medicine, but they had also seen its unanticipated side effects. In the mingling of wonder and fear that characterized their memories, they reflected both the awe and the ambivalence with which twentieth-century culture responded to this extraordinary technology.

The event that began it all occurred on November 8, 1895, when Wilhelm

Roentgen discovered what he called "a new kind of light." Two months later, in January 1896, Roentgen revealed the X-ray to the rest of the world. The discovery of X-rays may be the only major scientific discovery that was entirely unanticipated, but which was nonetheless accepted immediately, universally, and without question. The X-ray fitted extraordinarily well into the technical and cultural aspirations of fin de siècle society. Born at almost exactly the same time as the motion picture, the X-ray, too, thrived on advances in photography, physics, and chemistry. But even more than movies, X-rays validated suspicions that the cultural avant-garde had begun to articulate—that much of what was presented as useful, good, beautiful, and permanent was deceptive and ephemeral.

Aside from the chance discovery of X-rays, the development of various methods of imaging followed a common path. Within days of Roentgen's announcement, in a process that was never coordinated but would be repeated often, doctors, engineers, physicists, and chemists raced to improve the scope and quality of the images. The original X-ray tube was crude, its powers of penetration limited to exposing bones and foreign objects inside the body. Better focus seemed an obvious refinement, and within months patents were filed in Europe and North America addressing the problem. Throughout the twentieth century, this pattern of independent simultaneous discoveries and multiple patents was repeated in improvements to X-ray apparatus and in the development of CT, MRI, PET, and ultrasound.

With astonishing speed, people got used to seeing their insides displayed as snapshots in black and white or in moving images on a screen. This unprecedented familiarity with our own anatomy separates the modern view of external and internal from that of previous eras. That earlier, opaque world so full of mysteries on every level—anatomical, sexual, and mental—began to dissolve when X-ray mania swept the West.

It is hard to imagine how wonderful the X-rays seemed in the euphoric winter of 1896. One enthusiast described the experience as "the mind walk[ing] in among the tissues themselves." X-ray images of the body helped shift social and moral boundaries. The idea of "private parts," of privacy itself, began to change, and has continued to change throughout the century, depending on the kinds of images, and the responses of the people being imaged. No matter how the "new light" of X-rays was explained—as invisible rays or particles or as something supernatural—it changed the world.

A great deal of the intellectual effort of the last hundred years has been spent visualizing what was once invisible. Consequently, what used to be private—the brain and genitalia—is now public, an unexpected trade-off for the privilege of visually penetrating the deepest recesses of mind and body. Things that had been opaque, like skin, were now transparent, and what had been hidden could now be known. What had seemed a surface disappeared, and volume stood out as a mist of overlapping layers. The black and white images of the early X-rays simplified interior spaces that, until then, had been seen mostly by surgeons—bloody, messy, and confused with a multiplicity of colors and textures. The reality of the X-rayed body was redefined as a receding series of gray-toned planes.

Naked to the Bone tells the history of medical imaging from Roentgen's discovery in 1895 to the present, as imaging affected our entire culture. While this book traces the technological developments and their consequences in medicine, it also explores the impact that this new way of seeing has had upon society at large. Citizens of the twentieth century often sensed that their world differed in kind from what came before, and that science and technology are responsible for that difference.

Certainly there were negative aesthetic and economic effects from earlier aspects of the Industrial Revolution. Railroads cut ugly trenches through the countryside, leaving clouds of filthy coal smoke in their wake; the steam-powered mills in Massachusetts polluted once pristine rivers; and dislocation and unemployment followed the mechanization of factories. A hundred years after X rays entered public discourse, we are used to the notion of invisible effects that are remote in time and space from visible causes—like the ozone hole in the atmosphere, or chemical pollution. But a century ago people did not suspect science. The X-ray was the first technology that taught us, collectively, to hold our breath, waiting for the next shoe to drop. But the lesson came slowly, and the contribution of X-rays to making that break with the past, while more subtle, perhaps, than the impact of the automobile or airplane, is equally profound, interesting, and controversial.

The book falls naturally into two parts, corresponding roughly in time with the two halves of the century. The first part traces the history of the single technology of X-ray imaging; the second, the array of new competing technologies that arose after World War II when television and computers began to contribute to medical imaging.

In the first part, the emphasis is on the refinement of the technology of the X-ray and the immediate consequences of its discovery. As the machines improved, physicians gradually pushed back the veil in front of the internal organs, revealing first the living skeleton, then the stomach, intestines, gall bladder, lungs, heart, and brain.

These technological advances often came from several independent, different places at the same time, triggering discord over attribution of credit, laurels, and dividends. In any event, the actual market success of particular improvements was more a matter of historical accident than of any technological imperative.

As scientists, engineers, and physicians worked to make the X-ray machines more effective, the new technology stepped onto the stage of history. Part I also describes the ways X-rays figured in historic events, from political assassinations to world wars, and examines the ways X-rays changed the practice of medicine, the rules of evidence, the vision of artists—indeed, the self-perception of an entire culture.

Hard on the heels of physicians, lawyers introduced X-ray evidence into the courtroom and the crime lab. Throughout this book, courts play the role of candid camera: they fix the instant at which each new technology is accepted or doubted, codifying the rules for its acceptance as a legitimate way to convey reality.

Part I surveys the hold X-rays had on the imagination of the era. From pulp fiction to the fine arts, writers, artists, and movie-makers played exuberantly with the idea of seeing through bodies with invisible rays, of looking for secrets beneath the surface. They made their audiences reconsider what it was they were seeing.

Doctors live in society, as do chemists and physicists, and so it is not surprising that not long after X-rays had been shown visually to penetrate living flesh, the insights of these scientists were available to the educated and professional classes. They, in turn, reconsidered what it was they were seeing, and what vision itself meant. Inevitably, with doctors and lawyers seeing the world differently, the rest of the public gradually shifted its perceptions about intimacy and privacy.

Yet for all the rapid exploitation of the applications of X-rays, a curious aspect of radioactivity's introduction into modern life was the willful denial of its unanticipated side effects by so many of its champions. Before 1945, although radiation from X-rays had killed and maimed doctors, technicians, factory workers, miners, and some patients, too, few people associated X-rays with catastrophe. In truth, deaths directly attributable to X-ray exposure were probably very few in comparison to the thousands of deaths before 1945 from industrial accidents or killer diseases like polio and tuberculosis—diseases which X-ray diagnosis helped ameliorate.

However, from the year of their discovery, X-rays were associated with cancer. The machine that could spot lesions before they were visible to the naked eye, the machine that could cure some tumors, could also, it seemed, cause them. At the same time that Part I recounts the progress of X-ray technology, it also tells a darker story. The growing shadow of fear provoked the adoption of radiation safety standards, and an effort to quantify and regulate dosage. The X-ray was the first technology to come with a built-in time bomb. The shock of this realization tore at the fabric of faith in all technology—and that was perhaps the biggest change the X-ray made in twentieth-century sensibilities.

Part II deals with the second stage of the imaging revolution. Thomas Hughes suggests in *American Genesis* that the convergence of two new technologies can cause a revolution.[1] This is precisely what happened when X-rays met computers and produced CT, MRI, PET, and ultrasound. Each of these scanners reconstructs cross-sectional slices of the interior of the body, or creates three-dimensional volume images.

Unlike the X-ray, which had arrived full-blown to a surprised society, the computer developed from the 1940s on, gaining momentum as its hardware shrank from tubes, to transistors, to chips. Although computers were used commercially from the early 1950s, their potential for reconstructing images was only apparent after the 1970s. And even then, their improved capacity for speed and memory happened faster than the new breed of fortune-tellers who called themselves "futurists" dared to imagine.

Medical imaging has always combined research in basic science with engineering know-how. Not surprisingly, there is only one amateur in the early history—a patient who devised a way to image his own tubercular lungs—and none in the second half of the century. The interplay has involved collaboration between highly trained scientists, mathematicians, engineers, and doctors. This was not the place for the tinkerer whose exploits delight the history of less sophisticated instruments.

Although they evolved pretty much on their own for at least a decade after 1950, all of the daughter technologies benefited from the technological advances of World War II. Developing concurrently, each gained from the experiences of the others, borrowing from their use of computer algorithms or their achievements in marketing, for example, or exploiting their limits. Their histories differ until they collide with the advent of the computer.

As computerized imaging techniques entered the clinic, each at some point offered a way to detect malignant tissue. By the late twentieth century, the notion of "seeing" the seeds of cancer was tightly connected to the possibility of cure or remission.

In Part II these technologies are chronicled according to their appearance in the marketplace. CT scanning startled the medical world in 1972 with the image of the cross-section of a living brain. A decade later MRI, a creative application of the chemistry of nuclear magnetic resonance, was operating in clinics in Great Britain and the United States. Then came PET, a specialized form of nuclear medicine, itself a subspecialty with a long history of therapeutic applications. Because this is the story of imaging, nuclear medicine is only described in its remarkable, and relatively new, efforts to capture metabolic action in the living body. The discussion of the history of ultrasound, which has become part of contemporary pregnancy monitoring, and mammography, a special kind of X-ray diagnosis designed exclusively for women, uses particular patients to track a general trend. A discussion of the impact of all these new imaging techniques on culture underscores the way technology affects the entire society, not just those who manufacture, use, or are diagnosed by the machines.

Naked to the Bone recounts the impact that X-rays and its daughter technologies have had on diagnosis. It is not about radiation or ultrasonic therapy, although occasionally therapeutic applications figure in the narrative. In the hall of radiation horrors, most of the casualties of medical imaging have been people who were receiving treatments, although, as readers will discover, exposure to excessive diagnostic X-rays also took a toll.

The translation of computerized data from printed figures to a television image is as great a technological revolution as harnessing X-rays was in the nineteenth century. But the application of computers to imaging devices, despite the extraordinary difference between films of bones and colored representations of three-dimensional views of the inside of the brain, did not shatter cultural standards the way the introduction of X-rays did. That revolution, the revelation of the inside of the living body, occurred only once, in 1895. Although the technologies of imaging have expanded remarkably throughout the century, the removal of the scales from our collective eyes occurred just this once.

Twentieth-century culture accepted the dissolution of opacity with equanimity. The idea of X-ray vision became commonplace and reshaped the sensibilities of artists as well as of juries and judges, who hammered out new definitions of evidence and even of crimes, and of the medical profession, which used imaging technologies to attract patients, insurers, and corporate investment.

Although X-rays were discovered in Germany, they were rapidly explored by physicians and engineers in the United States. No technology in the twentieth century has evolved in national isolation. Ideas and skilled minds moved with the great migrations and carried new technologies across national borders. But a disproportionate amount of the technical innovation in imaging occurred in the United States, which benefited economically from the two great wars of the first half of the century. The size and structure of the American medical market shaped these technologies, which absorbed contributions from other countries without ever losing their American stamp.

The imaging revolution began with the stubborn determination of a somewhat pedestrian German physicist in November 1895 to explain a strange luminescence which ought not to have been there. It evolved into a continuing search for ways to capture visually smaller and smaller parts of the human body. This ongoing search has revolutionized the science of biology and the practice of medicine. How this happened, how it affected the nature of medicine, the law, and our culture as a whole, its grandiose promises and apparent betrayals, are the multiple and interrelated stories that comprise *Naked to the Bone.*

Part I

The X-Ray Years

One

The Discovery of X-Rays

Seeing Is Believing

On a hot, humid July morning in 1881, President James A. Garfield arrived early at the old Baltimore and Potomac depot on the corner of Sixth and B Streets in Washington, D.C. He had left his wife, Lucretia, with two of their four children the day before at what we would now call the "summer White House" in Long Branch, New Jersey, and returned to Washington before he was to head north again to Williams College in Massachusetts, where hundreds of students and parents anticipated seeing the president, a distinguished alumnus, receive an honorary degree. The waiting room at the station was almost empty when he arrived and, concerned about the time, Garfield checked with a policeman. Not to worry, Officer Kearney assured him, he had ten minutes before the 9:30 train was due. We know this because the policeman later testified in court that he had moved on, then turned abruptly at what sounded like a firecracker in time to see a bearded man fire a second time before anyone could interfere. This would be the last presidential shooting before the discovery of X-rays.

In a matter of seconds the district health officer, Dr. Smith Townsend, who happened to be nearby, was at Garfield's side, cutting through the president's gray traveling suit to probe the bullet hole with his bare index finger. Dr. Townsend estimated that the bullet, which had entered from behind, had turned right at the kidney and lodged somewhere in the small of his back. They would not know for sure until the inevitable autopsy.

The president was calm enough in the chaos that followed to ask to be taken back to the White House. Someone yanked mattresses from a nearby Pullman car and piled them into an express cart for a makeshift ambulance. By the time the president had been carried back up Pennsylvania Avenue, the south bedroom of the White House had been turned into a hospital. Despite Townsend's prediction, Garfield, a vigorous man of forty-nine, rallied. Soon he was sitting up and sipping fluids.

Half a dozen doctors collected in the White House, all stymied because they couldn't find the bullet. They pondered the president's condition and monitored his progress with state-of-the-art instruments—stethoscopes and thermometers. They were obsessed with the bullet: without knowing where it was, they couldn't decide whether to leave it alone or try probing blindly. The hidden bullet dominated national news while White House physicians argued publicly. Editorials all over the country demanded "Where is the bullet?" In an age that had seen the invention of the telephone and telegraph, the public demanded that someone find a way to detect a bullet lodged inside the president's body.

But even sophisticated people who were getting used to letting doctors look into their eyes with ophthalmoscopes or listen to their hearts with stethoscopes had no reason to imagine that they would *see* the bullet. When they said "locate," they meant some kind of metal detector.

Listening for the Bullet

A week after the crime, Simon Newcomb, the physicist-astronomer who headed the Naval Observatory in Washington, mused at a news conference that it might be possible to locate the bullet by the process of electrical induction. But he immediately dismissed the idea as too complicated to make workable in time.

Alexander Graham Bell, the Scottish inventor who had won international fame with his telephone, disagreed. Convinced that a machine that combined induction with some aspects of his telephone could save Garfield, he wired Newcomb to say that he thought he could rig up such a machine quickly. The next day, Bell left his home in Boston and, with his assistant Sumner Tainter, took a train to the capital.[1]

Bell was then at the peak of his popularity. In 1881 his Bell Telephone Company had become the first corporation ever to gross a million dollars in a single year. Bursting with confidence when he arrived in Washington, Bell recalled for the press a remarkable "induction machine" he had seen three years earlier in London, an apparatus that could generate an electrical field around a man. With such a machine, Bell asserted, an operator could pass an exploring coil over someone, like a divining rod seeking hidden water: the moment the coil passed over metal it would trip a mechanism to signal its find. The machine would literally get a ringing response from a lead bullet.

Bell drove directly from the depot to the White House, then a parklike oasis in the mosquito-ridden swampy city. (Over the next three weeks, four staff members would come down with malaria.) Washington was less developed than Boston or New York City, but like most other American cities it had gas lighting and indoor plumbing for the well-to-do, empty lots awaiting development, and very few paved streets.

To protect the president from the oppressive heat, his staff moved him to the north bedroom where Simon Newcomb, with the help of the naval engineers, rigged up what may have been the first electrical air-conditioning system. (It lowered the temperature twenty degrees by forcing air over six tons of ice blocks in the White House basement. The air was then dehumidified and conveyed through the hot-air registers.)

As the president lay sipping iced champagne, Bell and Tainter went to work. Starting from scratch, they scavenged equipment from all over town: huge induction coils that the physicist Joseph Henry had left to the Smithsonian, twenty enormous Bunsen elements that were used to ignite the gas lamps in the Capitol, and an electric motor from the Western Union Telegraph Company. The capital, like the rest of the nation, was decades away from providing electric power to every wall of every building. With this jerry-built arrangement, Bell and Tainter first experimented on themselves by holding bullets in their mouths, clenched fists, and armpits, taking turns passing a coil over their bodies and

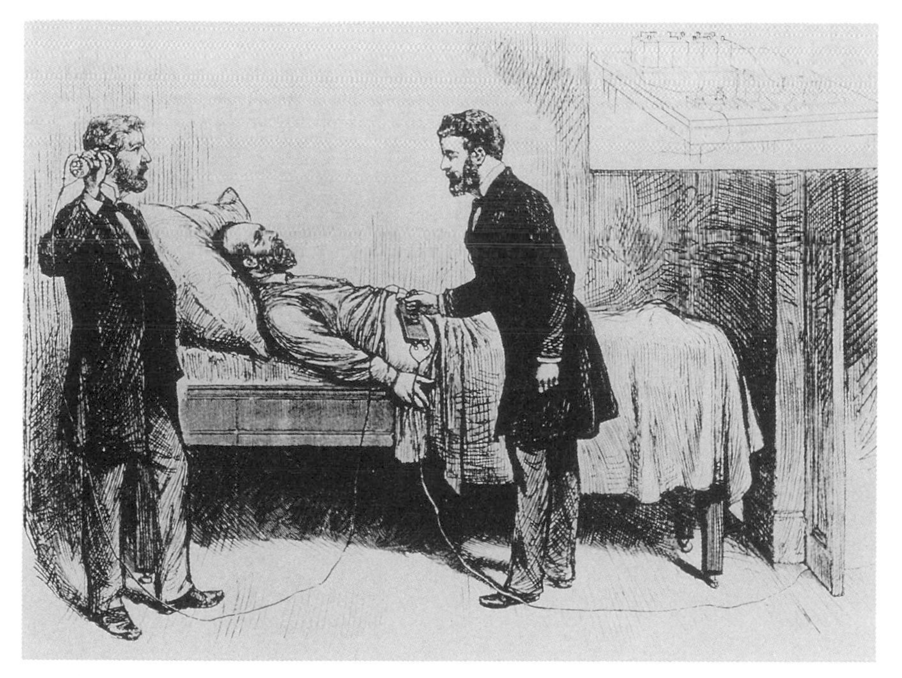

1. Alexander Graham Bell with President Garfield (1881). Bell devised a sound induction device to locate the bullet lodged inside Garfield's body. The upper right-hand corner shows a sketch of Bell's machine. Courtesy of the Archives Center, National Museum of American History, Smithsonian Institution.

listening for a faint telephonic click. Bell fine-tuned his machine by firing bullets into slabs of freshly slaughtered beef and experimenting with a bullet-ridden corpse whose build resembled the president's.

On July 26, twenty-five days after the shooting, Bell wheeled his apparatus into Garfield's bedroom. Under the gaze of five doctors, he moved the coil slowly over the dying man's body. For one instant he seemed to hear a signal, but the source turned out to be unsuspected metal coils inside the presidential hair mattress.

The idea was sensible, but the method was crude. It would be another thirty years before anyone successfully used sound waves to locate hidden objects (and then the objects would be icebergs after the sinking of the *Titanic* in 1912), and another fifty years before sound waves would be able to capture a picture of anything, including a bullet, inside a body.

President Garfield succumbed on September 19, eighty days after the attack. On the following day, an autopsy showed that the bullet had in fact turned left, 180 degrees away from Dr. Townsend's estimated path, and was lodged to the left of the vertibrate near the pancreas. The reputations of Townsend and the rest of the medical team plummeted.

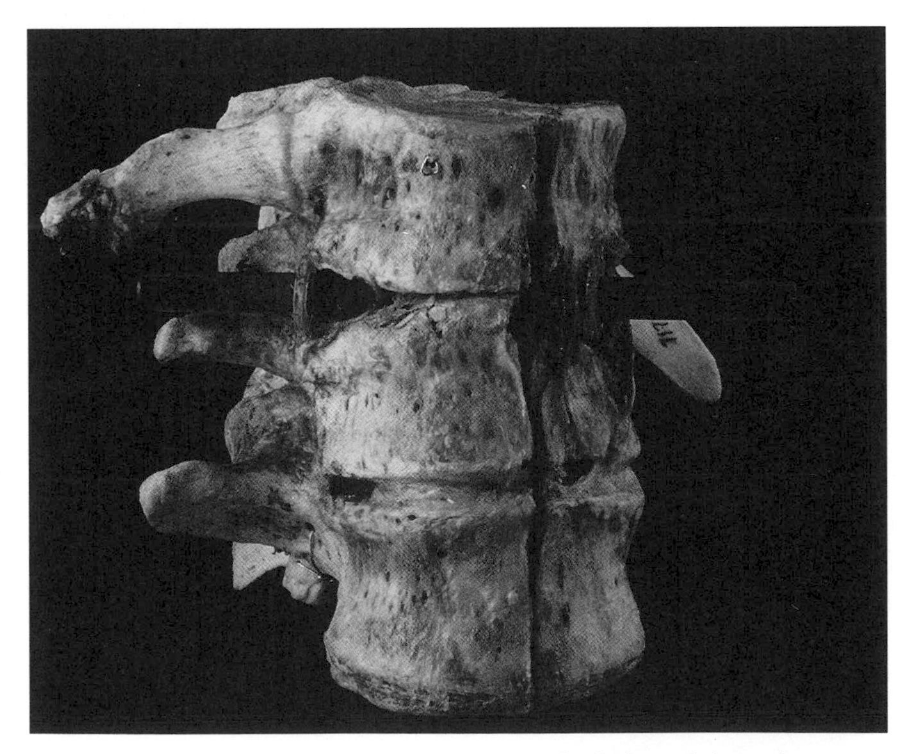

2. Bullet in President Garfield's spine. The bullet was finally located during the autopsy. Courtesy of the National Museum of Health and Medicine, Armed Forces Institute of Pathology, Department of Defense.

From Bell's point of view, however, although the patient died, the experiment was a success. Discounting his failure to locate Garfield's bullet, Bell patented his machine, which he described the following summer to the American Association for the Advancement of Science as "Electrical Experiments to Determine the Location of the Bullet in the Body of the Late President Garfield and upon a *Successful* Form of Induction Balance for the Painless Detection of Metallic Masses in the Human Body" (my italics). The nation hailed his patriotism. In November 1882, the Supreme Court of the District of Columbia granted the Scottish inventor American citizenship.

An unacknowledged competition was underway in the last decades of the nineteenth century between the domestication of sound and of light. With the invention and almost instant commercialization of the telephone in 1876, sound seemed to take the lead. For the first time in history, the human voice could be transmitted miles from the mouth of the person speaking. Edison's phonograph, in 1877, was an accomplishment of a different order of magnitude.

The phonograph was the first invention to capture a transient sensual experience, the first, it seemed, to conquer time. After listening to a demonstration, the writer Edward Bellamy published a short story in *Harper's Monthly*, "With the Eyes Shut." Bellamy's hero, traveling west by train from Boston and unable to read because of motion sickness, is rescued from boredom by a vendor renting gadgets uncannily like a modern Walkman, complete with earphones. The traveler listens to a book as he watches the passing scene and then discovers, after arriving in remote Colorado, that everyone in Denver is walking around with these gadgets in their ears. Moreover, in the short time since they had become "listeners," these westerners had forgotten how to read and write.

Bellamy suggests that hearing is the sense of the future, and coming none too soon to rescue eyesight, which "was indeed terribly overburdened previous to the introduction of the phonograph, and now that the sense of hearing is beginning to assume its proper share of work, it would be strange if an improvement in the condition of people's eyes were not noticeable."[2]

In the early 1890s sound seemed to be the door to a technology explosion. In medicine the stethoscope had become a staple in the physician's black bag, and percussion of the chest had become a routine method of sounding out disease. The possibilities of recording sounds on a phonograph inspired other writers of futuristic fiction as well as psychologists and linguists. (In 1900 the Anthropology Society of Paris founded a "glossophonographic" museum, and the Vienna Academy of Science started a phonographic archive.)

Neither Bellamy nor any of his contemporary fantasists predicted the technological possibilities of sight. They did not foretell moving pictures, and they certainly did not imagine a machine that could take pictures through solid matter, much less penetrate human skin to get a picture of the bones beneath. There is no reason they should have.

The idea that rays exist that penetrate the body had been around for ages. As far back as the thirteenth century the philosopher Roger Bacon had noted that "no substance is so dense as to prevent rays from passing. The rays of heat and sound penetrate through the walls of a vessel of gold or brass."[3] There were also spiritual rays that emanated from the body to the outside world, portrayed by artists as the spectacular halos painted around the heads of saints and the holy family. But nowhere did artist or philosopher suggest that any rays, whether passing from the outside in or emerging from the soul out through the skin, could reveal everything beneath the skin to the human eye, much less leave an impression on something else, like a shadow on a wall or a permanent imprint on glass or film.

What appears to be the only recorded prediction came in a talk delivered to a small group of physicians in Philadelphia in 1872 when the physician James Da Costa satirized the state of medicine by describing a future in which "Dr. Magnet, who is a very accomplished physicist, steps forward: 'If you will permit me, I will make you transparent.' And by means of a modified, portable Ruhmkorff coil [a kind of generator], and an instrument with lenses dexterously passed into the stomach, the fair patient is really rendered transparent."[4]

Looking back, it is hard to understand how deeply opaque the world, and the human body, seemed to everyone before 1896. This was an era when heavy window drapes were drawn each night and lace curtains hung during the day to shield those inside from the eyes of strangers. This was a world where men and women wore several layers of clothing in all seasons and entered the ocean to swim covered from neck to knee. Clothes concealed the skin, and the skin concealed the secrets of the heart. It was a world where full-length mirrors were a luxury, and few people ever saw, much less examined, their own naked bodies. Skeletons, which could be seen only after death, quite reasonably symbolized death.[5] It is a historical irony that the discovery of rays that could penetrate clothing and skin and leave an image of living bones appeared in the most inhibited period in Western history, an era whose name *Victorian* has become synonymous with extreme sexual repression and bodily shame. This era was drawing to a close in the mid-1890s, and the discovery of X-rays was one of the nails in the coffin of Victorian prudery.

Getting Pictures

The opacity of the Victorian world found validation in photography, a technology that had evolved slowly through the course of the nineteenth century. Conceptually, the idea of capturing images on film or glass was a continuation of the age-old human predilection for capturing portraits in paint, pen, or, for the less facile, of tracing silhouettes. Because of the time necessary to get an impression on the earliest photographic plates, the subjects of these portraits look frozen, like children playing "statues." People posed, and although the discomfort was probably negligible in comparison to having to return for repeated sittings for paintings, sitters may have felt that, rather than help capture an instant of time, they had been asked to hold time still.

The first photographic efforts involved chemists who discovered how to capture images on emulsion-covered paper or glass by using a camera obscura, a box with a pinhole to admit light, which had served as a draftsman's aid since the days of Da Vinci. Major advances occurred almost simultaneously in France, where Joseph Niepce and a painter, Louis Daguerre, "fixed" an image from a camera obscura by adding mercury to the silver compounds already in use, and in England, where the chemist Fox Talbot fixed his images on sensitized paper. Talbot, inspired by Daguerre, also invented a way of getting a positive print from a negative without destroying the negative. Talbot's techniques offered a convenient alternative to the cumbersome glass plates that photographers had had to soak in liquid emulsions immediately prior to exposure whenever they wanted to take pictures.

When dry plates entered the market in the 1870s, photography became simple, cheaper, and more commercial. By the mid-1880s, Kodak was selling a camera that amateurs could use. Photographers began recording images that had theretofore been too small, too fast, or too far away to see and capture. By adapting cameras to microscopes and telescopes, they got pictures of subjects as remote in size from each other as human sperm and Saturn's rings. By the 1890s photographs had become the standard recorders of objective scientific truth.

Clever photographers soon developed "slow motion" imagery that enabled naturalists and physiologists to document movement too rapid for the human eye. "Chronophotography" (developed independently by the physiologist Etienne-Jules Marey in France and the artist Eadweard Muybridge in the United States) used multiple pictures to record action, either with a set of cameras that took pictures in rapid sequence, or with a single camera that snapped pictures rapidly. Both approaches produced a series of images that could be analyzed mathematically. Glass plates still produced the clearest pictures, but celluloid film was becoming popular for cheap cameras: it was lightweight, more convenient, and flexible enough to move quickly across the lens to produce a series of motion-study shots. These series of overlapping images became a convention, first among artists like Picasso and Braque, whose images sometimes look like double exposures but are often serieslike as has become the standard among comic strip artists.

Movements that could be slowed down, frame by frame, by photographers could equally well be speeded up to simulate real-time motion. The challenge of creating moving pictures was taken up simultaneously by several inventors. Which one succeeded first is still a matter of controversy. The French have two candidates: Marey, and Auguste and Louis Lumière. Americans favor Muybridge and Thomas Edison. Marey (who had earlier invented a sphygmograph, a device that measured the pulse by tracing a zigzag line) believed in the superiority of visual presentations over words. He experimented with moving pictures by having a single camera take a series of shots rapidly in succession (as compared to Muybridge, who used a series of cameras located near each other, which were tripped to snap in rapid sequence). Edison's invention, the kinetoscope, worked like a stereopticon, a favorite Victorian parlor toy, in the way it was used by only one person at a time, who would gaze into the device's eyepiece to see pictures flipping by so rapidly as to give the impression of a motion picture.

The Lumières alone produced a combination camera and projector that displayed a moving picture onto a screen before a hall full of people. On December 28, 1895, they presented the first motion pictures to an audience at the Grand Café on the Boulevard des Capucines in Paris. Moving photographs on flexible celluloid film were part of the wonderful world of consumer gadgets that the growing middle classes enjoyed in the early months of 1896.

Americans embraced the future, delighting in the novelty of capturing their experiences in tangible form that they could enjoy repeatedly—an evening listening to operatic arias, snapshots of a summer vacation. On the eve of the discovery of X-rays, everything was in place: the cameras were loaded, the projection booth ready to go. But no one was prepared for a device that would change the face of medicine, law, the arts, and the way ordinary people perceived their own bodies.

Pure and Applied Science

When it happened, the world proved astonishingly receptive to this radical shift of perception. Overnight, much of what had seemed solid only the day before was shown to be translucent, even transparent. The public already respected the scientists who explained the miracle. They had listened in wonder to the physicists who were exploring the properties of electromagnetic fields. They had nodded in apparent understanding as these great men explained the mysteries of invisible rays and particles.

The connection between electricity and magnetism had been summarized mathematically by the 1860s by the British physicist James Clerk Maxwell in a set of equations that expressed theoretically the experimental facts about electricity and magnetism acquired in the preceding decades by giants like Faraday, Henry, and Ampère. The solution of Maxwell's equations implied the existence of electromagnetic waves that would propagate from a point just like the water waves that ripple away from a center when a pebble is plunked in a pond. Calculations predicted that these waves would travel at the speed of light, a prediction that suggested to a number of physicists that light waves might be electromagnetic waves, too.

A favorite experiment among the mid-1890s physicists was to send currents through small, pear-shaped glass tubes under various conditions. One very popular tube had been designed by an English chemist, William Crookes, in 1876. A Crookes tube included a metal plate, or *cathode,* at one end and often another metal plate, an *anode,* at the other end or outside of the tube. Crookes figured out how to pump most of the air out of the tube, leaving a near-vacuum inside, which made the cathode last much longer. When voltage was applied to the plates across the evacuated tube, particles which were soon dubbed cathode rays (and would soon be identified as electrons) moved through the tube in a straight line: the rays made the tube glow and made the wall opposite the cathode turn green.

The exploration of electricity, magnetism, and light, which was at the core of cathode ray research, happened in two different kinds of places: the research laboratories that entrepreneurial inventors like Bell and Edison set up in connection with their companies, and the laboratories at universities. Researchers in industrial laboratories were expected to look for practical applications, while university-based researchers were supposed to be devoted exclusively to a search for the laws of nature. In fact, a good deal of theoretical research occurred in industrial laboratories, and practical applications came out of the universities, laying the foundation for the new field of electrical engineering. However, a number of academic physicists adamantly refused to have anything to do with practical research, and Wilhelm Conrad Roentgen was one of them.

Roentgen, familiar in photographs at the time of his discovery of X-rays as a slim man with a full black beard, had held a chair in physics at the University of Würzburg for seven years in 1895. The son of a Dutch mother and German father, he had lived in Holland from the time he was three until he left Utrecht, without a secondary school degree, in the wake of a confrontation with school authorities over his refusal to identify a schoolmate who had drawn a caricature of a teacher. Without a degree, he could not enter a German university but went, instead, to the new Polytechnic in Zurich. There he got a diploma in mechanical engineering and became the protégé of the physicist August Kundt, who supervised Roentgen's Ph.D. in experimental physics and took him to Würzburg as his assistant. In Switzerland Roentgen met two of the people who would most influence his life: Anna Bertha Ludwig, whom he married, and Ludwig Zehnder, a fellow student who was something of a dreamer and against whose character and imagination Roentgen would define himself in letters and discussions for most of his life.

The Roentgens lived a quiet life in Würzburg, raising an adopted niece and enjoying annual hiking vacations in Switzerland. His friends and family remembered Roentgen on these trips as forever moving about with a big box camera and a black cloth over his head. He was a man who always kept visual evidence of where he had been and of what he had seen. Not surprisingly, he also kept photographic equipment in his laboratory.

On November 8, 1895, Roentgen was fifty years old, head of his department at the University of Würzburg, and hard at work investigating the properties of cathode rays. He was using several tubes, including a variation of a Crookes tube designed by a younger colleague, Philipp Lenard. Lenard had found, using his own refinement of a small aluminum foil window in the Crookes tube, that some cathode rays escaped through the aluminum foil window and that he could detect the escaped rays on a fluorescent screen. The rays would make the screen glow when it was set as far as eight centimeters outside the tube, but no farther. Lenard's observations prepared Roentgen for what he was about to see. He had remarkably sharp vision, and it may have been that his excellent eyesight allowed him his brilliant insight.

That particular evening Roentgen, following Lenard's technique, wrapped the tube in black cardboard to prevent distraction from the interior luminescence, turned off the lights, and turned on the Ruhmkorff coil with which he

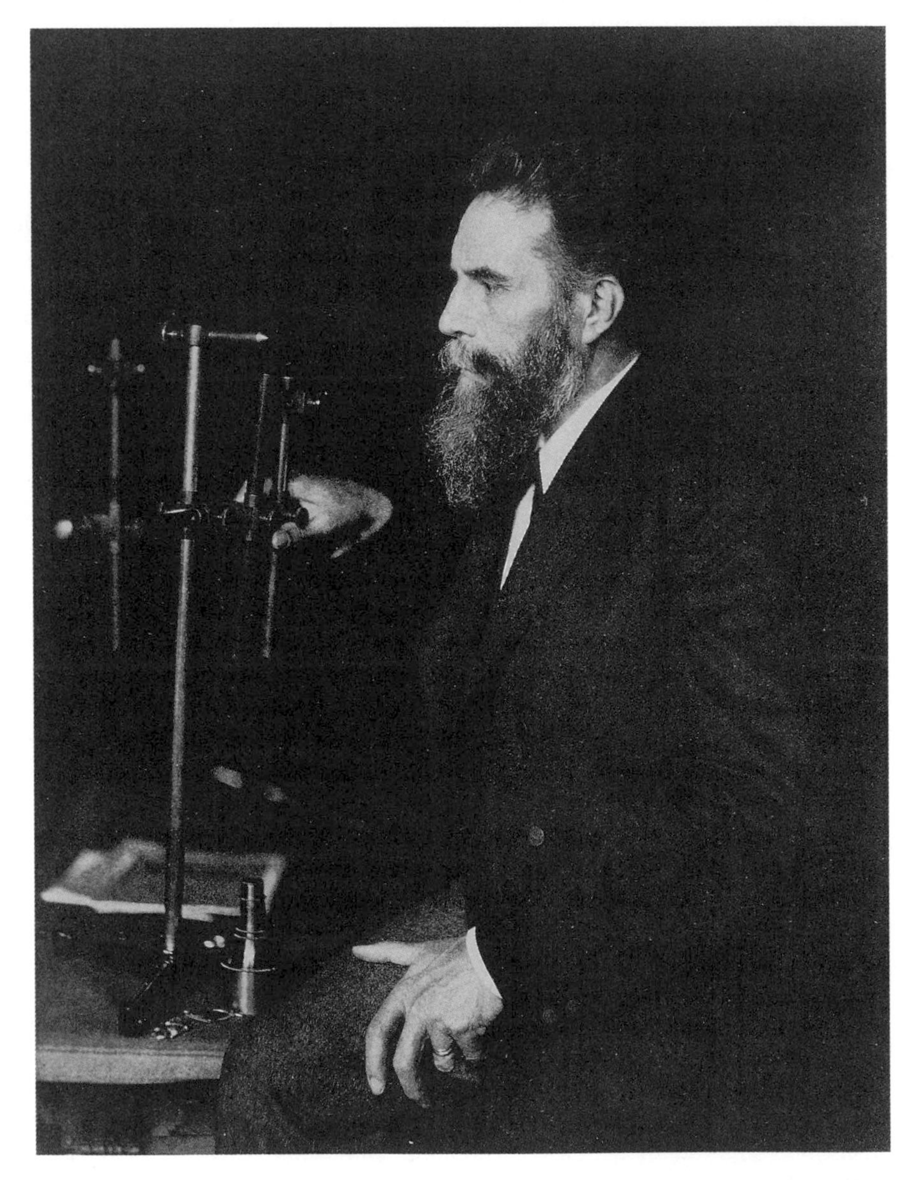

3. Portrait of Wilhelm Conrad Roentgen (1845–1923). This photograph of Roentgen was taken in 1906 while he was director of the Institute of Physics in the University of Munich. Courtesy of the Burndy Library, Dibner Institute, Cambridge, Massachusetts.

generated electric current. By chance, a cardboard screen like the one Lenard had used (it was coated with barium platinocyanide, a fluorescent material used frequently at the time to develop photographic plates) lay on a chair a few feet away. Once his eyes had grown accustomed to the dark, Roentgen noticed a soft glow coming from the screen. (Roentgen was colorblind so did not see that it was green.) He stopped for a moment. The glow, in the shape of the letter "A," came from a screen several feet away on which a student had apparently written after dipping a finger in the liquid barium platinocyanide.[6] It was the kind of glow he had expected to see if he had put the screen just a few centimeters from the tube. But there was nothing he knew of, including Lenard's rays, that could cause fluorescence at such a distance. Puzzled by the phenomenon and unable to explain it, he dropped his original plan and began to investigate the strange luminescence.

He disconnected the current and the fluorescence disappeared. The glow returned with the current. He repeated the experiment over and over until there was no doubt. The screen was glowing in response to something emanating from the tube. Neither cathode rays nor any other rays he could think of could account for the phenomenon. He checked his equipment and recharged the tube. The glow recurred.

Roentgen explored the phenomenon until late into the November evening. When he finally went upstairs to dinner (he lived in the institute) he was so preoccupied and distracted that almost immediately he returned to his laboratory. He did not reveal his discovery to his two assistants but spent all of his time for the next seven weeks alone in his laboratory experimenting and photographing the results. Legend has it that Frau Roentgen quietly slipped in with hot meals, then left him to his obsession as he mumbled that he was working on something so new that the world would think him mad.

To Roentgen, science was a calling, an almost religious obligation to expand knowledge of the natural world. The way to get that knowledge, he believed, was through experiment, and not by constructing a theory about the nature of the universe. When in the next months reporters deluged him with questions about his discovery and asked specifically what he had thought when he noticed the strange rays, he replied, "I didn't think, I investigated."[7]

This was probably disingenuous, but it reveals what Roentgen believed he should have done. An experimentalist, he rejected the notion that scientists begin with a working hypothesis so that their results fit into a grand system. He detested what we would call "overarching theorizing," the search for a unified theory. In a series of avuncular letters to his old classmate, Zehnder, who kept slipping off the German academic ladder in physics because he insisted on creating grand hypotheses, Roentgen tried to get him to change his ways. Roentgen suggested that Zehnder work as he, himself, had done throughout that crucial November and the rest of the winter. That is, he should systematically explore a single phenomenon from every possible angle and with no preconceived idea as to where it would lead.

Roentgen started with the remarkable ability of the rays to pass through opaque objects and leave a mark on a fluorescent screen, and soon established that they could also leave a shadow of some objects that were inside the ostensibly opaque ones, such as coins inside a wooden box. He proceeded to examine the rays methodically with everything he had on hand in the lab, and anything else he could get his hands on. He explored their effect on fluorescent materials and noted that when no rays got through, the image on the fluorescent plate was dark. When the rays did get through, the plate was white. When the rays hit a photographic plate, he found, as have all radiographers since, that he did not have a photographic image of the subject, but rather, the image of its *shadow.* These photographs proved crucial.

The pictures, with which we are so familiar today, provided visual proof for everything he claimed. He began by measuring the brightness of the fluorescent screen when he held a book between it and the Crookes tube, and the brightness of the screen without the interposing book. There was no difference. He tried to see if the rays would pass through a slim book, and a thick thousand-page volume; a single playing card, and two solid decks of cards. All proved transparent to the rays. So did thick blocks of wood, a sheet of vulcanized rubber, and a piece of tin foil. He separated those substances that stopped the rays, such as lead, from those they passed through.

Then he held his own hand to the invisible light—and became the first person in the world to see the shadow of his living bones.

Bones, Roentgen discovered, stopped the rays, as did glass made from lead. He took out a magnet and found that it could not deflect these rays as it could cathode rays. Nor would a prism refract the rays the way a prism would have bent visible light. Roentgen concluded that the rays were entirely new, and so he dubbed them "X," for X the unknown.

As 1895 dwindled away, Roentgen decided it was time to share his discovery. On December 22, he finally brought his wife, always patient but now very puzzled, into his confidence. He invited her into his lab and asked her to lay her hand on a photographic plate, then focused the rays on her for fifteen minutes. He made multiple prints of the X-ray of Bertha's left hand, her wedding ring apparently "floating" around the bone of her finger.

Shortly after Christmas, Roentgen sent a "preliminary" report to be published in the *Proceedings* of the Physico-Medical Society of Würzburg. He called it "On a New Kind of Rays," and to prove his assertions, he included several radiographs, one of which was the picture of Frau Roentgen's skeletal hand. The society would not meet until after the Christmas holidays, but the report was published with the date December 28, 1895. A mathematics-free paper, it may have been the last to reveal a major discovery in physics that was accessible to the general public.

What Roentgen had discovered were rays invisible to the eye. Research by many physicists over the next twenty years would reveal that X-rays are electromagnetic waves of very short wavelength—between .01 and 10 nanometers (one millionth of a meter). By comparison, visible light, which, as had been suspected, also turned out to be an electromagnetic wave, has a characteristic wavelength between 3,500 and 8,000 angstroms, an angstrom being equal to .0001 nanometers or .0000000001 meters. Later research would show that, like visible light,

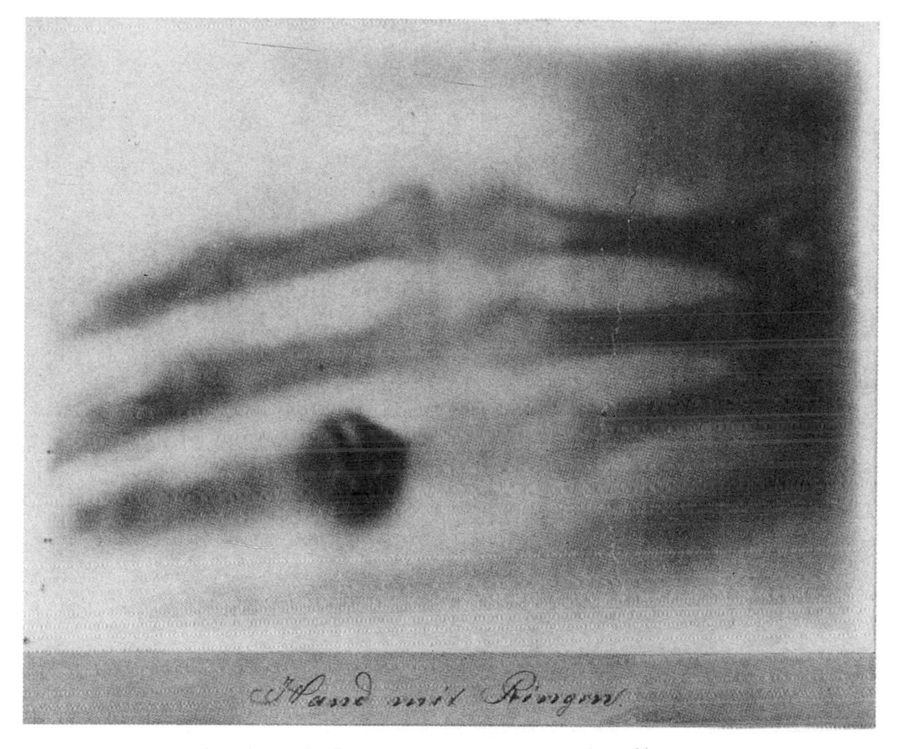

1. Frau Roentgen's hand (1895). Roentgen mailed eight copies of his paper along with this picture, among others, on January 1, 1896.

X-rays can be understood as a stream of particles, called photons, but that X-ray photons are far more energetic than the photons of ordinary light. In Roentgen's day, what most characterized X-rays was their obvious ability to penetrate and pass through opaque objects and to leave an impression on a photographic plate.

Whenever an X-ray encounters a photosensitized plate or film, it leaves a minute black dot. When an X-ray picture is taken of a subject, millions and millions of X-rays are aimed at it. Some of the rays will make it all the way through in a straight line, from the cathode ray tube, through the subject, to leave their black imprint on the plate. But most of the rays do not have such a direct path.

Some X-rays are stopped entirely when they encounter a substance that absorbs them. A white spot on the plate records their failure to get all the way through. This white image is, in effect, the *shadow* of the object that absorbed the X-rays. Lead will absorb all the rays, and other metals and bone will absorb a great many, so they show up as white silhouettes on the radiographs. Rays that are stopped and absorbed along the way are said to be *attenuated.* Still other rays ricochet off tissue and bounce off in random directions, to hit the film somewhere off their original straight path. These make gray blurs on the film and decrease the contrast of the attenuated rays. The proportion of attenuated rays to random rays is what is known as the signal-to-noise ratio. The *signal* is the recording of a real image; the *noise* is the proportion of exposed surface of the plate that has been hit by random rays. Even in the simple X-rays made at the end of the nineteenth century, researchers noticed the confusing blurs and began trying to figure out how to enhance contrast. The effort to improve the signal-to-noise ratio has been a major preoccupation of imaging technology ever since.

Many people initially dismissed X-rays as a mere adjunct to photography. The English biologist Alfred Russel Wallace mentions them in *The Wonderful Century,* a book he published in 1901 summing up the nineteenth century's accomplishments, only to dismiss them as a curious photographic trick.[8] Roentgen resented this assessment, but the photographic record was crucial to the rapid acceptance of X-rays. Without what we now call a *radiograph,* there would have been no dramatic evidence of the discovery.

Roentgen acknowledged the value of the camera to his investigation. "In order to find a law connecting transparency with thickness," he kept taking pictures.[9] Eventually he concentrated on the human body, for the rays penetrated layers of clothing, hair, and flesh and kept going, blocked only by calcium. That is why they left the shadow of bones on the photographic plate.

When on New Year's Day, 1896, Roentgen slipped several copies of the *Proceedings* into the mail, he included the radiographs that had accompanied his original submission. He sent them to the great scientists of his day, which to Roentgen meant Arthur Schuster and Lord Kelvin in Britain, the mathematician Henri Poincaré in France, as well as to his friends Zehnder in Leipzig and Franz Exner, a former colleague who was then director of the Physical Institute in Vienna. (No one in North America received a reprint.) Exner showed the paper and pictures at an informal meeting of a group of physicists, one of whom, Ernst Lechner, mentioned it to his father, who edited the Viennese newspaper, the *Neue Freie Presse.*

Recognizing a good story, the senior Lechner ran it on the front page on Sunday, January 5, 1896. The text was fine; the illustrations, especially Frau Roentgen's hand, caused a sensation. A British reporter in Vienna cabled the story to London where it appeared the next day in the *Chronicle,* and from there the news traveled, complete with picture, to newspapers across the continent and across the Atlantic.

The response astonished Roentgen. He became an instant celebrity. Within days of the Viennese paper's scoop on January 5th, X-rays won headlines wherever newspapers were printed. The reprints Roentgen mailed on New Year's Day took on a life of their own. A copy, hastily translated, reached the *New York Sun* on January 6 and the *St. Louis Post-Dispatch* the following day. Four days later it was picked up by the *New York Times* and on the twelfth of January by the *Times* of London, which had initially dismissed the news as some minor advance in photography.

By January 31 Roentgen's description of the rays, translated into English, was published in *Science* magazine. On February 22, *Electrical World,* a popular magazine for amateurs, inventors, and engineers, announced that there wasn't a Crookes tube to be bought anywhere in Philadelphia. X-ray fever remained throughout all of 1896, during which 49 serious books and 1,044 papers were published, as well as cartoons, verse, and anecdotes galore about the wondrous new rays.

The excitement pushed Roentgen into the spotlight. He patiently explained his discovery to the press and within a month was able to give visitors a well-rehearsed tour of his lab and a demonstration of the rays. But his own interest in X-rays was almost exhausted. He published a second paper on March 9, 1896, and final reflections in May 1897 in "Further Observations on the Properties of the X-Ray." He then left the subject forever.

He could not, however, regain his privacy. Honored in his homeland, he rejected the offer of a title but did accept the directorship of the Physical Institute in Munich, where he moved in 1900 and remained for the rest of his life. He was honored by scientific societies in England and France as well, and when the Swedish industrial giant Alfred Nobel left part of his fortune to endow prizes for outstanding scientific accomplishment, Roentgen received the first prize awarded in physics, in 1901.

The Nobel honor was marred by discord. The acrimonious Philipp Lenard never forgot that Roentgen had borrowed one of his tubes in 1894, or that Roentgen had not acknowledged Lenard's role in developing some of the techniques that led to the discovery. Lenard had been exploring fluorescence using cathode rays before Roentgen, even seeing the same strange glow, and he had published the results of his research in October 1895. The difference was that Lenard had neglected to pursue its origins, or to document the phenomenon with photographs. For years after the discovery, Lenard insisted that X-rays were simply a kind of cathode ray with new properties, and not a different phenomenon, and in this he was wrong.

Whatever they were, Lenard demanded credit for their discovery. Some glory came his way: throughout 1896 X-rays were often referred to as "Lenard-Roentgen rays," and the two physicists shared English and French prizes. But Lenard wanted more than equal billing; he wanted first credit. During celebrations at Glasgow University in the summer of 1896, one of Lenard's defenders maintained that the whole thing had been in Lenard's mind all the time. To which one of his British hosts reportedly replied that Lenard may have had Roentgen rays in his own brain, but Roentgen got them into other people's bones.

Indeed, we know now that when the first Nobel Prize was being considered, the committee put forward both names for a shared prize, but the academy, whose reasoning process is unknown, chose to honor Roentgen alone. Further fueling Lenard's fury was the decision in the German-speaking world to rename X-rays "roentgen rays," and the proliferation of elaborations on Roentgen's name, calling the pictures "roentgenographs" or "roentgenograms," and practitioners "roentgenologists."

In 1901 Roentgen recoiled at Lenard's rancor. He could not know that Lenard's reaction, if extreme, would be emulated many times, if not as blatantly, in the coming years by other image-making entries in the Nobel sweepstakes.[10]

Lenard received a Nobel Prize of his own in 1905 for his work with cathode rays, but he still smarted at what he considered the initial snub and used the platform in Stockholm to denounce their 1901 decision. For the rest of his life he discredited Roentgen whenever he had the chance, and Roentgen became so embittered that he left orders for all of his papers concerning X-rays before 1900 to be burnt, unopened, after his death in 1923. Lenard lived another twenty-four years. As one of Hitler's pet laureates during the Third Reich, Lenard denounced not only Roentgen, who was not Jewish, but all other physicists who, Jewish or not, he accused of doing "Jewish science." In his last interview in 1945 he still complained that the X-ray had been his "baby" and that Roentgen had been only the "midwife, the mechanism of its birth."[11]

The intervening years have brought evidence that Lenard's was not the only near miss. Earlier still in 1890 at the University of Pennsylvania, the physicist Arthur Goodspeed had demonstrated the properties of a Crookes tube to a visiting photographer who had left a couple of coins atop a pile of unexposed photographic plates. When the photographer later developed the plates, he had found them fogged with two small circular shadows. Unable to explain the images, he filed them away, only to remember them six years later. Goodspeed always claimed that the first roentgenograph was, thus, taken unknowingly in Philadelphia on February 22, 1890.

Roentgen's plate had also been exposed to X-rays by chance, but, whether or not his excellent vision contributed to his success, his accomplishment was more than a matter of a chance observation. Roentgen's genius lay not merely in noticing the new phenomenon, but in the experimental manner in which he documented graphically and in clear, simple phrases observations that would otherwise have seemed incredible.

The discovery of X-rays marked the beginning of a new epoch in science and medicine. They provided a tool with which physicists would explore the structure of matter, and doctors the interior of the human body. On a different level, they shifted the scales of the senses, making visual images, which they helped redefine, the dominating venue for exchanging information in the new century.

The Public and the Rays

From the start X-rays triggered a craze unlike any that had come before. In the clear light of hindsight, we can now recognize that X-rays brought with them a new fear of technology. By the end of the nineteenth century, the Industrial Revolution had generated an aesthetic revulsion within the middle classes at the ugliness of fuming factories, slag heaps, and overcrowded slums. Nineteenth-century opponents of technology could blame machines for unemployment and factories for destroying family life. But, in truth, human greed was more to blame for these problems than any technology as such. X-rays, however, introduced the possibility that an apparently benign scientific gift held an ugly surprise. Before the discovery of X-rays, science was a matter of

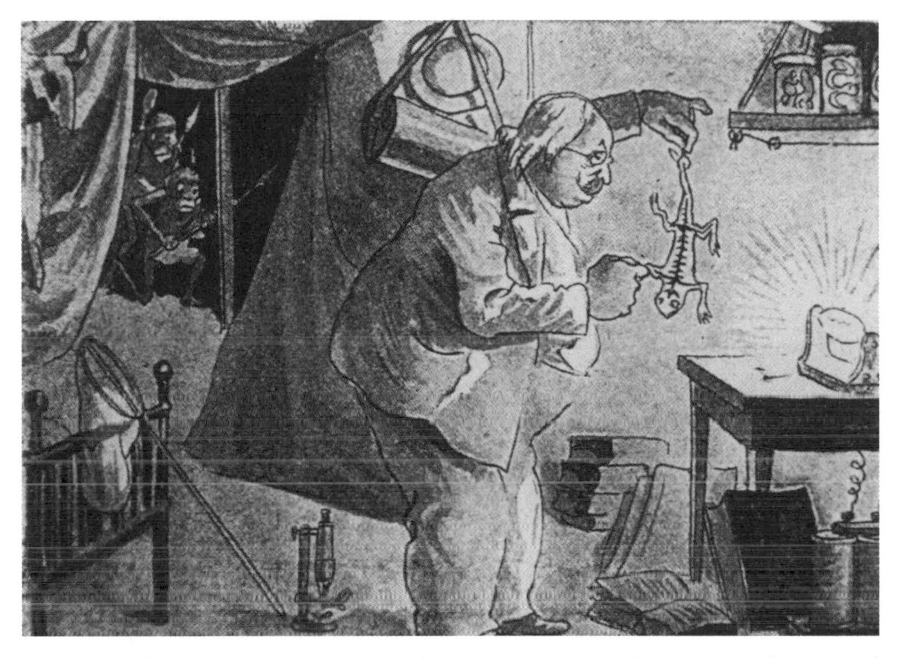

5. "The Wondrous X-rays or A Scientist's Adventures in the Desert." From a Danish cartoon of 1897, an example of the worldwide popularization of X-rays in the wake of the news. The story explained: "Employing X-rays, / he just has brought to light / the internal parts of an animal, / studying it consciously. / Alas, Alas, poor man! / Death is lurking outside the tent!" From *Illustreet Familie-Journal,* Copenhagen (August 29, 1897). Courtesy of Leif Gerward, Technical University of Denmark.

immediate causes and effects, close in time and space. You turn a switch on, and you get an electrical shock. You drink arsenic, and you get sick. With radiation, engineers, doctors, and eventually the rest of society were about to learn that technology could carry a long, deadly fuse—a lesson that would be repeated with chemical pollution. But in 1896, the fascination with X-rays was broad, swift, and undiluted by fear.

Many of those who read Roentgen's paper in early January 1896 immediately replicated his experiment, and even those who didn't have the paper easily figured out exactly what he had done. It wasn't difficult, once you knew there was something to look for.

Within weeks X-rays seemed to be everywhere. X-ray Boy's Clubs sprouted in the United States, and X-ray slot machines were installed in Chicago and Lawrence, Kansas, where, for a coin, you could examine the bones in your own hand.[12] In New York, Bloomingdale's brought in customers with demonstrations conducted by Herbert Hawks, a Columbia University senior who did research for his physics professor, Michael Pupin. In Paris, M. Dufayel, the owner of his own chain of department stores, alternated public demonstrations of an X-ray machine with demonstrations of the Lumière brothers' new moving pictures. There was no hint of danger.

The mechanics were simple. Anybody could cobble together an X-ray machine, and just about anyone did. A man in Rochester, New York, wrote to a prominent New York City doctor about his wife's hip, and the doctor asked him to send X-rays first so he could consider the case. The husband went out and bought the parts, then set up an X-ray machine in his basement where his wife lay for over ten hours of exposure so he could get a picture good enough to send. The picture may have been fine, but in his next letter he asked the doctor how to treat his wife's burns.

The rays had obvious medical applications, but they also appealed to constituencies beyond the health care community. There were the tinkerers, subscribers to *Electrical World* and *Scientific American*, who were simply fascinated by the possibilities of building better electrical gadgets. Earnest students of X-rays included psychologists and parapsychologists who studied psychic phenomena —including forays into the "fourth dimension," psychic auras, and extrasensory perception. There were also physicists who continued exploring the electromagnetic spectrum.

Within days of receiving Roentgen's letter, Henri Poincaré read a translation of Roentgen's paper to the French Academy of Sciences in Paris and wondered aloud if X-rays could be produced by ordinary fluorescent or phosphorescent substances. Antoine-Henri Becquerel, a professor of physics, was inspired to try exposing uranium compounds, which were known to be phosphorescent, to sunlight. In a famous scientific "accident," Becquerel, who had been waiting for a sunny day to expose his uranium rocks, had given up when the sky remained overcast and stuck the uranium rocks in a drawer along with some photographic plates. Days later, on the first of March 1896, he found that the plates showed an image of the rocks. He had discovered natural radioactivity (although the phenomenon would not be named until 1898). The uranium produced emanations that resembled X-radiation in their ability to cloud photographic plates and inability to be refracted, but that were unlike X-rays in the fogginess of the impressions they left. Becquerel's discovery did not trigger anything like the excitement of Roentgen's, although it was tremendously important to the development of physics and what would eventually lead to the nuclear age and nuclear medicine.

Other physicists focused their research on observations known to Roentgen, that a magnet placed next to a charged Crookes tube deflected cathode rays but not X-rays. This phenomenon suggested to the English physicist J. J. Thomson a better way to understand cathode rays. In 1897 he measured the ratio of their electrical charge to their mass and determined that the individual particle had a mass smaller than the atom's. He called it an *electron*. Roentgen had already noticed that, when X-rays pass through gas, the gas became a conductor of electricity. Thomson's work explained that the X-rays knocked some electrons loose from some of the atoms or molecules in the gas, leaving behind positive ions (atoms stripped of one or more electron). It was soon understood that the high voltage Roentgen had used to accelerate cathode rays, which are streams of charged particles, caused the electrons to slam into the wall of the Crookes tube. In the process of being captured by atoms in the glass, some of these particles were converted into elementary particles we now recognize as X-rays.[13]

Radioactivity would soon become the heart of research that had been triggered by Becquerel's discovery. Two other Parisian physicists, Marie Sklodowska Curie and her husband, Pierre Curie, were looking for a subject for Marie's doctoral thesis in 1896. Pierre had an established reputation from the elegant work he had done some years earlier with his brother, Jacques, discovering the phenomenon of piezoelectricity; this is a form of electric polarity in crystals, from which the brothers constructed an electrometer to measure current. Marie would eventually use this device in the work inspired by Becquerel's discovery. But in 1896 she was just beginning and was pleased that she had found the perfect problem for her dissertation.

Working together, Marie and Pierre Curie isolated minute quantities of what they had been sure were there—two new elements from eight tons of the uranium ore, pitchblende. These elements emitted many times the radiation of uranium, a quality she soon dubbed "radioactivity." They called these new elements *polonium* (after Marie's birthplace, Poland) and *radium,* and determined their atomic weights. For this work the Curies shared the Nobel Prize in physics with Becquerel in 1903. The American journalist Israel Zangwill dubbed radium "a pocket X ray," and called Marie Curie a secular saint—"Our Lady of Radium." After Pierre's death in 1906, Marie continued on her own, and in 1911 won a second Nobel Prize in chemistry. Still only halfway through her career, she would eventually play an important role in the dissemination of X-rays as a diagnostic tool.

Some scientists looked at the new discovery from a metaphysical perspective. Sir William Crookes, the designer of the tube bearing his name, saw nothing inconsistent between his interests in physics and in spiritualism. He attended seances regularly and conducted experiments to test the veracity of occult forces. In these pursuits, Crookes, like Roentgen, used photography, applying the new dry plate process to spectral analysis of chemicals, as well as to capturing the images of specters in the form of ghostly apparitions. There was nothing out of keeping in the scientific world of the first part of the twentieth century between Crookes's tenure as president of the Society for Psychical Research in 1897, and his presidency of the Royal Society from 1913 to 1915.

The world of X-rays and spiritualism was also the world of Sigmund Freud and Havelock Ellis. In a sense, the X-ray collaborated with these iconoclasts to break the long silence surrounding sexuality. Taking arms to defend the status quo, a New Jersey assemblyman is supposed to have introduced a bill forbidding the use of X-ray opera glasses,[14] and a London dry goods company offered ray-proof (presumably lead-lined) underwear. Playing off these sensibilities, a pamphlet advertising X-ray machines in 1896 came with red-tinted glasses and the sketch of a demurely dressed young woman on the cover. Looked at through the glasses, the viewer saw past her clothing, past her "private parts," right into her "sexual" skeleton.

The X-ray threatened to expose the two holiest sanctums of the human body—the sex organs and the brain—and in the process demystified both.

For X-rays did not stop at a woman's "hidden" genitalia, but probed deeper into the very untitillating spectacle of her pelvic girdle and spinal column. A generalized fear of exposure was revealed in the spate of cartoons and doggerel that filled newspapers and magazines. Emily Culverhouse summed up popular apprehensions in 1897:

> An Englishman's body belongs to himself,
> But surely that proverb was made
> Before Dr Roentgen's impertinent rays,
> With furtive, adumbrate, and mystical ways,
> Our structures began to invade.
>
> 'T is an "habeas corpus" of uncanny source,
> A forerunner of agencies evil,
> A gruesome, weird, and mysterious force,
> (But clothed in a garb of science of course)
> A league between man and the devil.
>
> For a steady gaze thrown on the sensitive plate.
> With a one-ness of theme and conception.
> And fixing our minds in a uniform strain.
> Will picture the image begot by our brain.
> And reveal our most inmost perception.
>
> Who among us is safe if this can be done,
> Who can bear such a scrutinization?
> Scant courtesy, too, our friends would afford.
> When they find that our actions are often a fraud.
> And our words but mis representation.[15]

Women's bodies were especially singled out as territories suddenly open to exposure. Women raised in an atmosphere of sexual repression shrank from the lustful gaze of X-rays: their husbands and fathers jealously feared that something privy to them would now be visible to strangers. There were also fears that women, tempted by the possibility of seeing past the clothing of other women, would succumb to the temptation to look at themselves, and worse. Conservative adherents of Judaism, Islam, and Christianity hid women's skin behind clothing. In some cultures even faces were veiled, but at the turn of the century many women were casting all of these covers away. In North America and Europe young cyclists had traded heavy petticoats and skirts for bloomers, and dancers and health faddists of the new avant-garde were tossing off Victorian constraints. Personal space, until then defined by clothing, was being redefined, and the X-ray was a natural progression in the trend. Skin became just another wrapping, something to be removed to reach what was more valid beneath it.

The transformation began with medical advertisements which almost immediately depicted white-bosomed women in front of X-ray screens, their lungs and rib cages boxed separately from the dissolved layer of satiny skin.

NAKED TRUTH

(as well as Motor Points) about MICA PLATE Static Machines, demonstrate that:—

1.—Mica does not collect moisture and therefor our machines generate every day in the year, rain or shine.

2.—Mica Plates are not breakable and so our machines may be run 2,000 revolutions per minute, tripling and quadrupling their generating capacity.

3.—Our Machines are more staunch and workmanlike—made for wear and high speed.

4.—The current derived from high speed is more sedative and effective in relieving pain—most efficient for X Ray work.

5.—Our Machines cost the Doctor less than one half what any other machine of same generating capacity cost.

6.—No other machine can do the same work.

R. V. Wagner & Co.
308 DEARBORN ST. CHICAGO

6. "Naked Truth" (1899). Advertisement by R. V. Wagner & Sons for static machines demonstrates the disappearance of privacy with the female body. Courtesy of the American College of Radiology.

These early advertisements, like medical advertisements today, used mostly female models. Women were a group to be serviced medically (they lived shorter lives on average than men until the mid-twentieth century), even as they did the serving. When the French physician Charles Bourchard invited his colleagues to a demonstration of X-rays in the fall of 1896, he used his elderly housemaid as a subject. He exposed the woman's bared breastbone to the view of strangers with no apparent concern for her privacy, perhaps because she was simply a domestic, a member of a social caste who was there to be used, when not being useful. Bodily privacy remained a middle-class privilege for another half century, but the X-ray would be one of the tools that led many people to discard it as no longer relevant.

Even at that time, modesty was only a sometime thing. Men and women routinely gazed at idealized naked women on canvas and in marble. The art of the Academy in the 1890s featured statuesque figures like those of Puvis de Chavannes. The rebels, who would soon become an orthodoxy of their own, included Whistler, Degas, Seurat, and the whole school of impressionists. Their figures, dressed or nude, were an exaltation of flesh tones and textures. Photography, which was moving from the realm of the enthusiastic amateur to the serious professional, seemed to be the ultimate recorder of reality. Within a decade, the educated artist's eye would incorporate the gifts of X-ray vision, and the visual arts would be transformed forever.

X-Rays in Court

For arousing the public interest immediately, nothing beat the appeal of bullets. X-ray images of bullets lodged in hapless individuals answered, belatedly, those 1881 editorials. Doctors and prosecutors could point at foreign objects inside a body and make a case. The X-ray became an instant forensic tool, and its use in court would soon set legal precedents.

At about the time the Roentgens were celebrating their last quiet Christmas outside the limelight in 1895, young Tolman Cunnings was losing an argument in a Canadian bar to a fellow named George Holder. Holder had a gun; he fired and hit Cunnings in the leg. At Montreal's General Hospital, the staff couldn't find the bullet and let the wound heal around it. The bullet remained hidden, and Cunnings, still in pain, brought charges against Holder at the Court of Queen's Bench in Montreal in February 1896. He would find justice, he announced to the press. "Professor Roentgen's new photographic discovery will be used in evidence."[16]

Cunnings's lawyer had contacted John Cox, a physics professor at McGill University. At McGill on February 3, Cunnings sat beside a table in Cox's physics lab with his leg tied with bandages and towels to a block of wood that leaned against a sensitized photographic plate. Cox turned on an electric current to a makeshift X-ray machine. After Cunnings sat still for forty-five minutes, Cox examined the plate and declared the experiment a success. Cunning's doctor then used the radiograph to excise the bullet. Cunnings brought the bullet, along with the X-ray picture of it still inside his leg, to court. Holder

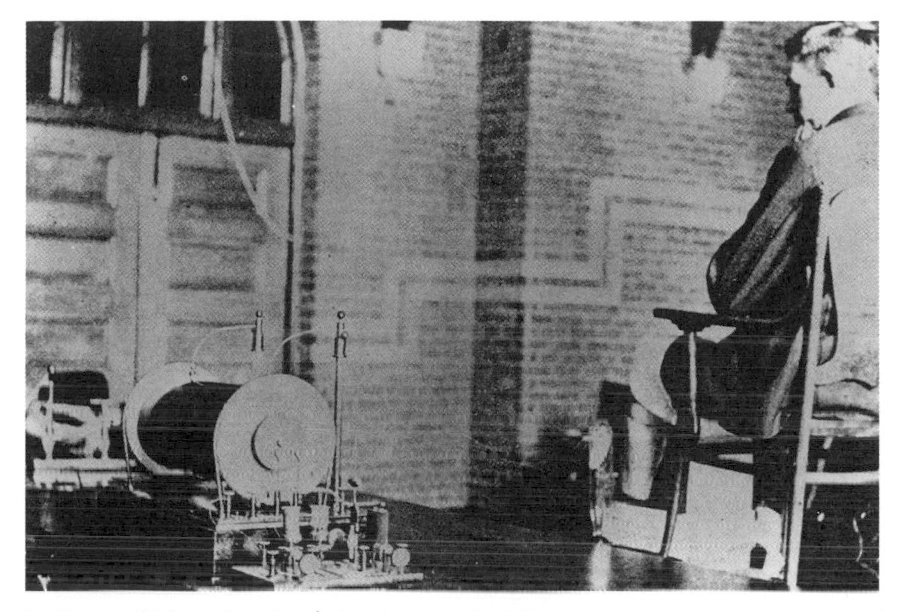

7. Picture of Tolman Cunnings being X-rayed at McGill University, January 1896. Courtesy of the American College of Radiology.

was convicted and sentenced to fourteen years in prison. Only two months after X-rays had become public knowledge, they were accepted as evidence in court.

Second only to bullets for courtroom drama were broken bones. Their milky images on a dark radiographic background were brought to the attention of the law in Denver, Colorado, in April 1896. James Smith had fallen off a ladder while painting a wall at his home earlier that spring. (When not fixing his house, Smith was reading law.) Three weeks after the accident, pain in his hip took him to W. W. Grant, a renowned surgeon who had performed the first appendectomy in the United States. Grant diagnosed a contusion and prescribed exercise. But Smith's leg never stopped hurting, and he soon noticed that it had become shorter than its mate.

In midsummer, six months after Roentgen's announcement, Smith had found two lawyers and a photographer to take his case. The photographer, who had been making X-ray pictures ever since he had heard about the possibility, produced an X-ray image of Smith's hip after eighty minutes of exposure. The picture revealed an impacted fracture at the head of the femur. Then as now the medically accepted treatment for a fracture, as opposed to a contusion, is rest.

From the start, it was obvious that X-rays were on trial, not Dr. Grant. No experts questioned the surgeon's competence, but experts did testify to the validity of the X-ray image.

Owen E. Le Fevre, a mining mogul turned judge (with a large head covered with white hair, a clipped white mustache, and pink face) was eager to set jurisprudential precedent. Both sides agreed that an X-ray image is *not* the same as an ordinary photograph. Grant's lawyer solicited the opinions of several judges who had refused to accept X-ray plates as evidence "because there is no proof that such a thing is possible. It is like offering the photograph of a ghost, where there is no proof that there is any such thing as a ghost."[17]

To counter this testimony, the radiographer and lawyers brought X-rays into court. They set up a shadow box with a small hole at one end and a candle casting a shadow upon a screen at the opposite end. They first showed the shadow of a hand to the judge and jury, and then a radiograph of the same hand. Then they displayed X-rays of other objects including a clock, a normal femur, and finally the X-ray plate of Smith's damaged femur in the region of the hip joint. They offered members of the jury pictures of the bones in their own hands, and then requested that the X-ray picture be admitted in evidence.

Grant's lawyer argued for three hours against their admission. No one had actually seen the broken bone; an X-ray of a bone was unlike an ordinary photograph that captures a scene that someone had seen because no one had ever seen the actual living bone. Therefore, the X-ray picture ought not be introduced.

Judge Le Fevre saw it differently:

> We have been presented with a photograph taken by means of a new scientific discovery. . . . It knocks at the temple of learning; what shall we do or say? Close fast the doors or open wide the portal? Rather let the courts throw open the doors to all well considered scientific discoveries. Modern science has made it possible to look beneath the tissues of the human body and has aided surgery in telling of the hidden mysteries. We believe it to be our duty in this case to be the first, if you please to so consider it, in admitting in evidence the process known and acknowledged as a determinate science. The exhibits will be admitted in evidence.[18]

Smith won his case.

Judge Le Fevre's opinion typified the fin de siècle optimism many Americans felt about science in medicine. Science held the promise of progress; "scientific medicine" could only lead to better health. Few people recognized the impact that the gray and white, two-dimensional images would have on the way people see, or the psychological scars that would convince future generations that all technological gifts come with unexpected taxes.

Two

Medical Applications

The Living Body beneath the Skin

By the end of the second week of January 1896, four days after learning about Roentgen's discovery, Thomas Alva Edison had built himself an X-ray machine in New Jersey. It was easy. The glass tube that Roentgen had used to produce the rays wasn't very different from the electric light bulb Edison himself had patented in 1879.[1] And the X-rays, though remarkable in their ability to penetrate opaque objects and leave an image on a photographic plate, did not seem all that different from the light rays he had been experimenting with in his search for a better light bulb. Edison delighted in the discovery and was eager to explore ways to make the rays both practical and profitable. He would be among the first to realize that radiation was a two-edged sword, and rather than try to understand the problem, he removed himself from X-ray research entirely.

Edison on the Bandwagon

Edison was an American icon in 1896. He had risen from humble beginnings, gone to work at the age of fifteen printing newspapers for the Grand Trunk Railway in Michigan, and become a millionaire by the age of forty. His wealth came from a series of inventions, beginning with the electric vote recorder he had patented in 1868 and continuing with a list that included the incandescent light bulb, the phonograph, the kinetoscope (an early movie projector), and an electric fan. By 1896 he had corporate headquarters in West Orange, New Jersey, where a team of scientists and engineers developed consumer products in the nation's first industrial research laboratory.

Within hours of learning the details of Roentgen's procedure, Edison directed his team to construct a darkroom in the laboratory so they could explore whatever Roentgen had been exploring, only better. Edison succeeded on two levels. First there was the tube itself. By using thinner glass than an ordinary Crookes tube, he produced a tube that allowed more X-rays through faster; and he replaced the platinum wires inside the tube with electrodes made of aluminum disks.[2]

Next, there was the fluorescent screen and the question of what made it glow. Edison directed his assistants to test the substances at the top of his chemical storage wall and work their way down to find something that would reflect a sharper image than barium platinocynanide. His assistants systematically explored over eight thousand different chemicals; they painted coin-sized dabs of each onto thirty-six test circles on a cardboard square. The substances were graded according to the way they fluoresced when X-rayed. The search led to calcium tungstate. Edison immediately turned over the discovery to a

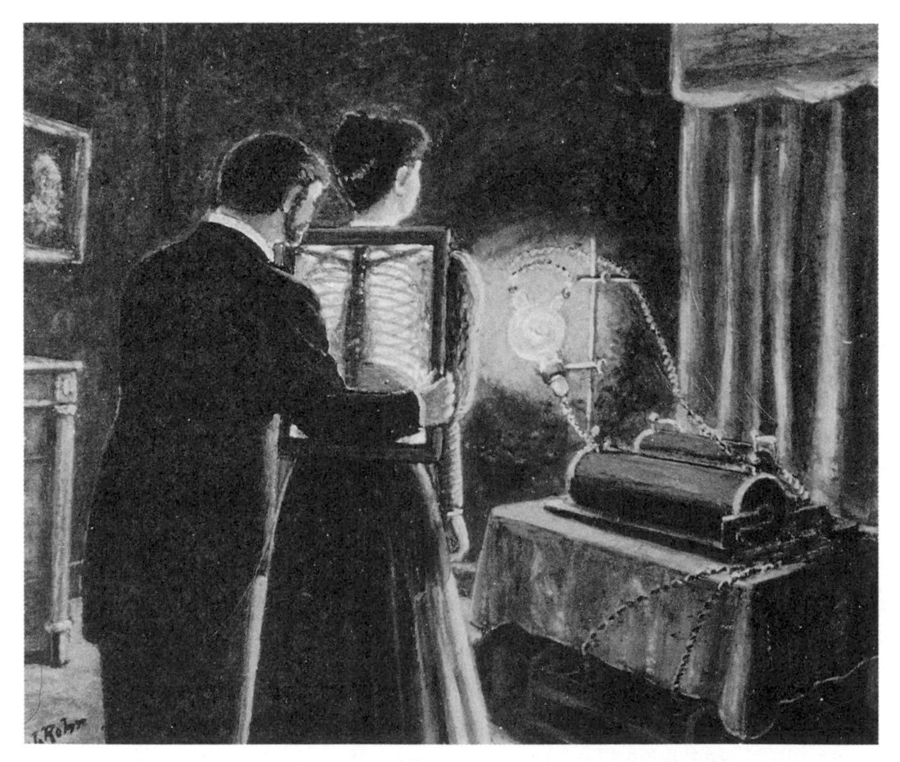

8. Painting by D. Jacques Rohr (1896) of fluoroscopic examination of a woman. The painting illustrates how doctors conducted fluoroscopic examinations. Note the X-ray tube, static machines, and electric coils. Courtesy of Dr. Guy Pallardy.

nearby manufacturer for marketing as a "fluoroscope" (he coined the term) under his supervision.

Edison did not patent this "fluoroscope," however, because variations on the theme of a real-time moving image on a fluorescent screen were already on the market—in Italy, where a Professor Salvioni had come up with a "crypto-scope" (secret image), and in Princeton, not far from the West Orange lab, where Professor Magie was already selling a "skiascope" (shadow image). But Edison's term *fluoroscope* became generic because his device was "user-friendly." The viewer leaned comfortably against a cushioned eyepiece and then looked with both eyes into a decorative wooden box covered by a dark hood at a calcium-tungstate coated screen. The viewer could see the living interior of another person's hand, or her own as it moved between the X-ray tube and the screen.

Hands were especially popular that first year. Everyone with access to a newspaper had seen Frau Roentgen's famous ringed finger, so it was reasonable in February for the prominent New York surgeon William Tillinghast Bull to want an X-ray of the hand of one of his patients. A wealthy New Yorker, Prescott Hall Butler had accidentally shot more than one hundred pieces of buck-shot into his own hand. Bull brought him to the Columbia University laboratory of the physicist Michael Pupin who, as a friend of Edison, had received a sample fluoroscope.[3] Doubled over in pain, Butler managed to unclench his hand just long enough for the surgeon to see it on the fluoroscope.

At this time, and for some years to come, most radiographs, as X-ray

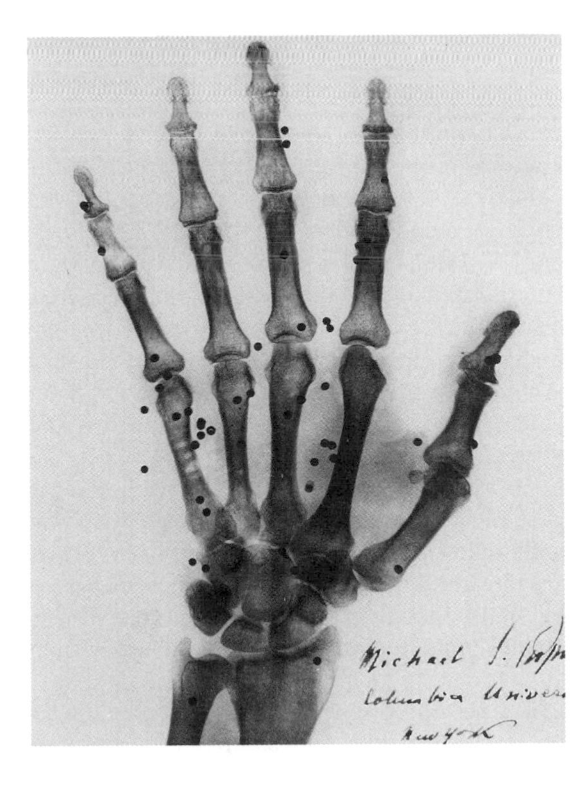

9. Radiograph by Michael Pupin of Prescott Butler's hand in 1896 revealing pieces of buckshot. Courtesy of the Burndy Library, Dibner Institute, Cambridge, Massachusetts.

pictures are called, took up to an hour's exposure. But as Butler clearly could not endure such a sitting, Pupin was inspired to make an instant improvement. He combined the luminescent screen of the fluoroscope with a photographic plate by placing the screen on the plate with the patient's hand atop the screen. The rays acted upon the screen first, and the screen's fluorescent light acted on the glass plate. As Pupin recorded, "A beautiful photograph was obtained with the exposure of a few seconds. The photographic plate showed the numerous shot as if they had been drawn with pen and ink."[4] Pupin's intensifying screen, as it was later named, was eventually adapted by many people, and Dr. Bull became the first surgeon known to have used an X-ray as an operating guide.

Delighted with the successful surgical outcome and the accompanying publicity, Edison declared "the appliance is for immediate use, and is a valuable aid to surgery and would be invaluable to a hospital. . . . With the roentgen ray you see here and the fluoroscope a surgeon can detect the nature of the fracture in a moment and set the arm accordingly."[5]

We have the picture and his testimony, but Pupin's intensifying screen with its high-speed exposure remained an anomaly for at least five more years. In the meantime, patients continued to endure long exposures. Nor did Pupin's picture convince a skeptical technical expert. The editor of the *American Journal of Photography* doubted that the X-ray was quite so wonderful. Instead of applauding Edison's feat, he decried his lack of academic credentials. "All of the above reads very nice, but still it smacks greatly of the sensational journalism, and until we have practical demonstrations by scientists of note and reputation who will show results, the glowing account of the fluoroscope will form a companion to the bright fairy tales."[6]

But it was sensational journalism that popularized X-rays in the first place, and the public responded hungrily to all news of the technology, as long as it was accompanied by a picture. The newspaper magnate William Randolph Hearst was never above creating a story if he couldn't find one "in the wild." Five weeks into the X-ray era, on February 5, 1896, he wired Edison: "Will you as an especial favor to the *Journal* undertake to make a Cathodograph [yet another name for a radiograph] of human brain."[7] Edison accepted the challenge, only to acknowledge defeat a few weeks later. He did try, but the opacity of the skull defeated his ingenuity. Hearst's challenge to capture an image of the human brain in the act of remembering, seeing, experiencing joy, and slowly dying, would not be fulfilled for another eighty years.

Ignoring the setback, Edison prepared to introduce his fluoroscope at a gala extravaganza in April at the annual Electrical Exhibition in New York City's Grand Central Palace, then on the corner of Lexington Avenue and Forty-third Street. The display was carefully arranged on the assumption that this would be a once-in-a-lifetime adventure for the thousands of expected visitors, and that they would want to see their own bones, not those of the stranger ahead of them in line.[8]

To accommodate them, Edison set up a display in a darkened room on the third floor of the Palace, directly above the exhibition restaurants. Familiar with

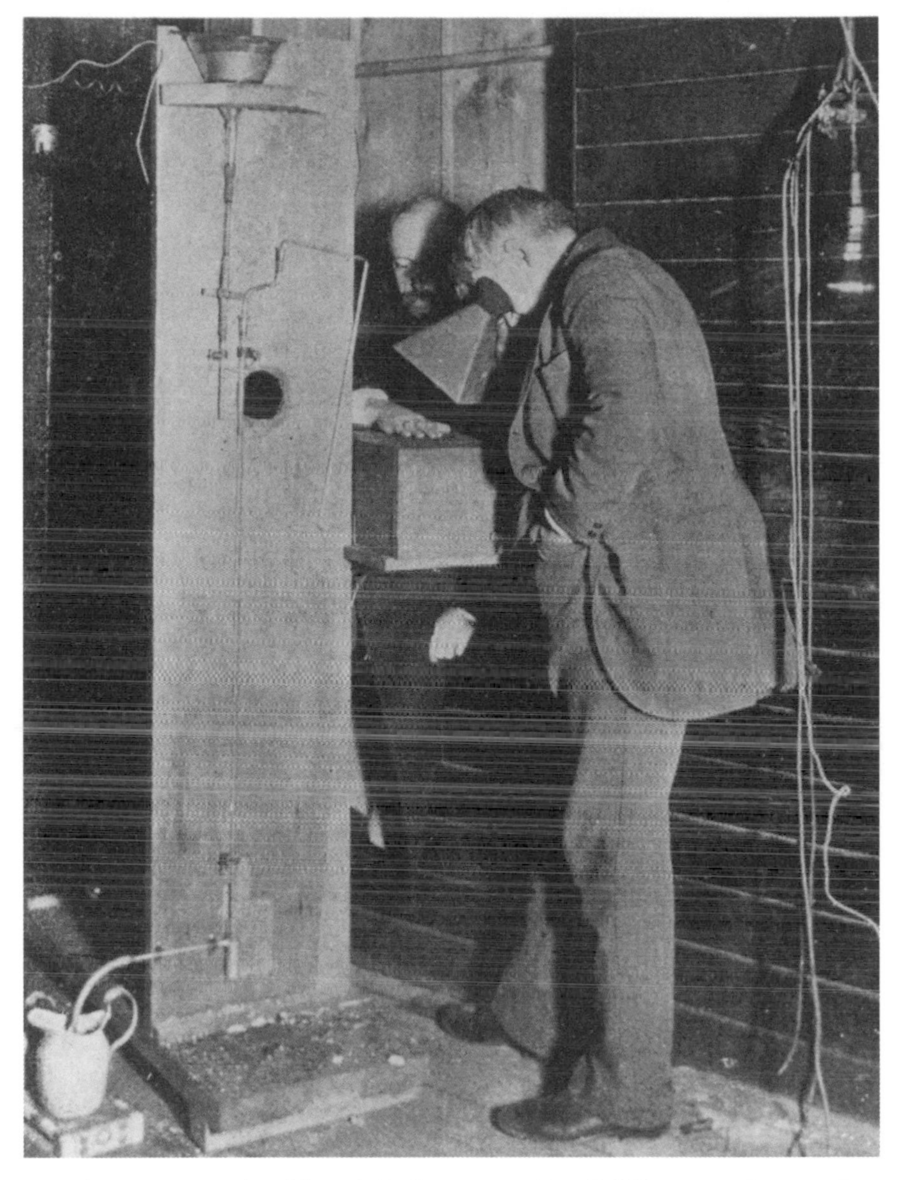

10. Edison examines a hand through his fluoroscope. (From E. P. Thompson, *Roentgen Rays,* New York, 1896.) Thomas Edison devised this X-ray machine to allow visitors at the Electrical Exhibition in New York to view their X-rayed hands. His assistant, Clarence Dally, holds his hand over the box containing the X-ray tube. Courtesy of the Burndy Library, Dibner Institute, Cambridge, Massachusetts.

the market for electrotherapeutics, a medical specialty that at that time mixed the bells and whistles of charlatans with respectable procedures that included an early version of electroshock therapy for hysteria, Edison's team contrived to establish a supernatural atmosphere, an aura of the occult. Inasmuch as the fluoroscope had to be seen in the dark, he described the experience as occurring "in Egyptian darkness, lit only by two blood-red incandescent lamps."[9] One at a time, visitors were admitted into the darkened room, given a coin hidden inside a glove to clutch so that they could see through the eyepiece their own finger bones and the now visible coin.

Some people reportedly flinched when their turn came and refused to look. Others crossed themselves and hurried on, sharing Frau Roentgen's reported reaction, that she was seeing her own death.[10]

Edison soon agreed that Frau Roentgen was probably right, although not as she had meant it—as a foreshadowing of the inevitability of death. Within a few months reports that exposure to X-rays caused hair to fall out or inflamed the skin were rampant. Edison had noticed some reddening around his own eyes (and stopped experimenting with X-rays himself) and strange pitting on his assistant's skin. As the most famous inventor of his day, Edison lent enormous prestige to the X-ray's debut. First on the X-ray bandwagon, he was also one of the first to jump off. Having perfected his fluoroscope and marketed a full line of X-ray kits (complete with a device for generating current), he turned his attention to other projects.

Medical Applications

The development of the apparatus was left to medical manufacturers. Edison had been absolutely right about the importance of the rays in medicine. But although the market grew steadily, it did not turn into an instant gold mine. In spite of the fanfare and attention in the popular press, the X-rays were not adopted as widely as, in retrospect, would have seemed likely. Conservative and suspicious, most physicians only resorted to X-rays when they felt threatened by malpractice suits—less frequent then than now and less remunerative, but already very much a part of the medicolegal landscape.

There were, however, important exceptions. A small but influential number of physicians, many at university-associated medical schools, fell under the spell of the new machine. A few had degrees in physics or engineering and, like their heirs who are now working with contemporary magnetic resonance imaging machines and computerized scanners, they lobbied their hospitals to buy and install the best machines available to get pictures of the interior of the human body. By the turn of the century these X-ray buffs were meeting to compare notes and discuss the finer points of the various instruments that flooded the market.

They were apostles of "scientific medicine," a movement that had begun in American medicine in the 1870s as news of the discoveries in European laboratories encouraged some American doctors to turn the art of medicine into a clinical science. They wanted the clinic where patients were treated to become more like a laboratory, with controls and planned procedures. Then they would be able to predict the outcome of treatment. "Like a laboratory" to these doctors also meant using machines. The X-ray was the answer for physicians who wanted to convince colleagues that technology was more than a novelty, that it could introduce a new approach to diagnosis.

They honed their diagnostic skills with a procedure they called "retrospectography." The process, which was used in the United States until about 1913, began with a doctor circulating X-rays of a patient without an accompanying diagnosis. The person who had taken the picture, whether physician or technician, would then attend the operation, if one was deemed necessary, or the autopsy, if the patient died. There X-rays would be made of the affected organs and the radiologist would be told what the right diagnosis should have been. Only at this point would the original plates be examined to see how a better diagnosis could have been made. The retrospectographers also built up a library of images illustrating difficult diagnoses, and they circulated radiographs to a range of specialists. It was the first time physicians could get a consensus of opinions about a patient's treatment. Later, academic physicians would show X-rays before and after surgery and describe the results to their colleagues and students.

This approach, however, contradicted the nineteenth-century medical view that disease is unique to each patient. For retrospectography to make sense, doctors had to consider patients as in many ways interchangeable, reproducible, and quantifiable, with the disease viewed as separate from the diseased.[11] If this were the case, then patients could benefit from the combined wisdom of a group of doctors who had treated similar cases. This was a strong argument. At the time, doctors were still thinking in terms of idiosyncrasy—the idea that disease is unique to the patient who happens to be peculiarly susceptible to a specific condition.[12] That was the opposite of scientific medicine, where like causes were assumed to produce like symptoms. This apparent dichotomy disappeared by the last third of the twentieth century when genetics research pointed to inherited genes as the cause of certain "idiosyncrasies," such as the inability to process sugar or digest certain foods.

Military doctors were early converts to scientific medicine as it applied to machines like the X-ray. They saw the utility of the new technology for removing bullets and shrapnel and setting bones in young, otherwise healthy patients. The British army installed X-ray machines in its London hospitals in 1896, but the first nation to use X-rays on the battlefield was Italy. In May that year, many wounded Italian soldiers who had been sent to east Africa in an effort to annex Abyssinia were X-rayed in field hospitals. By 1897 the British had their chance to test the rays in skirmishes in the Balkans and in Afghanistan, where field-type X-ray units were carried by Indian porters for two hundred miles. That same year they sent X-ray units to Egypt and transported field units to the front during the Nile campaign. There, in the heat of the Sahara, soldiers were detailed to pedal reconstructed bicycles that activated portable electrical generators.

Using the new technology, army doctors immediately investigated the mysterious *pied forcé,* a foot injury that had been endemic in all infantries. They discovered it was a subtle fracture of the second metatarsal bone caused by prolonged marching. Once the doctors understood the cause, they could treat soldiers already injured and prevent new cases.

The American military was well prepared in 1898 when the United States declared war on Spain. The U.S. Navy installed three Edison portable X-ray units on three hospital ships off the Cuban coast. Those injured in the Pacific theater, the Philippines, were brought back to San Francisco where they were hospitalized at the Presidio.

Wartime use of X-rays gave the specialty of surgery a boost. Operations to remove bullets and shrapnel after seeing them in radiographs produced dramatic results, and, because the patients were otherwise in good shape and usually recovered, they made the specialty look good. (The fact that soldiers were usually thinner than the general public helped—slim bodies yielded better X-rays.) The case was different for those physicians who used X-rays to peer into the chest cavity and found malignant-looking tumors or tubercular lungs. They could diagnose sooner and with more precision, but even as imaging techniques became more and more refined, they were often at a loss for effective treatment. Thanks to antisepsis and anesthetics, surgery was already on the rise from the bottom of the medical hierarchy. The X-ray completed the trio of discoveries that pushed it to the top. The famous Mayo brothers were among the first members of the surgical profession to install X-ray machines in their clinic. With the X-ray, surgeons could confidently and consistently repair many of their patients.

The novelty and apparent success of radiography-based surgery during the Spanish-American war was documented by the surgeon general, George M. Sternberg. Seriously wounded soldiers from the Philippines had been shipped to San Francisco, and especially complicated cases were sent to the studio of Elizabeth Fleischmann on Sutter Street. Like many of the first practitioners, she was not a doctor. Her only exposure to medicine had come from living with her sister and brother-in-law, a doctor.

Fleischmann's parents had emigrated from Austria to Placerville, in Gold Rush country, where her father worked as the local agent for the Wells Fargo company. By 1880 the gold rush had ended and the Fleishmanns moved to San Francisco. There, news of the remarkable rays reached the Fleischmann home in January 1896. Elizabeth immediately quit her clerical job to enroll in a six-month course in electrical science at the Van der Naillen School of Engineering and Electricity in San Francisco. Within the year she had set up shop.[13]

Like all radiographers at the time, Fleischmann worked on referrals from doctors, getting pictures of foreign objects such as pins and bullets that were lodged inside her patients. However, she soon became expert on bone injuries. During the war with Spain, her radiographs, taken from a variety of angles so as to locate the injury more precisely in space, were forwarded to Washington as examples of remarkable definition. The surgeon general noted the "nice adjustment of the ray according to the density or character of the object when she desires to photograph, which is an art in itself," and he made a point of meeting her on a tour of his West Coast facilities.[14]

The frequency with which X-rays were used seems to have depended on where in the United States the machines happened to be. Although the Pennsylvania Hospital in Philadelphia was among the first to install an X-ray machine and have at least a part-time physician to handle the pictures, a careful examination of patient records from 1897 through 1927 indicates that the X-ray was more symbolic than useful for diagnosis or research for the first five years. Even as late as 1912, patients with fractures severe enough for surgery did not routinely get an X-ray taken before entering the operating room.[15] Although comparable studies have not been made of other hospitals, the number of X-ray machines in the American West suggests that they were used more frequently there. Among the majority of physicians at the turn of the century, however, radiographs remained curiosities not directly related to what they would automatically do when confronted with an emergency.

Bullets in Buffalo: Another Presidential Hit

An emergency of headline proportions occurred at four in the afternoon on September 6, 1901, in Buffalo, New York. That Indian summer afternoon, newly reelected President William McKinley stood shaking hands inside the Temple of Music at the Pan American Exhibition, about to deliver an address.

The assassinations of two presidents within twenty years had ended the casual comings and goings of the head of state. After Garfield, security arrangements and secret service agents had become part of the presidential burden. Maybe it was the unusual heat that afternoon, but whatever it was, the presidential guardians did not notice the tall man who had wrapped a white handkerchief around his right hand, and who had pushed his way to the front of the crowd. Then two shots rang out, and the recoil blew the handkerchief away, exposing a gun.

The first bullet hit a metal button on the president's coat and was deflected into the ground. The second entered his abdomen about six inches below the left nipple, and proceeded through the stomach until it lodged inside a muscle next to his spine.[16]

Within seven minutes McKinley was inside an electric ambulance en route to the exhibition hospital. Ostensibly, he couldn't have been in a better place to get medical assistance. The Pan American Exposition was a showplace of modernism, featuring indoor toilets and telephones connecting all the buildings. At night more than 200,000 watts of electrical light bulbs lit up the "city of the future," which included the exhibition hospital that doubled as a first-aid station.

The hospital boasted separate men's and women's wards, a dispensary, a kitchen, and one operating room, which contained a white enamel operating table and flasks of sterile water. A single window let in light. There was no gas fixture, probably a precaution against ether exploding near a flame, and no electric power. The thousands of electric light bulbs, strung up like Christmas lights, were decorations.

Altogether separate from the hospital was a Science Hall which had an X-ray machine with its own dry-cell battery on display.

In the moment of crisis, the exhibition director had to act quickly. His first decision was choosing a doctor. Of all the surgeons available in Buffalo that afternoon, he chose Matthew Mann, an obstetrician with an excellent reputation. The director reasoned that gynecological surgery would have made him familiar with the lower abdomen. He did not know that Mann had never operated on a gunshot wound. Summoned, Mann had no choice but to operate. The next decision was where and when. Rather than waste time moving McKinley to Buffalo General Hospital where there was an up-to-date operating room, Mann decided to operate immediately in the exhibition hospital. He may have remembered the disgrace that ruined the careers of Garfield's doctors who, by delaying surgery in their fruitless search for the bullet, were still held responsible for that president's death.

No one suggested using the X-ray machine in the Hall of Science. Instead, racing to catch what remained of daylight, Mann began operating at half past five. His task was difficult. He had rushed to the exhibition grounds without his black bag and had to make do with the handful of knives and saws in the exhibition clinic. Worst of all was McKinley's enormous belly. By seven, halfway through the operation, someone had rigged up a metal tray to deflect the remaining September sunlight onto the patient. When it was almost dark, an eight-watt electric light was finally hooked up. Mann tracked the bullet's path and sewed up the stomach walls which it had pierced. The operation was taking a long time, too long, Mann decided, and not enough light was left for him to go for the bullet.

After surgery, McKinley was taken to a private home where, for the first few days, he seemed to be improving. Thomas Edison dispatched Clarence Dally, his number one X-ray assistant, to accompany his best new X-ray machine from New Jersey to Buffalo. As the train sped north, an independent group in Buffalo set up a sort of presidential look-alike contest in preparation for Dally's arrival. Fat men lined up in the hope of being selected as the stand-in to test the X-ray for the president. When the X-ray team arrived, Dr. Vertner Kenerson, who boasted the same fifty-six-inch waistline as the president, had been selected. Kenerson went to the house where McKinley was supposedly recuperating and, in a room just below and across the hall from the president, lay on his side with a light in front of him and the fluoroscope behind for the twenty minutes it took to get a picture showing "the entire interior arrangement."[17]

The president himself was feeling better and his doctors were so sanguine that they advised Vice-President Theodore Roosevelt to remain with his family on Long Island. McKinley himself had asked to have an X-ray taken as reassurance that the bullet hadn't settled in any vital spot. But his doctors declined, not wanting to subject him to whatever movement he would have to make to get to the machine. McKinley stopped asking a few days later when his condition declined dramatically. Eight days after the attack, he was dead from gangrene. In the end, he never had an X-ray. Roosevelt, who had served in the army in Cuba, was sworn in as president. He would be the next chief of state to receive a bullet in the torso.

In this first decade of the X-ray, outside of the military, dentistry was the only specialty to adopt X-rays immediately into practice. The first dental X-rays were made in Germany in January of 1896 (with a twenty-five minute exposure time) followed, in April, by C. Edmund Kells of New Orleans, who presented the first dental X-ray clinic ever at a meeting of the Southern Dental Association in Asheville, North Carolina. Kells was a great publicist of dental X-rays in the course of his lifelong campaign against the indiscriminate extraction of teeth and for root canal surgery instead.

Kells was followed by William Morton in New York, who explained the clinical benefits of X-rays. Teeth, he demonstrated, are more dense than the bone surrounding them, so with X-rays dentists can see children's teeth before they have "escaped from the gums."[18] Beyond detecting decay, X-rays expanded the wonderful new dental specialty of orthodontics (for the X-ray pictures could predict growth as well as monitor the apparatus used to correct bad bites). Advertisements in dental magazines—artlessly revealing the state of dental technology—added that they could also be helpful for finding "the lost end of a broken drill."[19] Whatever they were looking for, by the late spring of 1896, British dentists routinely X-rayed their patients. A contemporary ad shows a bearded man telling a child that the roentgen rays show all is well because she uses the proper tooth powder.

Sleuthing with X-Rays

Thanks to those dentists who increasingly insinuated themselves into middle-class hygiene, X-rays soon served the dead as well as the living. Dentists accumulated the first archives of X-ray records that could be used for personal identification. They became, willy-nilly, the working partners of coroners. Personal dental histories, as recorded on film, could identify the dead and, in more and more instances, reveal how they had died.

The first use of X-rays in a murder is the tragedy of twenty-year-old Elizabeth Anne Hargreaves Hartley, a loom operator in the English mill town of Nelson, who was shot in the head four times by her husband; he then leaped to his death in a nearby canal.[20] Elizabeth Anne survived and lay conscious in bed until help arrived. The question of the day was whether the bullets could be found and removed in time to save her life. She was shot on April 23, 1896, well into the X-ray's first year, and it is no surprise that the local general practitioner wanted an X-ray. He asked the physicist Arthur Schuster, who lived nearby in Manchester, if he could locate the bullets.

Schuster was ill, but he sent two assistants to Hartley's small terraced house. A horse-drawn cab carried them and their cargo of three cathode ray tubes, high-tension coil, and glass photographic plates over Nelson's cobblestoned streets. The local municipal corporation provided the electricity through storage batteries. The whole apparatus was assembled alongside the patient in the small bedroom. The first picture, which took seventy minutes, located three bullets—one of which was lodged in the base of her brain. A second picture, taken a few days later, found the fourth. They were never removed. Elizabeth Hartley died two weeks after the shooting. With the culprit known and dead, the dramatic effort to use X-rays could only have been to locate the bullets in the hope of removing them to save her life. No one seems to have wondered if the X-rays had contributed to her demise.

The first time X-rays are known to have identified the dead occurred about a year later in Paris, in the aftermath of a calamitous fire on May 4, 1897.[21] The occasion was an annual bazaar run by leaders of fashion and philanthropy from all the leading Catholic charities.

Six thousand people thronged the gift boutiques that lined a mock street in "Old France" (with overhanging second stories and half-timbered construction) inside a temporary exhibition hall. The long hall had been decorated with painted flats and draperies. The only electricity was a line brought in for a kinetoscope. Without warning, the electrical wire from the kinetoscope shorted. Flames spread in twelve seconds to the fabric wall coverings and to the unvarnished wooden floor. Fire engulfed the whole bazaar in eight minutes, and then the roof collapsed. After twelve minutes, over two hundred of France's most socially prominent citizens had perished. The dead, piled up against the walls under the roof, were charred beyond recognition. In explaining the use of the X-ray after the fire, the vice-president of the Society of Hygiene reported that "knowing of the existence of a fracture in a person, who has been burned or mutilated beyond recognition, we can hope to identify him by the X-ray and conclude therefrom that a member found really belongs to the person supposed to have disappeared."[22]

The French continued to demonstrate confidence in X-rays in August 1897, when the government installed fluoroscopes for its customs inspectors at the Gare du Nord in Paris. This was the first in what would become a major non-medical, investigative application of X-ray technology.

A month later, in early September, X-rays entered the French courtroom following events in the village of Courbevoie, near Rouen, where a milkman (known only as "X" in the report) was shot after an argument at a café. Another customer, identified only as Jacques K, was an enormous fellow known as a nasty drunk. Apparently exasperated by the milkman's argument with the café's owner, Jacques pulled out a revolver and put it on a small table beside the bar. The milkman ran out of the café and down the street, only to be followed by the gun-toting Jacques. The milkman turned and kicked Jacques in the left shoulder, sending him to his knees. X stood watching, thinking the altercation over. Then he saw Jacques stand up, the revolver in his hand pointed toward X, and instinctively he raised his left arm to protect his head, covering his eyes. Within seconds, a bullet passed through X's arm and continued through his upper body until it lodged in his chest, He did not realize he had been hit, until he suddenly felt his left hand go numb. He examined his shoulder, found the wound, and reported the attack to the police.

Jacques denied having discharged any bullets at all, and as the only evidence rested inside the milkman's body, he declared himself innocent. Then the milkman's lawyer suggested he get an X-ray. And there was the 9 mm bullet sitting inside his chest, like a shadow of truth.[23] At this point Jacques changed his story. "Yes, he had shot, but only in self-defense." He claimed that the milkman had kicked him from the back and he had fallen on his face. Fearing being kicked to death, and still lying on the ground, he had taken a shot with his left hand, without even looking, to frighten the milkman away. But the radiograph indicated otherwise. The angle of the bullet revealed in the X-ray indicated that it had been shot by a right-handed person—because the victim's left side had been hit—and from above, not below.

Impressive as this sleuthing may have been, there is no record of another such forensic application until 1913, in Germany. This time the sleuth was a distinguished physician, an X-ray expert and inventor who was about to make his name synonymous with X-ray technology. Gustav Bucky, a prominent radiological physician, was brought in to reconstruct a crime—the disappearance of a man whose wife had spent four years of widowhood suffering not grief, but guilt. Four years after his disappearance, unable to bear it any longer, she confessed that, with the help of the hired man, she had shot and buried her husband. Now she led the authorities to the grave. X-rays established that the murder weapon had, indeed, been a shotgun and, from the location of a piece of shot in the cervical vertebra, that the man had been shot from behind. In the years to come, criminologists would become dependent on X-rays for reconstructing criminal acts.

The Love Nest in Elmira

A bullet in the head was a different matter, as was revealed in the aftermath of the Orme trial in upstate New York in the summer of 1897. On July 8, a familiar triangle played itself out in the village of Horseheads when George A. C. Orme, an elderly man with reportedly "intelligent" features, returned home unexpectedly in the afternoon to find his wife in the arms of their Italian boarder, James Punzo. Startled, Mrs. Orme struck her husband over the head with a large tin dipper. Orme drew the revolver he happened to be carrying, but the blood dripping from his forehead spoiled his aim. His first bullet struck his wife in the mouth and tongue; the second made a clean path into Punzo's brain. Mrs. Orme recovered enough to testify (although she found it difficult to speak) at Orme's trial. Punzo was taken to the hospital; he remained dazed for about two weeks, but then improved so rapidly that he was soon walking around the hospital grounds and chatting with anyone who would spare him the time. His scalp had healed over the bullet hole when the prosecutor decided to find the bullet with roentgen rays.

To nail Orme, the prosecutor needed proof of his homicidal intentions, and for that he needed the evidence of the bullet locked in Punzo's head. The hospital, too, wanted an X-ray in order to find and remove the bullet and thus escape any accusation of inadequate care. However, what began as an effort to protect the physicians from malpractice and provide conclusive evidence for the prosecution had a grimmer outcome.

Punzo was sedated with ether, and a Crookes tube was placed an inch and a half from his skull and left on for thirty-five minutes. Although "conditions were favorable for the working of the apparatus," the trial record tells us, the rays were not powerful enough to get a picture of the bullet. But they were strong enough to do in Punzo, or so the coroner decided when, thirteen days later, Punzo was dead. Testifying at the trial, he concluded, "We know no less what the X-rays are than we know what light, heat and electricity are. All we know of any of them is by their effects. And we know that instances are now being published from all parts of the country of most destructive effects of the X-rays. . . . In my opinion James Punzo came to his death from injuries to the brain caused by a gunshot wound, anesthetics and the X-rays."[24] Orme was acquitted and the X-rays indicted. X-rays were on the record as intellectually helpful, and potentially lethal.

The Other Shoe

The diagnostic advantages of the new discovery encouraged the medical world as well as the man in the street to ignore gossip about whatever it was that had actually killed James Punzo. The surgeon general's report three years later on the use of X-rays in the Spanish-American war glossed over the instances in which X-rays produced strange burns on the soldiers' bodies that did not respond to the usual application of lead and opium lotions. Discounting the possibility that the rays were responsible, Dr. Sternberg, the surgeon general, attributed the burns to the patients' "personal idiosyncrasy and low vitality."[25]

The complaints of burns were more than balanced by reports from physicians who had begun using X-rays as treatment for skin conditions including acne and large birthmarks. The fact of the matter was that, for the first years, doctors confused the benefits of ultraviolet light with X-rays (both were invisible) and assumed that X-rays, like sunlight, would act as a disinfectant and kill bacteria. It was not until they saw under a microscope that X-rays did not hurt bacteria that they had second thoughts. But they had already seen that X-rays did ameliorate acne and other skin diseases, at least at first. Moreover, within the next decade X-rays, and their companion radioactive source, radium, would sometimes prove effective treating some cancers. In truth, no one yet knew how X-rays acted on living tissue.

Danger had been noted as early as February 1896 when a child who had been accidentally shot in the head was brought for an X-ray to John Daniel, a physicist at Nashville's Vanderbilt University, and his colleague, William L. Dudley. Dudley wanted to be sure that the procedure was safe, so before X-raying the child, he experimented on himself. He tied a photographic plate to one side of his own head and sandwiched a coin between his head and the plate, then placed the X-ray tube a half inch away from his head on the other side and exposed the plate for an hour. He got no image. But twenty-one days later Daniel noticed a bald spot on Dudley's head where he had held the coin. There was a simple explanation: electrolysis was a popular method for removing unwanted hair, and Daniel chalked up the bald spot to the electric current used in getting X-rays. Dudley and Daniel, caught in the enthusiasm of the moment, rationalized the reaction into insignificance. But Daniel did think enough about the experience to write it down for the record.

From its first months as a medical novelty, there was evidence that the X-ray could be less than beneficent. Still, most people rationalized the side effects. Few suffered immediate burns, and the medical world had not yet caught on to the delayed effect of exposure. When Herbert Hawks, Pupin's student assistant at Columbia University who had earned pocket money demonstrating an X-ray machine at Bloomingdale's, suffered severe burns from his work at the store, he attributed them to the electrical effects of the generators. And Chester Leonard, at the University of Pennsylvania hospital, noted in July 1898, "The X-ray per se is incapable of injuring the tissues of the patients, and their dermatitis, which has been called an X-ray 'burn,' is the result of an interference with the nutrition of the part by the induced static charges."[26] But this kind of rationalization could not continue much longer.

That the effects were real and nasty was clear to Thomas Edison by 1902. He took the evidence of his own sore eyes and skin rashes very seriously and did not hesitate to tell the reporters who dogged his heels that he had too much more to accomplish in his lifetime to risk his health with X-rays. He mentioned personal experiences with his own health, but what shook him to the core was the agony of Clarence Dally.[27]

Dally had joined the Edison Lamp Works in Harrison, New Jersey, when he was twenty-four, just a year older than Edison had been when he started the company. Dally had been working with his father and three brothers, all expert glass blowers, sealing off incandescent light bulbs, when Edison transferred him to the West Orange laboratory in 1890. Six years later, immediately after Roentgen's communication about X-rays, Edison had enlisted Dally's help in experimenting with ways to use X-rays, which, especially at the start, meant holding a hand in front of the tube to make sure X-rays were being produced.

Dally had first noticed slight burns on his face, which were followed by the loss of his mustache and beard, hair from his scalp, eyebrows, eyelashes, and the backs of his hands and fingers. Eventually he lost all of his fingers and then his whole left hand—right-handed, he had been in the habit of using his left hand to hold the objects to be X-rayed. He was not alone. A gloved or amputated hand became the emblem of X-ray workers. Dally's first symptoms were swelling, reddening and pain. Dally tried switching hands, and he treated his burns with patent ointments. They didn't help at all, but he kept on working with X-rays, rising to become Edison's chief assistant.

By 1902, the burns had given way to oozing ulcers measuring three and a half by two and a half inches across, and Dally was in constant pain. He tried skin grafts, but they did not take. He had a malignant ulcer at the base of his little finger, and before the end of the year he had his left hand amputated above the wrist. Within months, a malignant ulceration had appeared on his right hand, too, and he had four fingers removed. Both arms were eventually amputated, one at the shoulder joint, the other above the elbow.

Edison sent Dally to one specialist after another, but amputation was all they could offer. As his condition deteriorated, the pain became so acute he could not even lie down. Edison was troubled by the attention Dally's illness had attracted. When asked by the press about the dangers of X-rays, Edison explained, "I'm sorry that the story has gone out that I have been made blind by the X-ray, for that is wholly untrue. I have suffered from it much more in other ways." Calling Dally into the room, he displayed him to the reporter. "The strangest part of it all is that all this is the result of work with the X-ray five or six years ago and now comes this result."[28]

Dally died in 1904. It had been an especially horrible end. "Dally had died by inches," having spent his last months sitting upright in constant pain. In June 1931, when at eighty-four Edison collapsed in his chair in the parlor of his West Orange home (to die four months later), he offered his doctor a list of symptoms but adamantly refused to be X-rayed. He never forgot Dally's agony.[29]

In 1900 in San Francisco the Army's radiographer Elizabeth Fleischmann moved out of her sister's home to marry Israel Aschheim. She retained her name and her radiographic practice, branching out into the burgeoning field of dentistry. When she suffered from apparently minor skin irritations, she attributed them to the chemicals she used to develop film. By 1904, all the fingers of both her hands were badly ulcerated, and like Dally, she had to have an arm amputated. But the cancer continued to spread, and she was dead by 1905. Elegized in the San Francisco newspapers as "America's Joan of Arc," she is the only woman included in the 1936 publication *American Martyrs to Science through the Roentgen Rays.*

By 1911 more than fifty cases of X-ray damage, including mutilation, sterility, and death, had been noted. But the public, on the whole, was unconcerned. People died of all sorts of accidents and disease, and fifty is not a large number. Besides, most of the victims were technicians or doctors who worked with radiation. (At a meeting of radiologists in 1920, the menu featured chicken—a major faux pas because almost every one at the table was missing at least one hand and could not cut the meat.)[30]

Dally's and Fleischmann's deaths were swift compared to some of their colleagues' drawn-out agony. Dr. Kells had lost his left arm by 1908, but continued practicing dentistry with a special instrument he invented to replace his missing hand. Thirty-five operations later, during which he was "whittled away inch by inch," and after publishing an autobiography as well as a standard text on the planting of teeth and receiving the highest honors in his profession, despondent with pain, he shot himself in the head in a New Orleans hotel room. It was May 1928.[31]

But the side effects were not always bad. Physicians could not help noticing that the rays they applied to get an X-ray image frequently eliminated pimples. For a short period of time in 1904 researchers in California and New York came up with the same appalling idea. In San Francisco, Robert A. Rees, an undergraduate at the College of Chemistry at the University of California, reported that he had successfully combined X-ray treatment with radium to bleach the skins of Negroes white.[32] Dr. Eldridge in Boston reported success with fifteen-minute sessions (over an unspecified period of time) during which he gradually turned a Negro white. And in Philadelphia, Dr. Henry K. Pancoast, "an X-ray expert" at the University of Pennsylvania, announced that he, too, "could turn the complexion of the blackest man to a beautiful, soft, creamy white color."[33] Dr. Dieffenbach in New York agreed that it was quite possible to "make a white man of a negro," but he suggested that, if the rays were applied to the whole body, not just the face, "the subject would probably be fatally burned."[34] The "treatment" disappears from the literature as the year ends, with no mention of the fate of these human subjects whose "conditions" may have been treated.[35]

Dieffenbach's warning about the excessive use of radiation echoes the coroner in the Orme case, who seven years earlier had indicted the X-ray in the death of Mr. Punzo. These warnings were drowned out by enthusiasts who disputed whether the "dermatitis" actually came from X-rays. Some believed that X-rays were a normal part of sunlight and so the burns that often followed exposure were just another kind of sunburn; others explained the occasional burns that some patients suffered as a result of electrical short circuits, a frequent though admittedly undesirable side effect in all "electrotherapeutics."

A Few Good Tests

X-ray burns were different from sunburns or burns from electrical shorts because they did not heal. But the public and physicians did not want to see the downside of exposure. For a while it was easy to attribute the burns, rashes, and hair loss to electric malfunction.

Not everyone was ready to make excuses. In 1896 Elihu Thomson, a physicist who had left the Harvard faculty to work at the General Electric Company in Lynn, Massachusetts, had a vested interest in electrical safety. He had developed an electrical coil for GE that, he was convinced, was not responsible for any burns. To prove that the X-rays themselves were responsible, he decided to experiment on himself, and began by asking "what part of my body

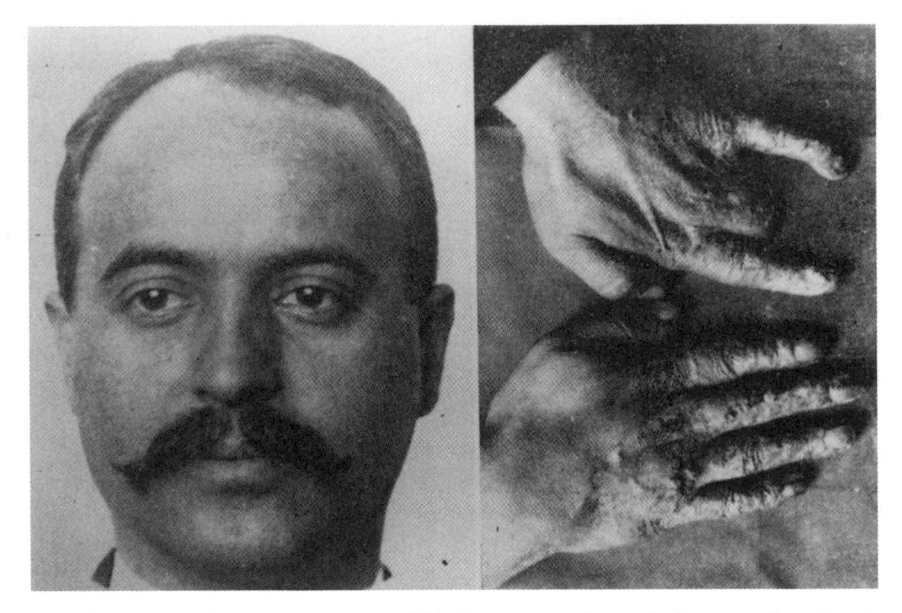

11. Mihran K. Kassabian (1870–1910) and his X-ray dermatitis hands. Courtesy of the American College of Radiology.

I could best afford to lose, and decided it was the last joint on my left little finger."[36]

He then subjected that joint for half an hour to radiation, holding it about an inch and a half from the X-ray tube. Nothing happened for a week. Then "that finger reddened, became extremely sensitive, stiff and to a certain extent, painful. After two weeks it continued to be sore and a large blister began to grow." He concluded that "there is evidently a point beyond which exposure cannot go without causing serious trouble."[37] He had hit upon the idea of maximum exposure, an idea that would remain part of the mythology about radiation for another thirty years.

At the same time that Elihu Thomson was experimenting with his own finger, a pair of medically trained brothers-in-law in Boston were independently experimenting with some of the burns and rashes associated with the new rays. The extrovert of the pair, Francis H. Williams, was a doctor with a degree in chemistry from the Massachusetts Institute of Technology. The introvert was William Herbert Rollins, a dentist with a medical degree from Harvard who was married to Williams's sister. Early in 1896 Williams got permission from MIT to experiment with its X-ray apparatus at night, so that is where he brought his patients with chest diseases from Boston City Hospital. Most doctors then were using the X-ray to explore bones, but Williams was using it to explore the chest, especially for signs of tuberculosis. Referring to percussion —the practice of tapping the body and listening to the sound—Williams noted, "We may now look where we have previously only been able to listen."[38]

As an undergraduate Williams had considered a career in physics. After graduation, he had joined an expedition to observe the rare astronomical phenomenon of a transit of Venus, then studied physics in Europe before returning to Harvard to study medicine. Roentgen's discovery brought together his two interests—physics and medicine. By April 1896 he had built himself an X-ray machine and presented a fluoroscopic demonstration of the bones of a hand and wrist to the local medical society.

By 1897 Williams had used the fluoroscope to examine patients with three visually distinctive kinds of lung disease—pneumonia, emphysema, and tuberculosis—and had also used the X-ray to find kidney stones. By the next year he had developed the use of a contrast agent, bismuth subnitrate, which was opaque to the X-rays and so outlined the internal organs it flowed through. He summed up all of his research in *The Roentgen Rays in Medicine and Surgery,* which he published in 1901. Yet even as he spent hours in the lab, he was aware of the side effects and was extremely cautious. "That I have escaped injury is due to an early recognition of the dangerous nature of x-light and to the precautions recommended in earlier papers having been taken."[39]

Those dangers had been underscored by his associate, William Rollins, a quiet man who had continued practicing dentistry by day despite his medical degree. He saved his passion for the X-ray for evenings at MIT. Rollins, an inventor who designed the earliest piece of American X-ray paraphernalia—a clip holding celluloid film that could be held firmly inside the mouth—had been severely burned during an experiment. After learning about Dudley's peculiar bald spot he collected reports of burns and rashes until he had a large enough number to suggest that they were the result of long-term exposure to X-rays. Certain that X-rays themselves were dangerous, Rollins devised a set of protective steps.

He reported in his "Notes on the X-Light" (published in 1904 in the *Boston Medical and Surgical Journal*) that certain injuries were reduced when he covered the fluorescent screen on the side nearest the eyes with a sheet of lead glass a centimeter thick, and coated the rest of the fluoroscope with lead paint. He also recommended moving the tube as far as possible from the patient (which was the opposite of the early practice of holding the tube flush up against the patient's body). These precautions notwithstanding, the core of the article described an experiment he had done three years earlier demonstrating the effects of X-radiation on guinea pigs. He had enclosed a strong male guinea pig in a metal box and suspended the box by insulators inside another grounded metal box for two hours a day, for ten days. The animal was examined and was healthy. He then exposed the animal to X-rays. On the eleventh day, the guinea pig died. By effectively separating the action of electricity from those of the rays, he was able to pinpoint X-rays as the malevolent factor. In further experiments with guinea pigs he demonstrated that X-rays in smaller quantities could blind, burn, or cause the female guinea pigs to abort. Rollins believed these results sufficient evidence to require protecting people from radiation, and he drew up a detailed list of suggestions for technicians, patients, and people involved in the manufacture of X-ray equipment. He urged everyone using X-rays to enclose the tubes in lead-lined boxes. He even devised a badge of film that, when fogged, indicated that the wearer had been exposed to an excessive quantity of X-rays.

Rollins never patented any of his devices, and while he did publish these results, his articles appeared in obscure journals and apparently went unread by those who could have used his advice. Rollins offered concrete suggestions to prevent the dangers of radiation, including the advice that its application be thought of always in terms of the smallest quantity needed to get the job done. His voice was quiet and his approach modest. As a result he was generally ignored. Today, however, the film badge is used universally by people working around radiation and minimum exposure has long been the rule.

Rollins also demonstrated the effect of radiation on rodent fertility (and suggested that the rays could be used to sterilize people, an idea that appealed to contemporary eugenicists who envisioned an improved human "stock" by weeding out the less fit). The ability of radiation to damage living tissue had been demonstrated in 1903 in Leipzig when the biologist George Perthes noted a correlation between the exposure of mouse cells to radiation and mouse reproduction, and in France the same year where four white rats exposed to X-rays developed skin ulcerations, after which two of the mice died, and one of the survivors developed a malignant tumor. Then in 1906, also in France, Jean Alban Bergonie and L. Tribondeau formulated the descriptive law that remained the working hypothesis about the effects of radiation through the 1930s. They said that the effect of radiation on living cells is greater in the earliest stage of cell division, that radiation affects reproductive cells more than other cells and causes the proliferation of cancer cells in proportion to their stage of development. Although this "law" has been replaced by more precise knowledge about the effect of radiation on reproduction, it is still by and large accurate. By the end of the first decade of X-rays in medicine, they were known to cause burns and ulcerations as well as sterility in male and female rodents, and by extrapolation, in all other mammals including ourselves.

This knowledge did not help Fleischmann or Dally, although they could have known about Rollins's work had it been published elsewhere, or triggered debate. There were forums where X-ray research was discussed; almost every European country had its journal of "roentgenology." Doctors and engineers eagerly published their experiences, including mention of unhealed sores and strange skin eruptions. But the naysayers were drowned out by the enthusiasm of the adventurers. Mostly doctors, they continued working without protection, assuming that the discomfort they suffered was the price for being in the forefront of a new enterprise.

Considering their symptoms part of the job, medical people ignored warnings. The attitude extended to scientists who worked with radium. Marie Curie handled radioactive substances barehanded for over thirty years, her raw and itching fingers a badge of honor. She never encouraged safety precautions in her lab, even after Pierre Curie and two physicians had demonstrated that even small quantities of radium gas (radon) could kill mice and hamsters. Even after Becquerel complained that a test tube filled with radium which he had carried to a London conference for them had burned his thigh, the Curies said nothing.[40] Decades later, after several close assistants had succumbed to anemias, Marie Curie still did not acknowledge the connection between radiation (both from X-rays and from radium) and leukemia and other blood diseases. Her biographer defends her, explaining that "there had never before been a poison quite like it: an unseen poison that acted on the body over many years and affected different people in different ways."[41] But this biographer concedes that Curie should have recognized the probability that precisely because radiation killed cancer cells, it would affect healthy cells as well.

As early as 1905 scientific reports from three countries noted that X-rays, while remarkable for their ability to get images of the insides of the living body, changed the tissues they passed through in ways that were unpredictable and often undesirable. The strange refusal to act on these reports may be explained by the fact that, while some effects were obvious right away in laboratory studies, many repercussions in human beings went undetected for as long as twenty years.

One of the first arguments used in defense of X-rays appeared in July 1897, in the *British Medical Journal.* "Deep Tissue Traumatization from Roentgen Rays Exposure" suggests that the average exposure lasted from twenty to forty minutes, but was sometimes as long as two hours. In remarking on a reaction in some patients akin to sunburn, the author concludes that "individual predisposition plays a vital part."[42] Blaming the patient instead of the treatment is a theme that continued to be sounded in connection with X-rays. People do respond differently, up to some degree of exposure. Beyond that, all succumb.

Paradoxically, X-rays that make the invisible visible were themselves the first invisible substances generated by scientists to profoundly affect human perception. We cannot see them, and we cannot always track the path of destruction they establish on a slow fuse. Whereas the first generation of X-ray explorers lived in a world where science meant progress, today we are aware of the potentially lethal repercussions of exposure to radioactivity and are apprehensive about the delayed actions of all sorts of invisible enemies from chemical pollution to dormant viruses to electromagnetic power lines. The combination of invisibility and delayed reaction is still hard to grasp. When the immediate benefits of exposure were life-saving—to the man in the street as well as the man in the White House—there was no question about making the choice in favor of the diagnostic image and ignoring a possible reaction decades in the future. It is easy to understand why so many people who ought to have known better reveled in the X-ray's benefits in 1912, and did not wait for the other shoe to drop.

Three

Technological Innovation 1897–1918

Building a Better Mousetrap

With the X-ray genie out of the bottle, the race was on to domesticate him. In the entrepreneurial climate of the turn of the century the very existence of the mousetrap was the impetus to build a better one. From 1896 through the end of World War I, doctors, engineers, and physicists took Roentgen's simple apparatus and refined it into a powerful, focused, efficient, ingenious, and increasingly safe device for peering into the living body. What had been touted as a photographic novelty in 1896 became a medical necessity. Competition grew keen over which improvements should be adapted and over who should control access to the X-ray's use. At the start, independent companies that targeted the new market prospered, often merging after a while with giants like General Electric but occasionally growing into a large presence. The race was an international affair, with companies having one foot in Britain, France, or Germany and the other in the United States. But it was never for amateurs. Almost all of the major improvements were made by doctors or engineers who were inspired by the increasing diagnostic value of X-rays, and by the demand created by the Great War.

Roentgen never patented anything to do with X-rays because he did not think of natural phenomena as something someone could own. But even if he had sought a patent, it is unlikely he would have been successful. All the equipment he used—induction coils, cathode-ray tubes, photographic plates—had been around for a while. What he had done was use these very ordinary laboratory staples to discover, and document, a phenomenon that several of his colleagues had already stumbled across, but either had dismissed or overlooked.

Although Roentgen never considered profiting from his discovery, most of those who refined the apparatus did. As early as 1896 and 1897, inventors went to court in the United States to stake claims to priority in both practical and conceptual innovations.

The companies that entered the market in these first two years included some players that are still in the game. The German firm Siemens was a natural contender; it had been in the electromedical business since 1847 and had provided Roentgen with his first cathode ray tubes. (Siemens became a publicly held company in 1897, and has entered partnerships and merged with other corporations several times since 1916.) In the United States the new General Electric Company, which included Edison's electric companies and the Thomson-Houston Company, went to work on X-rays on several fronts. At the GE research laboratory in Schenectady, New York, Elihu Thomson designed a better tube plus a high-frequency coil to power it, while in New Jersey Edison himself soon marketed both fluoroscopes and an X-ray kit that included induction coils, tubes, and glass plates.

Smaller outfits included Robert Friedlander, who started a company in 1896 with offices in New York City and Chicago. By 1905 Friedlander had twenty-three X-ray patents, including the first protective, lead-lined whole-body suit.[1] Another early competitor was Waite & Bartlett in New York, a company founded by Henry Waite, a physician who passed the firm on to his son, who was also a doctor. The Waites filed fifty-one patents, including those for the first shockproof medical and dental units. There was no Bartlett, just the name. Waite & Bartlett was taken over in 1929 by a relative latecomer to the X-ray scene, James Picker. Picker had emigrated from Russia to New York in 1901, where he took a job as a delivery boy in a pharmacy near Mount Sinai Hospital. Just five years later he had bought the store and introduced two services: a soda fountain and an agency for Kodak, whose fragile photographic plates the hospital was having trouble procuring. In 1915 Picker sold the pharmacy to devote himself to the X-ray supply business and immediately introduced the first printed price list and a policy of same-day shipping.

In the free-for-all economic climate of the end of the nineteenth century, not unlike the mood of the late twentieth century, big businesses hungrily merged with or devoured smaller businesses, but there was always room for "start-ups," like Robert H. Machlett's in New York City. Machlett, a third-generation glass blower, had emigrated from Germany to New York City in 1883, where he made glass apparatus for chemists and physicians in a small, upstairs shop on East Twenty-third Street. In 1897 he became the first commercial manufacturer of X-ray tubes in North America, which were all still hand-blown.

Queen & Company, a major Philadelphia importer of medical goods, crested early with its adjustable radiographic table and its self-regulating X-ray tube, which became standard in the United States. Newly incorporated in 1893, Queen saw a procession of talented engineers come and go, one of

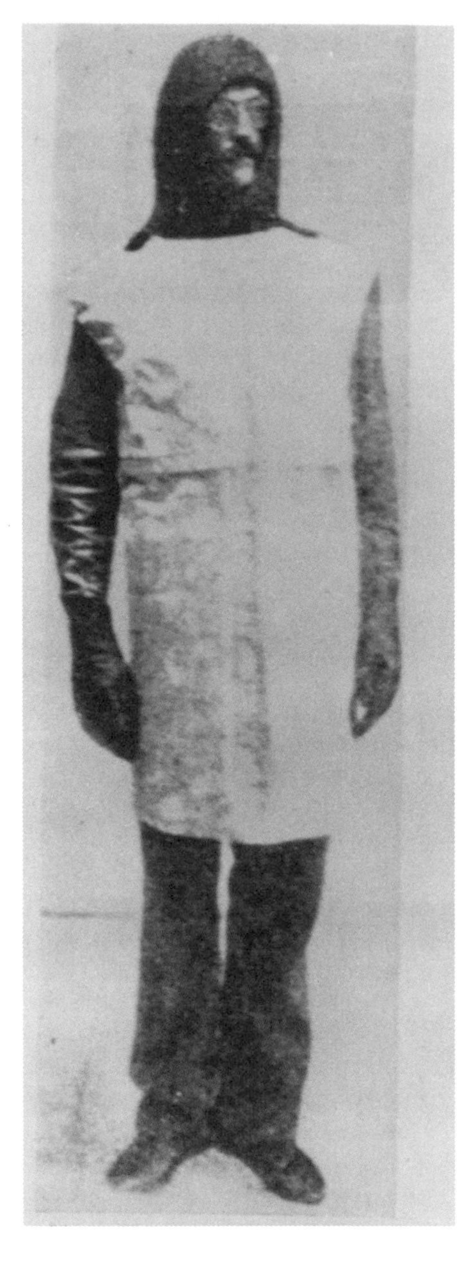

12. Friedlander X-ray protective suit (1907). This advertisement features the complete outfit (apron, hood, gloves, spectacles). It cost $30. Courtesy of the American College of Radiology.

whom left with the patent for the X-ray tube regulator. But selling a single product, even the best, was a bad gamble, and Queen left the X-ray business in 1912 when gas tubes were on their way out.

The fates of these early businesses seemed to rest on family, particularly sons: Waite had a son ready to take over, but Friedlander, who had been off to a brilliant start, founding and editing the *Archives of Electrology and Radiology,* died of radiation-induced burns in 1915 and his company died with him

Machlett, like Friedlander, also died from radiation-induced cancer—like so many glass blowers involved with X-rays, he tested his tubes with his own hand—but his company, Machlett & Sons, continued to grow after his death in 1926 and was still thriving in 1988 as an independent producer of X-ray apparatus.[2] There was a Waite in the line of succession to head Waite & Bartlett, and a young Picker, as well. Family-owned companies managed to hold out but few remain today. The Picker name survives as a division within the corporate body of the larger British-based General Electric Company (GEC Ltd). Today, the only names from the last century are General Electric and Siemens.

There was plenty of room for innovation in every area of X-ray production, from improving basic parts such as the X-ray tubes or the necessary adjuncts—glass plates, celluloid film, and fluoroscopic screens—to designing specialized furniture and film holders. Not every patent won the lottery. Losers include a 1902 patent for a coin-operated X-ray machine, and the 1898 "see-hear" device, co-invented by the Boston brothers-in-law Francis Williams and William Rollins, which combined a fluorescent screen with a telephone-like diaphragm (a kind of stethoscope) in order to register sight and sound simultaneously. It could be used, as Rollins demonstrated, by the operating physician to diagnose himself.

Competition, then as now, included expensive fights over patent infringements. Many such cases languished while newer technologies made the arguments moot. Inventors moved from company to company, as owners or employees, according to the luck of the market. So did sales representatives.

The Market

Technological progress was largely doctor-driven: sales representatives specialized in developing warm relations with doctors and hospitals, and when they changed employers, brought along a dowry of well-cultivated clients whose complaints about fragile tubes or poor photographic plates moved manufacturers to improve their products. As physicians began to specialize, they required instruments that could get a good picture of particular parts of the body. Manufacturers raced to satisfy their demands. And when the doctors did not think it worth spending money on a product—such as lead shielding to limit excess radiation from spilling onto patients, technicians, and themselves—these products, like Friedlander's suit, disappeared from the marketplace. Most of the early shielding devices, whether attached to tubes or worn as clothing, were bulky and awkward to use. Besides, most physicians wanted to believe that X-rays were benign and chose to avoid products that suggested the opposite.

By 1910, X-ray machines were being hawked in all forty-six states directly to dentists and doctors for their private practices, and to hospital administrators for their institutions. It was a difficult market. According to a survey by the *American Journal of Roentgenology,* 67 percent of hospitals owned their own equipment. Only 12 percent of the hospitals paid their X-ray experts a salary, so most of the doctors lived on patient fees.[3] Radiologists usually posted a fee table, and while it is hard to translate the numbers to contemporary costs, radiographs of eyes and teeth were about the same price, while pictures of the stomach, bowel, and pelvis cost twice as much, with an additional 50 to 500 percent for work done outside the laboratory, depending on the distance traveled by the doctor.

In the first years, photographers had had a large share of the X-ray curiosity market. Those who could afford it happily paid for images of their skeletons. Celebrities set the pace: the czarina of Russia rushed to have her hand X-rayed; Kaiser Wilhelm II of Germany opted for an image of his arm. The British prime minister and his wife had had their hands done, together, and Queen Emilia of Portugal sent her ladies-in-waiting to get their rib cages X-rayed to illustrate the evils of tight laces.

Once the novelty was over, though, the medical community eased out the competition from photographers and others. Laboratory physicists, of course, continued to explore the X-ray as a scientific tool, but their needs could be satisfied by rigging up gadgets in the lab. They did not require the capital-intensive organizations of mass production. Electrical engineers, like the distinguished A. A. Campbell Swinton in England, who made some of the finest early radiographs, and youngsters like Herbert Hawks in New York and Elizabeth Fleischmann in San Francisco soon found their autonomy challenged by hostile physicians. During the first years, engineers, scientists, photographers, and doctors all claimed the right to use X-rays. Each group reasoned that its members not only understood how the apparatus worked, but were needed to operate them. But the only people willing and able to invest in more expensive machines that could penetrate ever more profound depths of the human body were the doctors.

Consolidating Power

Some of the young photographers and electrical engineers who had grown fascinated with X-rays decided to become doctors. In Boston, Walter Dodd, the photographer at the Massachusetts General Hospital, began by taking X-ray images and went on to earn an M.D., and in New York, Eugene Caldwell moved from electrical engineering and X-ray photography to medical school, eventually becoming the chief radiologist at Bellevue Hospital. And from the Mideast Mihran Kassabian, who attended the American Missionary Institute in Caesarea, went to London intending to become a medical missionary. Detoured for a while by his interest in photography, he continued his journey to Philadelphia where he had just entered the Medical-Chirurgical College when news of the X-rays appeared in 1896. He was still working his way through medical school when war broke out with Spain in 1898, and he interrupted his studies to join the Hospital Corps of the American army. It was in Cuba that he first used X-rays, developing skills that led to his appointment as an instructor in electrotherapeutics on his return to Philadelphia. Degree in hand, he got an appointment at the

Philadelphia Hospital where he continued his work with X-rays. Then in 1907, he published the second major radiology textbook, *Roentgen Rays and Electro-Therapeutics.*

Kassabian joined the ranks of medical experts in America, France, Germany, and Austria (including Antoine Béclère, who had translated Francis Williams's text into French) who were determined to ensure that organized medicine controlled the new technology. Their campaign to push out photographers and engineers from their radiological organizations and publications was encouraged by the American Medical Association, which justified the exclusion of laypersons on grounds that only physicians understood the human body. The fledgling radiological community protested. The medical leaders of this purge did not bother to mention that by keeping control over the use of X-ray devices, their income from fees for medical and forensic referrals would be assured.

As doctors consolidated control, they campaigned to keep X-ray technicians subordinate everywhere: in hospitals and on the staffs of the newly founded X-ray journals and organizations. The very nonphysicians who had, in many instances, founded the journals, were no longer welcome as contributors. It was nasty, but swift. Within a few years there were no more X-ray "sittings"—a term used by artists and photographers—at "studios." Instead, patients came for "treatments" at laboratories in doctor's offices or in hospitals.

The struggle between technicians and physicians was petering out when dissent erupted within the medical profession itself. There were two different battles. The first was among advocates for X-rays as diagnosis, the second among those who used X-rays in therapies. Kassabian's textbook is a good illustration of the confusion about the benefits of the latter. As treatment, X-rays were initially classified as "electrotherapeutics," a specialty of turn-of-the-century medicine that used electricity in therapies ranging from hair removal to sexual rejuvenation. Respectable doctors used X-rays to treat cancer, tuberculosis, and infertility.

Doctors eventually accepted X-rays as a major contribution to the rationalization of diagnosis. They could see, and then compare, healthy and diseased views of the same organs in different people. The X-ray permitted groups of physicians to examine pictures of a condition before and after treatment. And, not to be dismissed, it allowed patients, for the first time ever, to see their own diseased organs and be included in a plan of treatment. With the appearance of radiographs, the ideal of an objective diagnosis became a major element in the transformation of medicine from an art into a science.

Despite these obvious advantages, the change within medicine was gradual. Anyone could buy and install an X-ray machine, and many general practitioners, surgeons, and obstetricians did just that. After the purge of technicians, tensions remained among physicians. Radiology had not yet begun to coalesce as a specialty. A six-week course in how to use the machine was all that an ambitious physician needed to declare himself a "roentgenologist."

There remained a small inner circle of physicians who had become obsessed with improving the quality of X-ray images and the possibility of getting images of hard-to-see organs. They spent long stretches of time absorbed with the apparatus and were looked on as odd, in somewhat the same way that people obsessively interested in computers were dismissed as "hackers" in the 1970s.

Fine-tuning the Machine

The fascination with X-ray apparatus is easy to understand. There was room for improvement all along the way, beginning with the source of the electrical power, and continuing with the stability of the X-ray tube, and the problems of speed and resolution in photographic plates and fluoroscopic screens.

By 1896 scientists knew that electromagnetism existed and how it could be harnessed, but they did not understand the nature of its waves, rays, or particles. Even as engineers harnessed electricity into power-grids that could serve whole cities, neither they nor those who focused the X-ray tubes and adjusted the machines that powered them understood what we take for granted today—the structure of the atom and its constituent parts. Nor did they understand the way human tissue can both benefit and suffer from bombardment with these particles.

All that was known in 1896 was that an electric current, energized to a very high voltage in a partially evacuated glass tube, produced mysterious "X" rays that when directed through an object left a permanent record of the internal structure of that object on a photographic plate.

As the tubes that produced X-rays improved, they became easier to control and so more useful. But they had to be powered, and it was not clear which was the best way to generate voltage high enough to produce X-rays. Although electric power was generally available in most American cities by 1900, service was so often erratic that most X-ray apparatus still came packaged with its own power supply.

Two different methods of generating current competed for attention—induction coils and static machines. Each had advantages. Coils were less bulky, usually produced higher voltages than static machines, generated higher energy, and produced better contrast in radiographs of deep-lying organs, like the gall bladder. But coils depended on mechanical interrupters which were both clumsy and noisy. Static machines, on the other hand, were more reliable, needed fewer repairs, and could be operated by either an electric motor or by hand (this was an advantage in remote rural areas). They were, however, sensitive to humidity, and primitive models sparked, filling the air with the distinctive smell of ozone.

Compounding the confusion over which to use and misconceptions about the safety of X-rays was the fact that the generators worked very differently from each other. For at least a decade, these differences provided an explanation, or an excuse, for the burns and unpleasant skin conditions that afflicted many patients and doctors after X-ray examinations. Defenders of X-rays insisted that the conditions resulted from exposure to ozone, electrical sparks, or short circuits produced by induction coils.

It did not help that poor insulation was responsible for burns and even an occasional electrocution. (Electrical hazards were not eliminated entirely until well-insulated "shock proof" cables were manufactured in 1930.) Through the intervening decades doctors, physicists, judges, and juries confused the real danger of electrocution with the equally real but just dawning understanding of the hazards of radiation. What seems obvious in hindsight would not be altogether clear until the electrical wrinkles had been ironed out of the machinery.

The first-generation machines were easy to sell because they were inexpensive and novel.[4] By 1900 there were at least two hundred diagnostic X-ray installations in the United States, Britain, France, Germany, and Austria. At the start of the new century, manufacturers were offering a broad selection of X-ray machines, many with real improvements over earlier models, and consequently more expensive. The market was almost entirely medical, and manufacturers competed to provide the equipment doctors seemed to want at prices doctors were willing to pay.

Just like a researcher today trying to decide which new imaging system to buy, George C. Johnston, president of the American Roentgen Ray Society, complained in 1909 that "the apparatus of today is obsolete tomorrow. There is a constant race between our pocketbooks and the inventive genius of the up-to-date manufacturer."[5] And in 1909, he was only talking about what, we know in retrospect, were cosmetic changes. The next important advance would be a replacement for the gas tube.

Gas tubes, which were basically unreliable, were the heart of the machines. Every professional photographer or "roentgenologist" carried three tubes for every one needed, on the safe bet that one or two would fail. A popular description of a gas tube was "a glass bulb surrounded by profanity." Gas tubes had three problems: no one knew how to measure the voltage that was passing across the tube, no one knew how to build tubes that could produce a steady voltage, and no one knew how to maintain the vacuum that produced a steadier beam of rays. When Roentgen demonstrated his original X-ray apparatus to an English reporter at his laboratory in Würzburg late in January 1896, he had used a pear-shaped glass tube that took over an hour to get an exposure. The hundreds of people who read Roentgen's original paper and followed his directions discovered for themselves that it was not always easy and seldom quick to get a clear image.

In March 1896, the first improvement was made by an Englishman, Herbert Jackson, who curved the cathode plate so that the rays were focused in a column that struck a platinum plate, the anode. This procedure, which channeled the X-rays in a line through to the target, prevented a good proportion of random rays from blurring the picture. This innovation reduced the blurring previously caused by random rays that reached the photographic plate.

Jackson's "focus tube" also shortened the time of exposure, but two-hour radiographic sessions continued to be commonplace for another five years (and for another decade in the offices of doctors who did not want to invest in newer, more expensive machines). In the United States, Clarence Dally often took over an hour to get a single exposure for Edison. Complete amateurs, like the physician in Willimantic, Connecticut, who purchased an X-ray machine early in 1899, had no hesitation about testing the tube by holding it five inches from his own groin for forty-five minutes.

When Edward Parker Davis, a practitioner at Jefferson Medical College in Philadelphia, made the first image of a living fetus in 1896, he exposed the young mother to the rays for an hour the first time around, and an hour and a quarter the second. Delighted with the pictures, he suggested that X-rays be used routinely in obstetrics "as it requires no exposure of the patient, no vaginal manipulation, and puts her to no essential discomfort." He added "there has not been the slightest evidence that the passage of the rays through the uterus has affected either mother or child."[6]

The kind of effect that we know now could have occurred, the development of leukemia in the child ten years later, was simply not part of the way people looked on medical cause and effect at the end of the last century, and it is doubtful anyone ever followed up on the mother or child. Few doctors made X-rays a routine part of pregnancy at this time, however, because there was little that could be seen until the last trimester, and it was an expense few people wanted to incur. The focus of medical attention was the mother, and since pregnancy was an obvious condition, there seemed little to be gained from making the woman endure the discomfort of a radiological examination. There was no cultural precedent for invading the privacy of the developing fetus.

Although the focus tubes (and there were many in the wake of Jackson's) helped shorten the exposure time and offered the operator some control over the amount of energy emitted and over which tissues were being penetrated, an enormous amount of radiation still escaped into the surrounding area. But focus and time-exposure were not the only problems. By the early years of the twentieth century it was clear that not only did the quality of X-ray images reflect the heterogeneous nature of the materials the rays passed through but that the X-rays themselves were heterogeneous. They have a range of penetrating power, some entering deep into the body, and some stopping at the skin. The so-called "hard" rays penetrate deep into the bones while "soft" rays stop near the surface. These soft rays were responsible for the burns or "dermatitis" that killed Dally, Fleischmann, Machlett, Friedlander, and Kassabian (who died of X-ray induced cancer in 1910). To get clearer diagnostic images, manufacturers improved the focus of the tubes by eliminating extraneous soft rays that could damage skin as well as extra hard rays that fanned out and blurred the picture.

Even with better focus, the glass tubes were a nuisance. Whenever these first-generation tubes were charged, they left a residue of gas on the inside of the glass. A certain amount of gas was necessary, but the residue built up and made the tubes "harden" (a term not to be confused with "hard" rays). The pressure of gas inside changed as the tube heated. If the pressure became too great, the fragile tube simply cracked. Every X-ray lab kept a large supply of extra tubes, and when X-rays had to be taken outside the lab, someone had to arrange to have an extra supply of tubes on hand, just in case.

The Great Leap Forward

Many of these problems disappeared in 1913 when William David Coolidge invented the modern high vacuum, hot cathode, tungsten-target X-ray tube. Coolidge was typical of a new generation of inventors. He had a Ph.D. and European training before he joined General Electric at its university-style research laboratory in Schenectady, New York, in 1905. There, working amid a cluster of Ph.D-trained physicists and engineers, he had been encouraged to pursue basic research (but never forgetting the possible practical applications). This suited Coolidge perfectly. He had grown up on a hardscrabble farm in rural Massachusetts where college had not figured as a possibility until he won a scholarship to Boston Tech.

In 1891, Boston Tech (soon renamed MIT) happened to be the only American institution besides West Point that awarded engineering degrees. Degree in hand, Coolidge went to Germany in 1896 to do graduate work. With a German Ph.D., Coolidge returned to teach physics briefly at MIT before joining GE, which was at that time a new kind of corporate laboratory that invested in long-term technical research. It was there that he began looking for better filaments for electric light bulbs, exploring tungsten, among other metals. Tungsten had a lot to offer, except that it was brittle. Coolidge discovered that by reducing the temperature at which the metal was worked he made it more ductile. Thanks to this discovery, GE introduced tungsten into its light bulbs in 1910.

Coolidge continued to find new uses for ductile tungsten, which soon replaced platinum as contact points in automobile ignitions. In 1912 Coolidge suggested to the American Institute of Electrical Engineers that tungsten replace the platinum anodes in X-ray tubes. It was ideal for the job, Coolidge explained, because tungsten has a much higher melting point than platinum but, at the same time, of all the metals, tungsten vaporizes the least and so leaves the walls of the tube clear of residue.

However, simply replacing the filament with tungsten did not solve the problem. It was only after conferring with another GE scientist, Irving Langmuir, that Coolidge realized he had to remove almost all the gas from the tube, leaving "not more than a few hundredths of a micron." The first time he tried it, the new tube emitted so many X-rays that Coolidge "unintentionally sacrificed my own back hair [apparently with no lasting effect. Coolidge died in 1975 at the age of 102.]. So I didn't like to practice on other living subjects. For further experiments I was, through the kindness of a medical friend, provided with a human leg which had outlived its usefulness."[7]

When the new Coolidge tube was ready for the clinic in 1913, it rated terrific on five counts: it could be accurately adjusted; it was stable; it reliably produced exact duplications of previous images ("the apparatus can be set for a given penetration, and by using the same milliamperage through the tube, a hundred roentgenograms can be made so nearly alike that it is impossible to tell them apart"); the tube was flexible enough to go from high to low penetration immediately; and finally, although this was certainly not the priority, its promoters noted that it was safer for operator and patient because there was less scattered radiation.[8]

The Coolidge tube was immediately popular in the United States, and GE led the market, to be joined in 1913 by other tube manufacturers who patented variations and improvements, or paid GE to use its patent. With this reliable new tube in hand, the next generation of radiologists would be able to measure radiation and control how much radiation was being produced. In Europe, however, there were few orders for the new tubes. Europe had gone to war, taking along only gas tubes in its medical paraphernalia.

At almost the same time that Coolidge revolutionized the X-ray tube, another improvement was in the process of being perfected that solved a different problem of the X-ray process. As X-rays enter the body, they ionize molecules in the tissue and this sets off a second wave of rays. Physicists understood that the blurred parts of most pictures came from these unfocused rays hitting the photographic plate or the fluoroscopic screen. It was also obvious that the volume of X-rays originally emitted from the tubes was enormous compared to the minuscule proportion that managed to go all the way through the subject and continue straight on to the photographic plate. (In 1920, the Eastman Kodak Research laboratory suggested that as much as 80 to 90 percent of all radiation reaching its film was causing blurring, and a mere 10 to 20 percent was carrying information.)

The blurring had been noted as early as 1896 by Arthur Wright at Yale, and in 1903, Otto Pasche, a physicist in Bern, Switzerland, suggested that placing something between the patient and the photographic plate could eliminate much of this scatter. He devised a system similar to one used in some cameras, but it didn't work.

It was 1913 when Gustav Bucky in Berlin solved the problem of scattering rays by inserting two metal grids, one between the patient and the tube, the second between the patient and the photographic plate. The grids were placed so that the primary rays that came directly from the focal part of the X-ray tube passed through them, so that the secondary rays that were emitted when the primary rays struck atoms in the patient's body were blocked. This process is called *collimating* the rays, literally forcing them into a column instead of letting them fan out every which way. Bucky introduced his invention at a meeting of the German Roentgen Society in 1913, and patented it in both Germany and the United States. His pictures were a tremendous improvement on ungridded images, but they were marred by shadows of the grid on the radiographs.

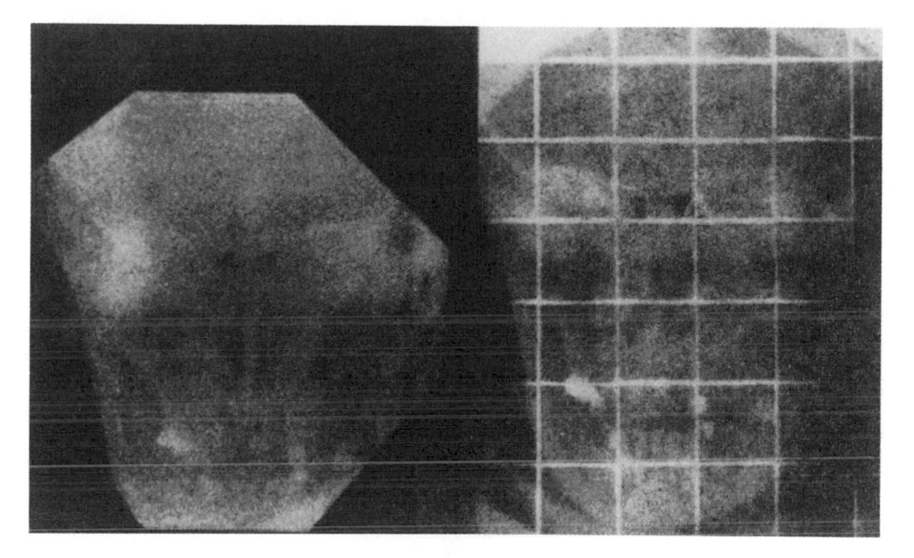

13. Radiograph of the face with and without the Bucky grid/diaphragm (1913). Initial example of the value of Bucky's invention. *Left,* without grid. *Right,* with grid. Courtesy of the *British Journal of Radiology.*

Bucky immigrated to the United States in 1923, but without his patent: he had lost all rights to it after World War I because of the forfeiture laws imposed on citizens of the Central Powers. He made up for some of his lost fortune by patenting elaborations of imaging technologies; and, when he confronted patent infringement suits—which was often—he drew on the help of his close friend Albert Einstein (an expert since his youth in the Swiss patent office) who emerged from behind his wall of privacy to defend Bucky's work. (Bucky returned the affection and, as Einstein's personal physician, was with Einstein at his death.)

Meanwhile, with the United States cut off from Germany, another inventor, Hollis E. Potter, picked up on Bucky's invention and augmented the grids, as he understood them from the American patent, by making them movable. Potter explained how what he called "vagabond" rays—rays that came from outside the focus point, or secondary rays—could be effectively eliminated by adding regular motion to the grid. Many radiologists had already observed that when something inside the body moves while being X-rayed, such as a fetus inside its mother, the radiograph shows no fetus at all! Following this principle, and after a great deal of experimenting, Potter devised a tubular instrument that worked on the operating principle that "invisibility is only secured when each and every portion of the sensitive plate is successively covered and uncovered by the grating for equal periods of time."[9] Any uncollimated X-rays are then suppressed.

An unplanned result of the Bucky-Potter grid, or diaphragm, was freedom from the cumbersome glass photographic plates. Without the grid, the larger

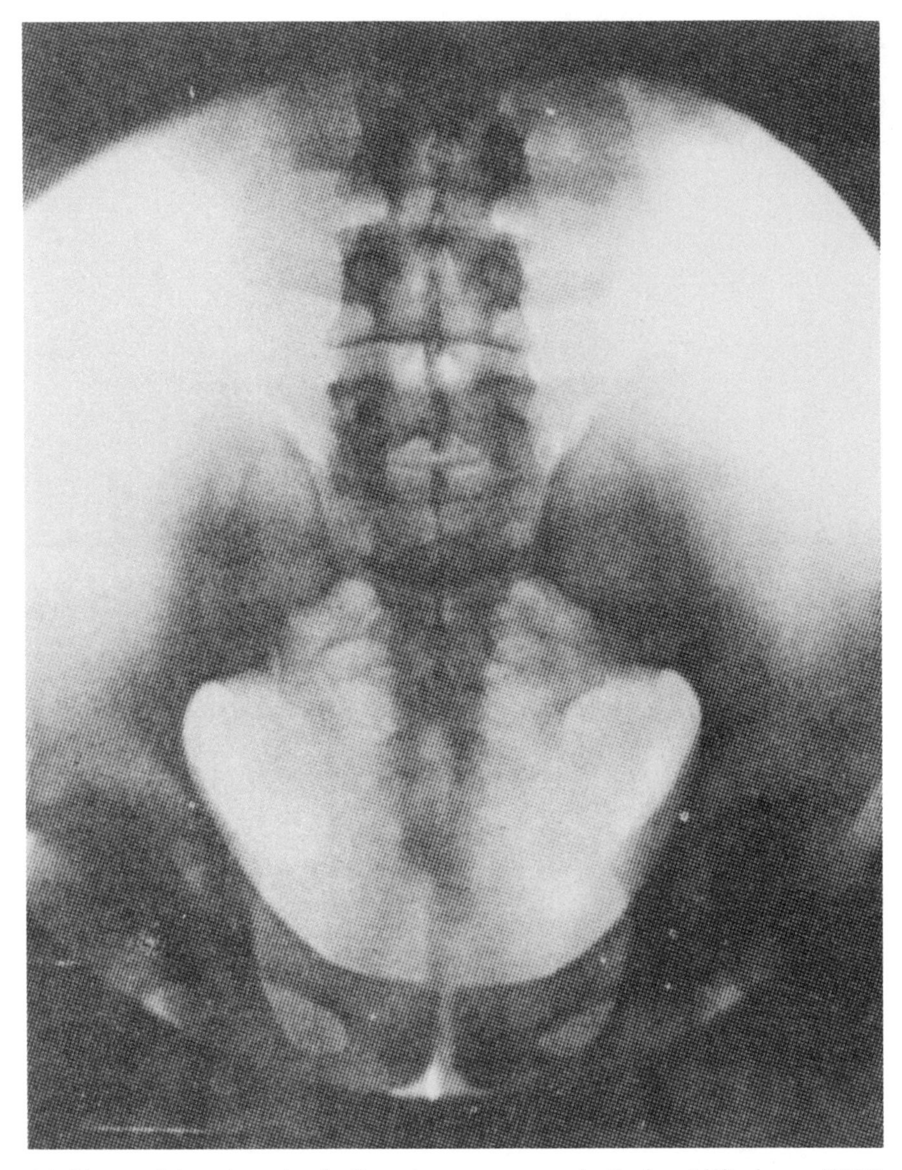

14. Picture of the spine using the Potter improvement on the Bucky grid/diaphragm (1920). (H. E. Potter, "The Bucky Diaphragm Principle Applied to Roentgenography," *American Journal of Roentgenology* 7 [1920]: 292–295.) Courtesy of the American Roentgen Ray Society.

the plate, the more the blurring. This phenomenon helped restrict early radiographs to small plates, usually four by five inches. The new grid opened the door to larger, finely resolved pictures. And because large pieces of glass are hard to work with, the Bucky-Potter grid also hastened the conversion to film, and to the familiar fourteen-by-seventeen inch radiograph—all a result of taking advantage of a new situation.

Still Better Pictures

Meanwhile, the technology of the X-ray image itself improved dramatically. Early exposures, like those Roentgen made in the last weeks of 1895, could take as long as two hours. This was clearly uncomfortable, unhealthy, and impractical. When it was simply a matter of having a picture taken in the manner of a portrait, a long exposure was tolerable. But for someone with an injury, sitting immobile for any length of time was painful and often impossible. As early as mid-February 1896, John Carbutt, a dry plate manufacturer in Philadelphia, developed an emulsion for his plates that reduced exposure time to twenty minutes. By 1906, most exposures were down to a few seconds for a hand and only minutes for thicker parts of the body.

Aside from the comfort of the patient, speed was essential for getting sharper pictures of the thorax, where the motion of ordinary breathing or the beating of a heart blurred the subsequent image. Barring a few exceptions, like Francis Williams, neither radiologists nor patients worried about the length of time they were exposed to what we now call ionizing radiation. It was not a matter of ignoring their patient's welfare or of being ignorant to the dangers of excess exposure. Most doctors adhered to the axiom that William Rollins had articulated—only the area to be treated or photographed should be exposed to "X-light." But, unbeknownst to the operators, unshielded tubes spilled radiation over the unprotected bodies of patients and doctors.[10]

The real demand for quick images came from physicians in a hurry to diagnose their patients. Most preferred looking at a fluoroscopic screen rather than waiting for a radiograph to be developed. Fluoroscopic images enabled doctors instantly to spot tubercular lesions or a collapsed lung, giving them the option of operating immediately, or medicating. The fluoroscope also allowed the physician to watch the heretofore invisible workings of the stomach and colon. Investigations using bismuth to enhance the visibility of the digestive process allowed physicians, by 1910, to "explore the human intestine from end to end. To their surprise, they found little resemblance between the position of the stomach of the living person and the position shown in textbook pictures, drawn from postmortem appearances. Generally vertical in the living, the stomach often became a horizontal, elegantly curved organ in the dead."[11] Moreover, in corpses the intestines seemed to be in a fixed position, while in living subjects fluoroscopic examinations revealed that they could be almost anyplace in the abdomen.

But fluoroscopy had drawbacks: aside from the fact that both patient and doctor were exposed to more radiation, the images on the fluoroscope screen were less detailed and less clear than radiographs. This discrepancy in sharpness between fluoroscope and radiography was puzzling, until explained by Antoine Béclère. Béclère was one of the first French physicians to embrace radiology, and he soon became the dean of the field. But he was not the very first, as he recalls in a memoir, for he did not see an X-ray demonstration until the summer of 1896 when he accepted the invitation of his colleague Charles

Bouchard. Bouchard had helped demonstrate the new device at a medical congress and had become an evangelist of the rays, setting up demonstrations in his own Paris household where he subjected everyone—family and servants—to the fluoroscope. When Béclère had arrived late at the apartment, and the elderly servant, who had been the subject, had already gone to sleep, Bouchard had no compuctions about awakening her and asking her to stand again in front of the tube.

To Béclère it was like a religious experience; he was "seeing the road to the promised land."[12] As the old woman stood quietly, Béclère watched her heart beating, her diaphragm rising and falling, and noticed a veil of tissue on a lung that had previously collapsed.

As soon as he could, Béclère installed an X-ray machine at his home-office in Paris, and when he could win support, established an X-ray facility at the Hôpital Ténon where he was *chef de service.* Soon he had systematically studied every medical use of the new machine, published a French X-ray text, and in 1908 established the first organized lecture series anywhere in the world for physicians interested in roentgenography.

But it was Béclère's expertise in ophthalmology that led him to understand the poor resolution of fluoroscopic compared to radiographic images. Using his knowledge of the eye and optics, he concluded that the problem was one of physiology, not physics. What the eye sees depends on how much light there is and how the eye accommodates to it. But film or glass continues to accumulate light after extended exposure and therefore can produce a more detailed image. The fluoroscope would remain a staple in the radiologist's armamentarium as a source of instant information, but it could not compete for detail with radiographs.

Fluoroscopic images could be better, Béclère explained in a paper published in 1899, where he showed for the first time that dark adaptation is a function of the retina, not a reaction to the dilation of the pupil as had been previously assumed. Two years later Francis Williams explained in the first radiology textbook that, if the radiologist lets his eyes adapt to the dark for about ten minutes, and wears dark glasses, he will be able to see better. There was a great deal of debate about wearing red glasses early in the century, but in 1916 the discovery of the sensitivity of the retinal rods in the range of red light gave a scientific basis to the practice. Red goggles were standard radiologist's gear until the development of image intensifiers in the 1950s made fluoroscopes viewable in ordinary light.

Physicians also benefited from couches and tables that could be turned, rotated, and slanted; screens that could be adjusted up and down; and elegant wooden holders for the glass plates. They also bought everything they could to enhance the radiographs, especially in their efforts to locate foreign objects. The first, and most successful, approach to pinpointing a deeply embedded object (like a pin) was an X-ray adaptation of a stereopticon.

Stereopticons were ubiquitous in middle-class homes a hundred years ago, like today's computer games. The images were made by a camera that had two lenses set about two inches apart—the distance between the eyes, so that each eye is presented with the image it would see if it were looking at the scene. When viewers looked at the double films through binocular glasses, they saw the same kind of three-dimensional picture that they saw in their daily lives. Stereoptic equipment was quickly adapted to X-ray cameras, and surgeons, especially, looked to stereoradiology as early as 1896 to get a better idea of the location of a foreign object. The drawback of stereoradiology was the fact that many radiologists simply found it difficult to see through a stereopticon. They chose, instead, to simply cross their eyes. Those who did this saw what looked like a glimpse through separate receding wings in a miniature proscenium theater, rather than a three-dimensional scene. But imperfect as they were, stereoradiographs helped surgeons get a better idea of the location of foreign objects. While stereoradiography never met medical needs, it suggested that images that created the illusion of three dimensions were worth striving for. The ambition never faded, but wasn't realized for another three quarters of a century.

With such a spate of refinements, it would seem that X-rays were routinely used in private practice and clinics. But this wasn't true. They were a novelty, a curiosity and a status symbol through the first decades of the new century. Consider the events surrounding twenty-seven year-old John Van Boskirk, who in May 1912, was putting awnings on the windows of the post office in Omaha, Nebraska, when the ladder slipped. Boskirk fell eighteen feet to the ground, and was treated for a sprained ankle at a nearby hospital. Seventeen days later, still unable to stand on the hurt foot, a new doctor in charge of his case, Dr. Pinto, suggested that he get an X-ray.

The picture was conclusive—he had a broken bone—and Boskirk sued. At the trial four doctors, one an X-ray specialist, testified that "the failure to have an X-ray picture taken as an aid to diagnosis at this time" did not indicate any lack of regular care.[13] Boskirk lost his case. Even while companies like General Electric produced better X-ray tubes and new ways of eliminating shadows, doctors outside major medical centers still looked on the device as an increasingly expensive gadget which they resorted to only at a patient's request, or, in some instances, as bait to attract a wealthy clientele.[14]

Beyond Broken Bones and Lead Bullets

In 1912 someone like Boskirk in Omaha might not have been entitled to X-ray diagnosis, but veterans of the war with Spain expected X-rays and sought them out. The celebrated veteran of San Juan Hill, the retired President Theodore Roosevelt, was campaigning that spring on the Bull Moose ticket in Illinois. Having memorized his speech, he folded it and stuck it in his pocket. The wad of paper saved his life: a would-be assassin aimed at his heart but the paper deflected the bullet's path so that it came to rest harmlessly in Roosevelt's shoulder. The ex-soldier knew all about X-rays, and he went immediately to Chicago, where he had pictures taken which showed that the bullet was lodged in muscle, where it stayed until his death seven years later.

As a rule, surgeons marveled at the X-ray. In October 1897 at the XIth Surgical Congress meeting in Paris, Professor Gross, from Nancy, had delighted at the ability of X-rays to locate foreign bodies, like bullets, in the pharynx, the esophagus, the trachea, and the lungs. He went on to describe how physicians could now see bone diseases, and concluded by calling radiology "a veritable autopsy of the living."[15]

What it meant to autopsy the living was spelled out the next year at Harvard when Walter Bradford Cannon mixed up a batch of food with bismuth subnitrate and fed it to a cat. He watched as the opaque food make its way through peristaltic contractions, coating the cat's digestive organs so they could be seen through a fluoroscope as digestion continued. Before long, bismuth and barium were the meals of choice for subjects of gastrointestinal observations. An autopsy of the living began with the digestive organs. The next part of the body to reveal its secrets was the arterial system, which was also breached by introducing a tracer. The first medium for this purpose was a toxic dye, which was injected first into a freshly amputated hand. Within the decade, however, experimental physiologists as well as physicians had a new substance that they could use to explore the living body.

The substance was radium. By 1898 Marie and Pierre Curie had separated two new elements from the uranium oxide they knew emitted radiation: polonium, which has a very short life, and radium. They understood that the invisible rays emitted by radium acted very much like X-rays, and Marie dubbed this phenomenon "radioactivity." The radiation emitted by these elements has shorter waves, more energetic waves, than X-rays (now known as gamma radiation), but it acts on photographic plates and on living tissue very much like X-rays, which lie adjacent to them on the electromagnetic spectrum.

Radium's impact on the public imagination echoed the excitement that greeted Roentgen two years earlier. The phenomenon was already familiar, but radium hinted of alchemy and besides, it had been discovered by a beautiful young woman. Radium, the Curies explained, emits radiation similar to X-rays, but does not produce a clear image on film or on a fluorescent screen. It did not make the visible translucent, but it glowed by itself and seemed a different kind of miracle. Rare and expensive though it was, radium was used by manufacturers for almost everything, from coating crucifixes so they would glow in the dark to lighting up cocktails at fashionable dinners.

The idea of placing radioactive materials inside the human body followed immediately on the heels of the Curies' discovery. In the excitement caused by the new substance, radium was used cavalierly in the theater and at private parties. One reporter suggested injecting radium directly into a living person's veins, literally lighting up the patient so a doctor could see all the internal organs without bothering with the intermediary of a fluoroscope. This was nonsense, of course. Others suggested administering the magic substance by mouth. However ingested, radium remained the major component of nuclear medicine for thirty years, largely as implants to treat cancer.

It may have been madness to suggest radium cocktails, but it was not crazy to search for substances for patients to swallow that would be opaque to X-rays and give a clear image of a working digestive tract—or a thinking brain. Radioactive agents to enhance the radiographic image would not become a major medical tool until after 1934 when new radioactive substances would be injected into the body and tracked by detectors.

But the idea was lurking in physicists' minds in 1911 when George Hevesy, a Hungarian researcher visiting the English physics laboratory of Ernest Rutherford, tried to separate lead ore into ordinary and radioactive isotopes—species of an element that have the same number of electrons but a different atomic weight. He did not succeed, but he understood that the radiation emitted by radioactive isotopes might leave a trail that could be detected with the right instrument.

Hevesy's work is an important reminder that X-rays continued to excite physicists as well as physicians. The physicists were fascinated both by the phenomena of the rays themselves, and their use as a tool for understanding the structure of the atom. Colleagues of Roentgen (but notably, not Roentgen himself) continued to investigate X-rays. And in 1912, Max von Laue, another German physicist, discovered that when X-rays passed through the planes of a crystal, the crystal acted like a three-dimensional grating that diffracted the X-rays, causing them to cast a pattern of the molecular structure of the crystal onto a film placed on the other side. This procedure, X-ray crystallography, would become basic to all chemistry in determining the structure of elements. The X-ray, Laue demonstrated, was much more than a medical instrument.

In England the following year, H.G.J. Moseley discovered that the X-ray spectra of the heavier elements vary in a manner that is mathematically related to the charge on their atomic nuclei. He was able to use this formula to predict the existence of the elements #45 and #63 in the periodic table (elements that were not actually found until the 1930s). The refinement of X-rays in the laboratories of crystallographers and physical chemists advanced more rapidly in the prewar years than improvements to the erratic tubes used to explore the human body. These forays into the structure of matter would eventually lead to extraordinary advances in X-ray imaging as well as to a new kind of image generated in nuclear medicine.

World War I

Moseley died on the beach at Gallipoli, a reminder that Europe's first "total war" shattered the world of science as well as nations. Especially in medical research, World War I caused a parting of the ways between physicians in the Central Powers and those in the Allied forces, including the United States. In the world of X-ray technology this meant that communications ceased between German factories, scientists, and doctors and their British and French counterparts. In America, the lively traffic between Germany and cities on the eastern seaboard trickled away as the United States moved from neutrality to join the Alliance against the Central Powers.

The war forced Britain and its allies to manufacture their own optical glass when they were cut off from their source in Germany. In addition to training craftsmen, they had to train radiologists. Antoine Béclère, by this time the uncrowned head of French radiology, taught 260 new radiologists, more than doubling the national supply, and Marie Curie gained new renown in her role of angel of mercy.

Widowed since 1906 when her husband and colleague, Pierre, had been killed by a carriage not far from their Paris laboratory, the Nobel laureate took it upon herself, with the aid of her seventeen-year-old daughter, Irène (who would one day win her own Nobel Prize), to transform ordinary automobiles into mobile X-ray vehicles. Marie Curie learned to drive to avoid being encumbered by a chauffeur. She personally escorted X-ray equipment to the front in railroad cars and loaded and unloaded them herself to make sure they arrived where and when needed. When she saw that the public health service was unprepared for war, she organized X-ray apparatus for the battlefront, and transformed her new Institute of Radium into a school for X-ray technicians.[16] During the battle of the Marne in 1914 she moved from one radiology station to the next and, with the help of the Red Cross, fitted up a touring motorcar that carried both a dynamo (worked by the car's engine) and an X-ray machine. As the war continued, she helped place two hundred radiologic installations near the French and Belgian armies, and she gave the army twenty more of her fitted touring cars, which were known affectionately as "petits curies." Between 1916 and 1918 she personally trained 150 female X-ray technicians.[17]

An ugly truth about modern wars is that, despite their toll in human mis-

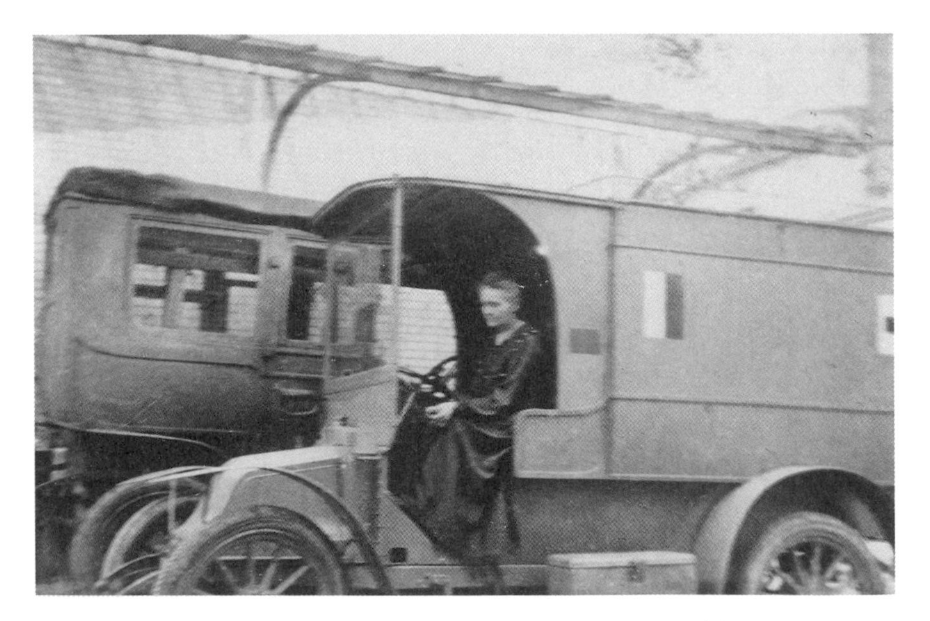

15. Marie Curie driving a "petit curie" during World War I. Courtesy of the Archives Curie et Joliot-Curie, Paris.

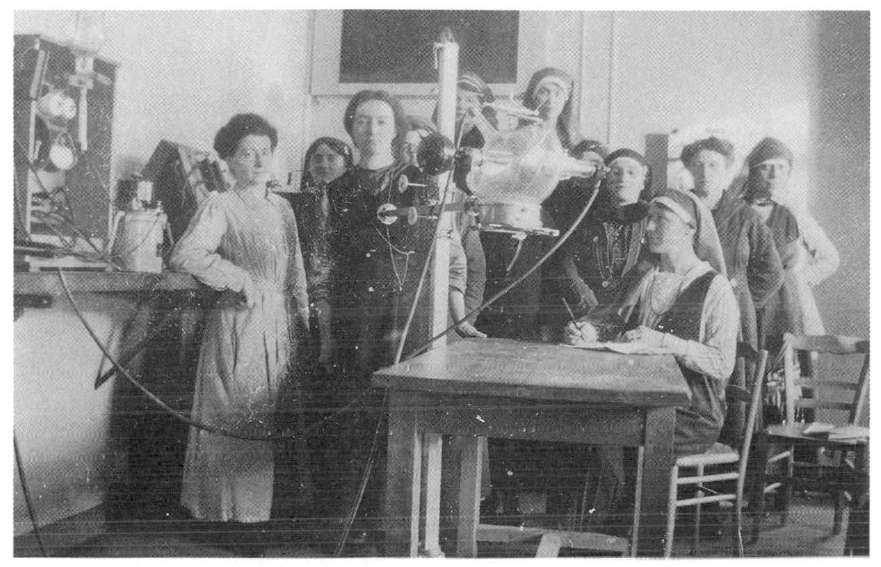

16. Marie Curie with seventeen-year-old Irène in the radiology laboratory at L'Hôpital Edith Cavell, Paris (1917). Courtesy of the Archives Curie et Joliot-Curie, Paris.

ery, they stimulated the growth of medicine. X-rays had been used on a modest scale in the skirmishes that punctuated the end of the nineteenth century, but the long duration of World War I, the numbers of people involved, and the variety of human devastation made the new portable X-ray models irreplaceable, and brought X-rays into the forefront of medicine.

For three years after Europeans started fighting in August 1914, Americans remained officially neutral. Even as observers, however, Americans were affected by the war, which ruptured first emotional and then commercial ties with the continent. X-ray manufacturers who had had German connections were suddenly on their own, and those with French and English representatives found their colleagues, who would eventually become allies, unable to concentrate on innovation in their preoccupation with the practical matter of getting cumbersome tubes, screens, and plates to the front. American industry waited in the wings for the signal to join in.

"Preparedness" was the catchword of 1916, and thanks to the radiologists' committee on "preparedness," within days of U.S. entry into the war in April 1917, X-ray experts had joined the Roentgenological division of the Army Medical Corps. Radiology training schools were set up from New York to Los Angeles, with two additional schools at the Medical Officers Training Camps at Camp Greenleaf, in Georgia, and Fort Riley, in Kansas. During the brief American foray into Mexico in 1916, the Army Medical Corps had introduced a portable X-ray unit operated by a gasoline engine which powered an electric generator. Self-contained, this arrangement was much easier to handle than the cumbersome old-fashioned induction coils used by the French and English to provide enough electricity to produce X-rays.

Under pressure to work more efficiently, the army asked William David Coolidge to develop a better and quieter X-ray apparatus; he rapidly designed a tube capable of rectifying (that is, of changing alternating current into direct current so that a constant voltage could be applied to the tube). A regular army ambulance was fitted with a fluoroscope and screen as well as facilities for developing films or plates. Army physicians went on to develop a mobile Coolidge tube for hospitals that could travel from bed to bed where patients were too ill to be carried to an X-ray unit.

Most important, this new portable equipment had few moving parts and was easy to repair. With demand from the front greater than the old crafts tradition could produce, the tube industry moved into mass production. The companies that supplied the war effort are still leaders in manufacturing medical imaging machines: Picker and GE in the United States, and Siemens in Germany, which had been licensed by GE to produce Coolidge tubes before the United States joined the Allies.

Coolidge himself had interests beyond the X-ray tube, and he turned to the problem of submarine detection. He invented a device for picking up sound waves from submarines hiding under water, but because the new X-ray tube already bore his name, the new device bore his initial and became known as the "C" tube.

The American army sought enlisted men who, before the war, had been X-ray technicians, electricians, or photographers, or who had worked in the factories that manufactured X-ray apparatus. The army trained them as trouble-shooters to repair equipment. They also took physicians who were general practitioners and instructed them on how to find bullets and shrapnel at special classes in military hospitals in the states and at special courses in Paris and Tours. American physicians established friendships with French radiologists and shared techniques and even terminology. These connections would influence international agreements through the postwar years.

The prewar American supply of five mobile X-ray units mounted on four-mule wagons grew in the fifteen months of hostilities to over seven hundred automobile units. With glass hard to obtain and transport, American radiologists turned to film. (But when glass plates became plentiful again toward the end of the war, many physicians rejected film, still highly flammable, for their old favorite.) At the time of the Armistice two hundred American doctors had been trained as X-ray diagnosticians. They were second only to surgeons in numbers and status.

By the end of the war, physicians in every participating country had experienced the benefits of X-ray diagnosis, and American doctors had seen the advantages of the Coolidge tube. Besides its greater reliability, the new tube emitted much less ionizing radiation. It would seem that everyone would want one. But Coolidge tubes were expensive. Even in America, where they were

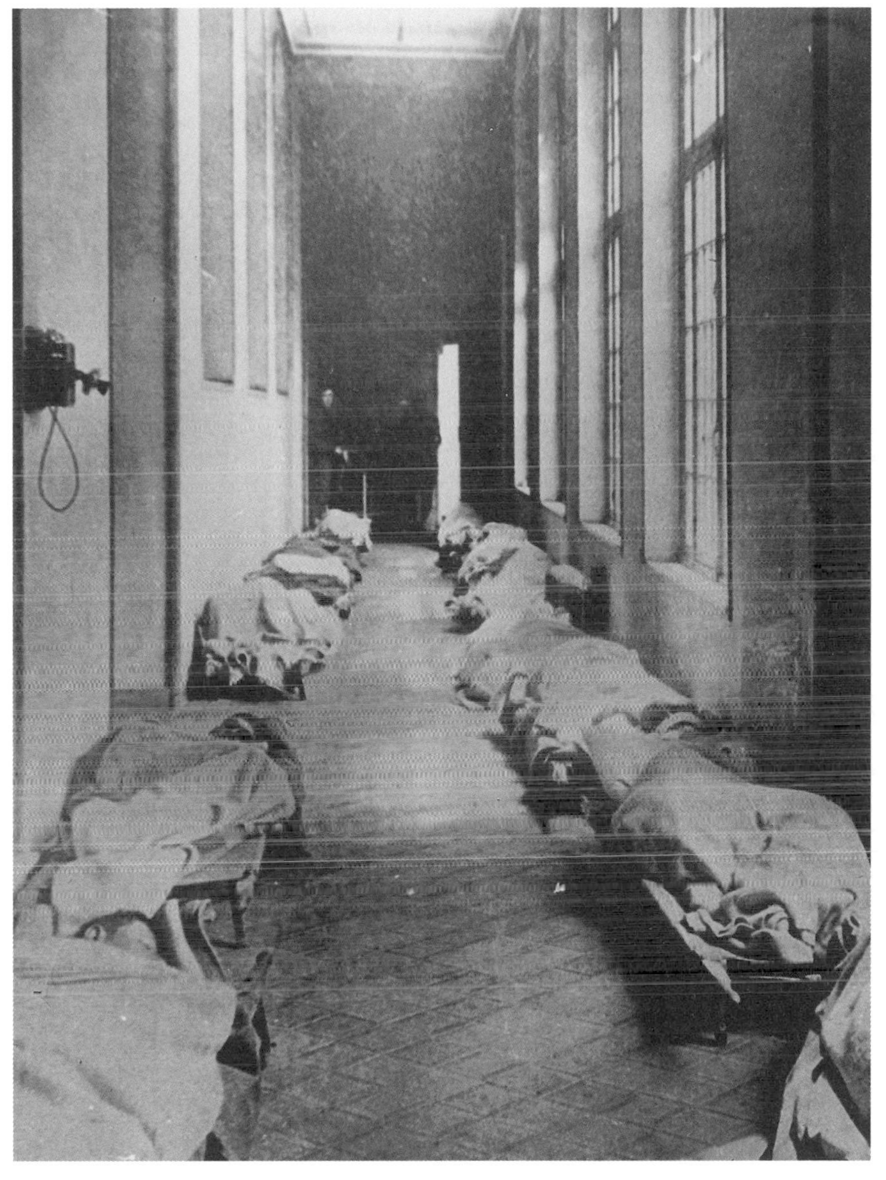

17. En route to the X-ray room. A corridor of a French castle, transformed into an American Army hospital during World War I. Courtesy of the American College of Radiology.

on the market by 1918, doctors continued to buy and use the old gas tubes. In cash-poor Europe, it would be almost a decade before most radiologists could afford the luxury. Meanwhile, they continued to use gas tubes and fluoroscopes, and they continued individually to endure excess exposure to radiation, and managed to rationalize their personal risk by denying the existence of any form of radiation that could not be cured with fresh air, sunshine, and rest. While focus tubes and Bucky-Potter grids were staples of X-ray machines everywhere by the early 1920s, it was another decade before the Coolidge tube routinely replaced gas tubes in the United States and Europe.

America didn't change overnight with the 1918 Armistice, but during the 1920s it sometimes seemed that way. The war years were a tremendous boon to American technology in general, and to imaging technology in particular. With demobilization, trained technicians and physicians flooded the civilian market, and military medicine became the standard for the newly minted veterans. Ordinary citizens now expected an X-ray as routine medical care.

Four

Medical Politics between the Wars

Setting Standards

Between 1917 and 1940 radiologists asserted and consolidated their position in American medicine. Awash in the legacy of good feelings generated by their successes on the battlefront, physicians joined international committees to investigate and respond to public fears about radiation. They were now able, with the help of scientists, to quantify dosages and set guidelines for exposure. In the 1920s, X-rays were firmly established as part of medical culture. Doctors used them to diagnose broken or fractured bones immediately, rather than to confirm their original diagnosis after treatment, and judges in the United States now ruled that failure to use X-rays in cases of possible fractures was medical malpractice plain and simple. With the help of the courts, radiologists took possession of the radiographs they made and interpreted. As a result, X-rays moved from the arena of mysterious, unpredictable rays that illuminated the hitherto unknown, to a new arena of inaccessibility defined by the need for explanation by an expert with esoteric training.

During the nineteen months that America was at war after 1917, more than two million doughboys arrived in France, and half of those who were hospitalized were X-rayed. The widespread marketing of Coolidge tubes coincided with American entry into the war and helped extend routine, high-quality chest X-rays to a broad population. What was a singular experience for each man—a memorable first time in front of an X-ray tube—was a cumulative experience for those physicians who peered into the chests of thousands of soldiers. To the doughboy the sight of the radiograph left a conviction that medicine was indeed scientific. And those who experienced medical care of any kind for the first time were determined to retain it. To physicians the impact was very different. They were startled to see that almost half of the recruits suffered from chest diseases which, had they been identified earlier, could have been arrested or possibly cured. Back in civilian practice, these newly trained radiologists crusaded to provide large-scale X-ray screening.

The Chest

Military doctors in 1898 had used X-rays almost exclusively to locate bullets, shrapnel, or shattered bones. Doctors in 1917 examined ostensibly healthy draftees and saw that the darkened lungs of farmers' sons and city boys alike showed the effects of cigarette smoking, which were noted in the record but not considered worrisome. They saw, too, that many young men had tubercular scars although stethoscopic examinations had picked up no hint of infection. Some of these soldiers never saw combat but went instead, and at considerable expense, to army hospitals. By the time of the Armistice, a whole generation of young Americans had had their chests screened for the effects of poison gas, or for the influenza that swept through Europe in 1918 and moved across the Atlantic the following year. And many were found to have active tuberculosis.

Pulmonary tuberculosis, an ancient disease, had been identifiable by auscultation—listening with a stethoscope—since the middle of the nineteenth century, and by microscope after the tuberculosis bacillus was discovered in 1882. Actually seeing the lungs with an X-ray machine was not easy at first. Lung tissue is softer than bone, and its image was hard to capture with the old-style

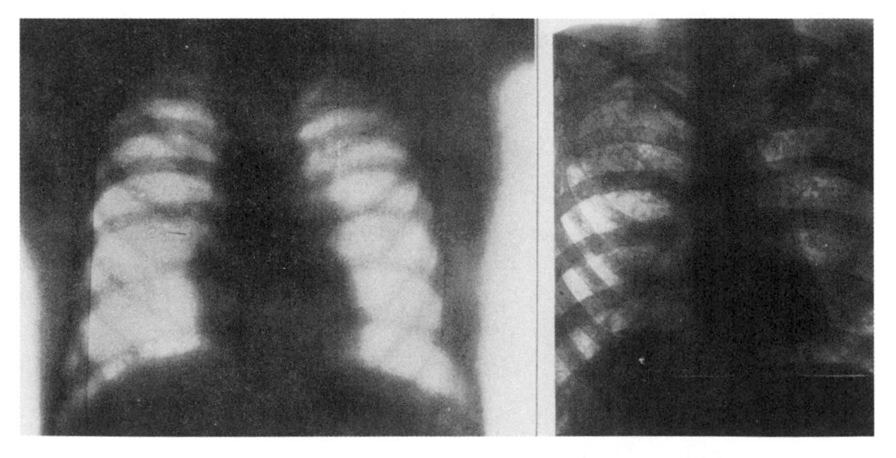

18. Chest X-rays (1902). *Left,* radiograph of normal chest (M. Kassabian, "Instantaneous Skiagraphy of the Thoracic Organs," *Transactions of the ARRS* [1903]: 95–100). *Right,* radiograph of tubercular chest (H. Hulst, "Skiagraphy of the Chest," *Transactions of the ARRS* [1903]: 88–94). Courtesy of the American Roentgen Ray Society.

gas tubes. Before the end of the nineteenth century Francis Williams, in Boston, and his friend and translator Antoine Béclère in Paris had campaigned for the use of X-rays to detect TB. But they had a hard time convincing colleagues. The rib cage obstructed the view, breathing blurred the picture, and it was hard to get patients to hold their breath long enough to get a still image. Williams and Béclère recommended using a fluoroscope instead, for while it was not as clear as a radiograph, they could watch the lungs in motion.

In the first decade of the twentieth century, however, the exposure necessary for chest X-rays had been cut to thirty seconds, and physicians could reasonably ask patients to hold their breath that long. The doctors now got excellent images and hailed the X-ray for the early diagnosis of TB. Once tuberculosis was detected, however, there wasn't much medicine could do. This was one of radiology's first encounters with the early detection of incurable conditions. It was one thing for doctors to diagnose deadly diseases in people who felt symptoms—that had always been part of the physician's job—but now physicians had to inform apparently healthy people that they harbored a terminal disease.[1]

Until the 1950s, the treatment of choice for TB was rest at a sanatorium. While sanatoria could not promise cures, they forced patients to rest while providing fresh air and abundant food. At the least, they removed patients from homes where they might infect others. X-ray pictures of diseased lungs became routine in America around 1913, but the American Sanatorium Association did not recommend chest X-rays until the mid-1920s.

This was when Thomas Mann dramatized life in the hot-house world of an alpine sanatorium in *The Magic Mountain*.[2] By this time thousands of American as well as European readers could identify with the hero Hans Castorp because the sanatorium and the experience of being X-rayed had become a common experience of the middle class. They could nod in agreement at Mann's evocation of the strange smell in the X-ray lab. "Ozone" is "our own private thunderstorm," Castorp notes. The technician gives Castorp a tour. "Lenses, switchboards . . . glass diapositives in rows set in the walls. Hard to say whether this was a photographic studio, a dark-room, or an inventor's workshop and technological witches' kitchen." And then the electrical generator is turned on, and "for the space of two seconds, fearful powers were in play—streams of thousands, of a hundred thousand volts, Hans Castorp seemed to recall—which were necessary to pierce through solid matter." Castorp is promised "a free copy; then you can project the secrets of your bosom on the wall for your children and grandchildren to see" —the X-ray offered hope that he would live to have children and see his grandchildren.[3]

Science Triumphant

These hypothetical children would have had their own X-ray experience, not of their chests but of their feet. A curious spin-off from America's embrace of the new Coolidge tube was a large surplus of Army portable X-ray units, especially fluoroscopes. Quick to improvise, and perhaps remembering the popularity of prewar X-ray slot machines, sales clerks found the ready-to-wear shoe industry an excellent market and initiated a love affair with the shoe fluoroscope. Shoe stores around the world purchased the Foot-O-Scope (which was marketed in 1920 by the United Shoe Machinery Corporation) or one of its clones. This do-it-yourself gadget turned ordinary shoe sales clerks into amateur podiatrists.

All over the world, people who grew up between World War I and the 1960s recall the joy of standing inside the machine, pressing the appropriate button (usually labeled "Man," "Woman," and "Child" although the X-ray dosage was identical) and staring at their wriggling toe bones. The Foot-O-Scope signaled the acceptance of X-ray machines in everyday life. Present in local shoe stores everywhere, they suggested that X-rays were safe and cheap enough so that just about anyone who shopped for shoes could see beyond the skin barrier.

Shoe fluoroscopes were advertised as an unofficial extension of scientific medicine to the young mothers who wanted to protect their children against flat feet and fallen arches. It was the machine that counted. The sales clerk didn't need a medical degree if he had such a scientific instrument. The shoe fluoroscope can be seen as a litmus test of popular confidence in X-rays as a simple, harmless, scientific machine. They remained a part of the furnishing of shoe stores for another forty years, as ubiquitous as the shoehorn.

Within two years of the Armistice, X-ray machines had become a staple in doctors' offices. Sinclair Lewis, who was the son and brother of Midwestern physicians, noted in *Arrowsmith*—a novel for which he received the Pulitzer Prize in 1926—that his young doctor-hero furnished his first office (before World War I) with a golden-oak sideboard and a "Roentgen Ray outfit." In a "society" practice in Chicago, Dr. Arrowsmith says that the clinic gave "over-many roentgenological examinations to socially dislocated women who needed children and floor-scrubbing more than pretty little skiagraphs."[4] Lewis's dismissal of X-rays as frivolous vanities to entertain the idle and enrich the doctor would echo through the century, gathering volume as X-rays evolved into the much more costly computer-reconstructed images made in doctor-owned imaging centers.

Yet Lewis's hero, albeit skeptical of the medical benefits of X-ray images, is tremendously supportive of X-ray therapy. From the early days of 1896 doctors had noticed that patients exposed to X-rays for long periods of time (which was almost all of them), were often cured, at least temporarily, of skin conditions like acne, and occasionally malignant tumors would shrink or even disappear. In the 1920s Marie Curie linked her Institute and a cure for cancer in her pleas for donations. There was a clear need to rationalize the mystery that surrounded both kinds of radiation. Solving the mystery was part of the impetus as well as the bonus for making medicine more scientific.

Scientific medicine meant many things in 1920, both to the medical world and to the public. It meant the laboratory detection of diseases like typhoid followed by a war against the errant bacteria. The idea was to treat the disease, rather than the patient. It meant being "objective," getting multiple opinions from groups of increasingly specialized physicians, including those who were expert at looking at radiographs. Scientific medicine had begun to mean controlled studies of treatments; *and* it also held out the promise of machine-generated miracles.

Machines embodied certain scientific virtues. They were objective. Everyone could see and agree upon what they saw, or so it seemed. Postwar X-ray machines, newly streamlined and hygienic-looking with tubes and grids for better focus and sharper pictures, became the gold standard of scientific medicine. And scientific medicine had come to dominate medical practice.

But there were holdouts in the medical community who objected to technology as a substitute for hands-on examinations and insisted that they themselves personally intended to treat symptoms, not X-ray pictures. They also distinguished between treating the patient and treating the disease, but believed—not without merit—that everyone responds differently to exposure to the same germs, or pathogens, and that everyone deserves a tailored medical protocol. Since all disease is particular to the patient, this argument runs, the way patients respond to any treatment is highly personal.

Idiosyncrasy was still a respected explanation for unanticipated responses to treatment. People *are* different. But while doctors of an earlier generation treated all conditions as unique to the patient, adherents of the new scientific approach were more selective, not only in considering the ability of bodies to generate good X-ray images, but also in judging the amount of radiation individual bodies could safely absorb.

When Mr. and Mrs. Goodrum brought suit for their daughter Mamie in 1918, this was the question at hand. Mamie had gone to St. Luke's Hospital in Little Rock, Arkansas, for a fluoroscopic examination of her back (no particular symptoms are mentioned) on the morning of December 3. She had another treatment that afternoon and a third the next day. For all three examinations Mamie was attended by a technician (Miss Green at the trial, and Mrs. Chamberlain by the time of the appeal two years later). Although the examinations were supposed to have lasted only four seconds each, Miss Green admitted that she had gotten carried away explaining the subtleties of the X-ray machine to Mamie's parents. In her loquaciousness, she had left Mamie exposed to X-rays for forty minutes. That is one hundred and twenty minutes within twenty-four hours. Mamie sustained permanent scars from her neck to her waist, and the Goodrums sued the medical practice of Runyan, Kirby, and Sheppard for damages.

St. Luke's had a resident radiologist at the time, A. G. McGill, a Tulane University Medical School graduate with advanced training in X-ray work. He testified that Miss Green—the technician—was as expert as he was himself, that in fact "one of the best X-ray men he knew of on the face of the earth is not a doctor" (the man who ran the Mayo Clinic's X-ray machine). Dr. Runyan, head of the staff at St. Luke's and the named defendant in the case, defended his staff in 1921 (when the case was heard on appeal), claiming that "the injury resulted without any fault on the part of the operator and without any defect in the machine itself by reason of the *uncontrollable nature of the X-rays.*"[5]

Mrs. Chamberlain testified to the nature of X-rays and the way she administered them. The usual thing, she explained, was to darken the room and wait until the eyes are accustomed to the dark, and then to turn on the current and look through the patient. But often, even before she turns on the current, she noted, patients frequently complain they are being burned. Knowing that is impossible, she always ignored them. She had often been X-rayed herself, she explained, and knew from experience that there is no burning sensation even while the current is on. So, while the plaintiff may have complained of burning, which Mrs. Chamberlain couldn't recall one way or the other, it would have made no difference to her because she wouldn't have paid any attention because she knew it was purely imaginary. Finally, it was acknowledged by her radiology colleagues both that *X-ray machines are idiosyncratic* and that "one person of a certain type and temperament would be susceptible to a burn while another person of a different type under the same circumstances would not be burned."[6] So, while the machine was unpredictable, it was the child's own fault that she was burned. The old logic of the idiosyncratic patient lost Miss Goodrum her case.

Mamie Goodrum's appeal provides a snapshot of how the public understood X-rays at the start of the 1920s. They admired the apparatus, the epitome of scientific medicine, all the while accepting it as unpredictable and unknowable. The presence of a scientific tool—the X-ray machine—assured the patient that there would be scientific results, but they did not expect the machine to be harmless. At almost the same time of the Goodrum appeal, a woman brought her daughter with an elbow injury to the Pennsylvania Hospital in Philadelphia for an X-ray. She was asked to hold the child's elbow. In the course of the examination, a wire from the machine sparked, burning mother and child and knocking both to the floor, spraining the mother's ankle.[7] The Board of Managers at the hospital were relieved that the family did not file damages, and seemed to have accepted this kind of incident as part of the unpredictable nature of X-ray apparatus.

Families like these most likely assumed that those in charge of the X-rays knew how to handle the machine, how to control the dosage, and what biological effects the rays would have on human tissue. But the medical community was just beginning to confront questions of dosage, quantification, and long-term effects of radiation exposure. Medicine had succeeded in convincing its consumer constituency that diagnostic X-ray images were, indeed, scientific. In the matter of radiation treatment, however, and the effects of radiation even during diagnostic procedures, the aura of the unknown and unpredictable was still present.

The New Medical Order

By the late 1930s, Mamie's treatment would have appeared outrageous and the Goodrums, most likely, would have won their case. In the early 1920s, however, general practitioners were just beginning to appreciate that they would have to look to experts for X-ray advice.

The practice of medicine had come a long way since James Da Costa addressed his students at Jefferson Medical College in 1872. Then he had speculated that, if medical progress continued at its present rate, it would soon be impossible for any individual to master everything. "Let us take a glimpse into this future. Madame is in her boudoir, reclining on the sofa, in expectation of her medical attendants," when a team of four arrives: one to get a history and a volumetric reading of every fluid in her body, a second to record her pulse and muscle contractions, a third who uses an "improved ophthalmoscope" to take photographs of her eyes, and finally Dr. Magnet who gets the equivalent of an X-ray.[8]

Da Costa had excellent foresight. The first medical board—a professional group that certifies that specialists are indeed expert—was established in 1917 in ophthalmology. It was followed in 1924 by otolaryngology, in 1932 by obstetrics and gynecology, and dermatology, and in 1934 by radiology. Specialization came with a psychological price. It exacerbated the trend toward separating the body into its constituent parts. Neurologists looked at the brain, cardiologists at the heart. It was as if the body itself was breaking apart. Specialists took pictures of the brain, lungs, intestines, or ovaries, reflecting a shift in medical attention. Terms like *cardiac* and *thoracic* became familiar to alert medical consumers as the general public also began to see their bodies as sets of parts to be studied and treated individually, rather than as a single organism.

As early as 1912, physicians at Pennsylvania Hospital had begun drawing pictures of their patients' torsos to illustrate problems, a phenomenon, it has been noted, probably attributable to the influence of X-rays, which made doctors think of their patients in visual, anatomically standardized terms.[9] This signaled a shift in medical record keeping, which began with an individual physician's freehand sketch and evolved into providing the physician with simple forms to be filled out that included a stamped, anatomical chart. The chest to be X-rayed was homogenized to a standardized size and shape, implying that patients with the same symptoms were standardized, like the stamped chart.[10]

Dr. Runyan at St. Luke's in Little Rock was typical of the physicians who had been lured out of private practice into hospitals equipped with expensive machines. American medicine was beginning to resemble the capital-intensive industry that we recognize today. The center of gravity had shifted, and getting an X-ray taken, more often than not, meant going to the hospital. Although private doctors continued to buy their own X-ray apparatus, as many still do, only hospitals could afford the improved, more expensive machines. By 1929 seven out of ten doctors had a hospital affiliation.

But the affiliation was often uneasy. Hospitals, having invested in expensive equipment, wanted to place radiologists on salary and bill the patients themselves. They had to pay a cadre of specially trained technicians as well, many of whom seemed capable of making diagnoses. Radiologists, of course, objected and parried that only physicians could practice radiology; hospitals could not establish radiology departments and bill for services because that would mean that an institution was practicing medicine, which is not permissible. Radiologists battled fiercely to remain independent, in terms of billing, from the hospitals whose facilities they used.

In Pasadena, California, Carl H. Parker, one of the city's first radiologists, followed a typical schedule. His physician son, Donald Parker, remembers his father spending mornings with private patients at his office on Colorado Boulevard, and afternoons at the city hospital (which would soon accept a bequest from the will of the railroad magnate Henry Huntington and take his name), and on occasion lending his expertise to the physics faculty at the California Institute of Technology down the road.[11]

Carl Parker, a graduate of Pomona College in Claremont, California, and Rush Medical School in Chicago, married and joined a practice in Pasadena in 1911. He had planned to spend a few years in general medicine, then move on to surgery. But Parker became interested in radiology and in 1916 went to Rochester, Minnesota, to take the Mayo Clinic's three-month radiology course ("the best in the country").[12] A couple of years later he honed his skills with a few months at New York's Presbyterian Hospital and in 1918 became head of radiology at Pasadena Hospital. He bought the most up-to-date X-ray equipment for the then-hefty sum of $6,646, but he maintained his private practice on Colorado Boulevard. He was wary of the new hospital environment for fear they would put him on a salary and eliminate his fee-for-service practice. Hospitals were the core of the new medical order and radiologists, still jostling for position within organized medicine, moved to make themselves irreplaceable in the new medical centers.

Getting Organized

By the early 1920s, Parker had a choice of joining two organizations devoted to protecting his interests. Radiology depended from the outset on experts, and even at the turn of the century there were plenty of them in California. Doctors, engineers, and technicians like Elizabeth Fleischmann established X-ray facilities in San Francisco and Los Angeles. When the American Roentgen Ray Society, the first American organization, had its inaugural meeting in New York's Grand Central Palace in December 1900, it had to decide whether or not to affiliate with the American Medical Association, already the most powerful medical organization. If the society went with the AMA, it would have to exclude all nonphysicians. But in 1900 no serious practitioner of radiology could imagine excluding the experts they had learned to depend upon, and so the Society went it alone for a while.

Within another decade however, as their self-confidence grew, radiological physicians grew more exclusive. Although radiological or "roentgenological" societies had formed in 1896 in almost every country in Europe, they began to exclude lay technicians and photographers—but not scientists—from their ranks.[13] The American Roentgen Ray Society elected the physicist Arthur Goodspeed its third president in 1902, but his election was a recognition of Goodspeed's special contribution.[14] They purged the organization of questionable practitioners in 1905, and announced their goal as the establishment of radiology as a separate and distinct specialty with the same standing and respect accorded to the established specialties of surgery or obstetrics.[15]

Time changes most things, including organizations, and by 1911 the Roentgen Ray Society had amended its admission requirements, making it hard for physicians west of the Alleghenies to join.[16] Not surprisingly, in 1915 Californians organized the Western Roentgen Ray Society, which eventually drew members from thirty-eight states. It changed its name in 1920 to the Radiological Society of North America—today the major organization for radiologists and nonphysician scientists. To symbolize its national identity, the RSNA held its 1921 meeting in Boston, the heart of the eastern establishment. Parker, a first-generation Californian but a second-generation physician proud of his roots in medicine and in the American West, joined the RSNA when he became fully qualified as a radiologist in 1923. At this time Albert Soiland, a Los Angeles radiologist, successfully campaigned the AMA to approve a Section Council on Radiology, limiting the practice to trained experts.

Bursting with confidence, some radiologists wanted a more elite organization, and that same year of 1923 they established the American College of Radiology. Limited at first to one hundred members and mostly ceremonial functions, it became an important voice in establishing the Board of Radiology in the early 1930s and grew even more important as it took on a political role during the Depression, when physicians began to feel threatened by changes in medical economics. Finally in 1939 the two once-contentious organizations, the American Roentgen Ray Society and the Radiological Society of North America, which had co-existed awkwardly, peacefully united along with the American Radium Society under the umbrella of the American College of Radiology, which took over the economic, political action, and practice supports for all its members.

Setting Safety Standards

Before war broke out in Europe in 1914, American doctors and engineers had participated in seven international conferences of medical radiology and electrology and were on good terms with their German and Austrian colleagues who had been leaders in the physics of radiation since Roentgen's breakthrough. The war dampened friendships just as it destroyed business connections. As soon as fighting erupted in August 1914, French and German medical associations not only stopped exchanging information but actively kept information from each other. Later, American physicians as well fell victim to anti-German propaganda (in the United States sauerkraut was renamed "liberty cabbage"). In Britain the *Archives of the Roentgen Ray* changed its name to the *Archives of Radiology and Electrotherapy* when they learned that Roentgen, then seventy years old, had sold his gold Rumford medal from the Royal Society of London in order to donate the proceeds to the German Red Cross. Long after treaties had been signed and blotted and Roentgen had died, British books described Roentgen, the Nobel laureate, as "Dutch" (his mother's nationality and his own as well until his first professorship) when they restored him to his pedestal in the scientific pantheon.[17]

Even after the Armistice the Allies continued ostracizing Austrian and German doctors, excluding them from international meetings of all sorts, including science and medicine. Americans joined with their recent wartime allies to keep scientists from the Central Powers from joining the International Council of Scientific Unions until 1926. Physicians were equally hostile. As late as 1923 Germans were excluded from thirty-five of the fifty international congresses held. This continued hostility was a problem when it came to the matter of establishing a uniform scale for measuring radiation. In X-ray therapy as well as imaging, differences between German and French approaches to tumor radiation were settled on grounds of patriotism, not science. Until the early 1930s, French approaches and definitions usually won because of the old wartime lineup. The winners got the spoils; in this instance, the right to determine how quantities would be measured in the international arena.

The most urgent matter before these congresses was determining uniform quantities of radiation and ascertaining which dosages were safe. The medical community was worried: doctors were dying. The death from aplastic anemia in 1921 of Ironside Bruce, one of England's most prominent radiologists, sent a chill through the public, now alert to the effects of radiation on blood.[18] Then in 1925 two French engineers who were exposed to radiation while preparing radioactive thorium for medical use in a suburban Parisian laboratory died, prompting a French weekly newspaper to run a front-page list of "The glorious martyrology of radium and X-rays."[19]

To protect themselves and retain consumer confidence, physicians, physicists, and X-ray manufacturers had to agree on safe levels of radiation and guidelines for products to shield both technician and patient from scattered radiation.

When General Electric marketed the Coolidge tube after the war, the apparatus was covered by a lead jacket and an array of contrivances designed to protect the radiologist as well as the patient. Americans had been especially sensitive to the dangers of radiation because of fatal incidents among the first generation of X-ray physicians and technicians. When it was still customary for doctors using fluoroscopes to use their own hands to test the image, American doctors noted the injuries among fluoroscopists and opted to take radiographs. In contrast, European radiologists economized by not using film on X-ray pictures and they risked exposure to radiation by conducting whole examinations by fluoroscope.

Physicians and their patients were not alone in their demand for uniform measurements and effective shielding. The experimental physicists not only recognized the problem, but offered a means to resolve it. By 1925, when the first postwar congress of radiologists met in London, physicists concerned with identifying and measuring the particles inside the atom had perfected ionization chambers. They could now detect and compare different degrees and kinds of radiation. In the next year, an instrument devised originally by the German physicist Hans Wilhelm Geiger was perfected. Geiger had worked in Manchester, England, with Ernest Rutherford before the war, and with Rutherford had built an ionization chamber to track and count individual alpha particles (positively charged particles emitted by some radioactive isotopes). Back in Germany in the mid-1920s, as a professor at the University of Kiel, he collaborated with Walter Muller to build a portable device known as the Geiger-Muller counter to detect and measure the intensity of radiation. This included radiation emitted by radioactive materials like radium, and from X-ray tubes.

The first order of business in London in 1925 was the definition of a *roentgen.* This unit of X-radiation was calibrated differently in France and Germany. The next item on the agenda was the *curie,* the unit defined as the quantity of radiation emitted by a gram of radium. The congress established an International Commission on X-Ray Units which was charged with presenting a report on both units at the next congress to be held three years later in Stockholm.

The Stockholm meeting of 1928 was the first major postwar radiological conclave, with representatives from several continents, including those from the nations that had lost World War I. The delegates went to work under mounting pressure from insurance companies and labor unions concerned with workers' compensation. They needed concrete advice—numbers, to be precise—about what constituted acceptable exposure to radiation. News about more deaths from radiation arrived from Norway, Holland, and the Soviet Union. And in the United States, Preston Hickey, editor of the *American Journal of Roentgenology,* gave the results of questionnaires he had sent to every American radiologist. Of the 377 who responded, 138 reported barren marriages, and those radiologists who had children reported almost twice the average abnormality rate. The evidence was impossible to dismiss. Too much was at risk not to respond to this indictment of radiation. On a practical level, life insurance companies had noticed the figures, too, and in Europe they, along with labor unions, had begun "red-lining" occupations connected with X-ray manufacture, declaring them risky.

There had been an embarrassing contretemps in the United States about who should represent American radiology in Stockholm. The ARRS and the RSNA were unable to agree on a representative, so each sent its own. In addition, and as a kind of liaison between the two, Lauriston Taylor, then a young employee at the National Bureau of Standards in Washington, entered the scene for the first time. He would remain a leading figure in radiation medicine for another forty years. His directive was to mediate between the other two representatives so as to represent the overall interests of American medicine. In the course of his long career in radiation standardization and control he would head the U.S. Advisory Committee until it was dissolved in 1946, at which time he became head of the National Committee on Radiation Protection and Measurement. Still employed by the Bureau of Standards, Taylor lent the independent advisory committee a quasi-governmental patina. He played a role in almost every area concerning radiation, public health, and public policy through the establishment of the Manhattan Project, the postwar years of nuclear testing, and the era of nuclear medicine, into an active retirement in 1963.

In Stockholm physicists, physicians, and engineers agreed on the American unit of radiation (identical to the German), which became the standard *roentgen.* It measured the amount of radioactivity that would produce one electrostatic unit of charge in one cubic centimeter of air at zero degrees centigrade and 760 mm pressure. A roentgen is the measurement of radiation emitted by an X-ray tube and directed from the tube into the target, usually a patient, in order to get an image. The French measure was adopted for the *curie,* the unit of radiation emitted from a gram of radium.[20] Both curies and roentgens measure the strength of radiation emitted from a source.

Like X-rays, radium emits ionizing radiation, but of a shorter wavelength than X-rays. It played an important role in the development of radiotherapy.[21] In the 1920s Marie Curie, through the Curie Institute in Paris, publicized the potential of radium for treating and curing cancer. The public confused the two sources of radioactivity for a long time. Both are used medically. Radium's reputation as a quasi-miracle elixir was promoted in the 1920s with an enthusiasm that is hard to recapture in the knowledge of the damage it inflicted on so many who worked with it—including Marie Curie.

Permissible Dosage

Measuring the quantity and quality of radiation was relatively easy compared to the next step, determining an acceptable level of exposure for people who worked with radioactive materials, as well as for those treated by them. Biological evidence gathered over almost thirty years indicated that different animals reacted differently to radiation. However, the evidence suggested that different parts of the same animal responded differently as well, and that damage to human beings seemed to vary with the kind of radiation (whether the rays were "hard" or "soft"), the length and the frequency of exposure, and which part of the body was exposed.

The Stockholm Congress handled this problem as it had handled earlier problems, creating an International Committee on X-Ray and Radiation Protection with representatives from the ranks of physics, engineering, and medicine, which was asked, like its predecessor committees, to report back in three years. In the meantime, there were proposals in Stockholm to identify radiation and measure its intensity by wearing either badges of film that slowly become clouded with increasing exposure or chemical badges that change color under bombardment by radiation.

That X-ray operators and radium workers were coming down with leukemia had been evident by 1911. And in Germany, which has a history going back to Bismarck of government-sponsored medical care, laws limiting exposure to radiation had been passed that year. France followed Germany, as did other European countries before World War I. Early in the century radiologists had learned about "X-ray dermatitis," whose skin eruptions looked like a rash or sunburn but could be the first sign of cancer. It had also been known for a long time that X-rays made laboratory mice and rats sick or sterile, and, in the case of pregnant animals, killed or deformed the offspring. But the fact that the reactions were often delayed, and that they were different in different species, provided lazy personnel an excuse to doff the clumsy shielding that got in their way when they used X-ray machines.

In an effort to convince people that some precautions should be taken, Arthur Mutscheller presented a compromise paper to the American Roentgen Ray Society in 1924. He reasoned that "there must be known the dose which an operator can, for a prolonged period of time, tolerate without ultimately suffering injury."[22] He suggested what he called a "tolerance dose," a specific number that could guide engineers in designing equipment and help physicians determine how much radiation they and their technicians had absorbed, preferably by a photographic film monitor.

Mutscheller's suggestion was aimed at protecting doctors from lawyers, and was made before the publication of research showing that exposure to radiation above a threshold level could wreak serious damage on reproductive organs, genes, and chromosomes. While Mutscheller never claimed that the tolerance dose was a threshold below which there would be no radiation damage, he did look on it as the amount of exposure from which the body could repair itself—if given a chance—because the body does, in many instances, do exactly that. Mutscheller acknowledged that there was no way to know how much radiation is safe for living tissue. The issues concerning threshold doses are still unsettled and continue to trigger honest debate about the role of radiation as an accelerator to the aging process. But the fact that excess exposure is dangerous was implicitly accepted by this time.

Elsewhere, researchers were getting a handle on the amount of radiation that was certain to be destructive, and aiming it deliberately and as narrowly focused as possible at malignant cells, but how much radiation the average person could absorb without ill effect was a mystery. In 1927, the biologist Herman Muller at the University of Indiana gave shattering experimental proof of X-ray damage *within* cells. By irradiating populations of tiny fruit flies, drosophila, Muller demonstrated that X-rays damaged their germ cells—the eggs and sperm that carry the animal's genes—and produced monstrous mutations.

Muller's work left little doubt that X-rays could have a like effect on human genetic material.

Although Muller did not extrapolate his results from fruit flies to people, he didn't have to. His experiments were a clear indication that radiation is harmful to all animals, including Homo sapiens, in their reproductive years. Harmful, but different for everyone. That difference, the lack of predictability as to who would suffer how much from what degree of radiation, was the reason physicians in 1928 suggested a ceiling on exposure to radiation. This first effort was measured in quantities called "erythema doses," the amount of radiation required to redden Caucasian skin. It was a foolish measurement, as it varied from country to country and, in the United States, was totally ineffectual for judging exposure in African-Americans. It implied, without any evidence, that dark skin was a protection against radiation.

The variation in skin dose was just one part of the legal loophole of the medical concept of idiosyncrasy, the term that seemed to cover the apparently whimsical character of the rays as they produced different reactions in different individuals. In the face of idiosyncrasy, there could be no real guideline about dosage. Consequently no fault could be assigned the radiologist or technician for what might look like an overdose, as shown by the ruling against Mamie Goodrum.

But most members of the radiology community found idiosyncrasy too broad a term, given their increasing knowledge about radiation. In 1928 the representatives in Stockholm considered Mutscheller's paper (which had been published in 1925) and offered it as a guide to what would be tolerable. It was never meant to establish a definite threshold figure, like the numerical figure at which water boils. Indeed, Mutscheller admitted it was an almost arbitrary amount of radiation he had arrived at from personal clinical experience. In any event, the suggestion was not adopted.

But Mutscheller's idea of a tolerance dose was exactly what the International Protection Commission needed. They proposed it again in 1931 at their next meeting, defining it as 1/100 of an erythema dose per month, or 2.2 rem.[23] With regular adjustments reducing the amount, the tolerance dose was accepted throughout the 1930s. During this period most physicians and scientists knew that the dose was arbitrary and that no one really knew what the suggested level of exposure really meant. It was useful nonetheless to have a figure—a level of radiation that both X-ray manufacturers and radiologists could live with.

The public never understood how arbitrary the tolerance dose was. The quantification of radiation into roentgens and curies and recommended dosages sounded scientific. The numbers sent a false message of safety. Giving a number to something fearful is a way of mastering it, like knowing the magnitude of an earthquake on the Richter scale. Pinning a number to a natural phenomenon provides an illusion of control. The illusion of control of radiation turned the arbitrary tolerance dose into a rigid maximum permissible level of exposure.

Throughout the 1930s, Lauriston Taylor's Committee on Radiation Safety met frequently with consultants from the leading X-ray manufacturers: GE, Kelley-Koett (which was eventually absorbed by Picker), Picker itself, Standard X-ray Company (a Chicago-based manufacturer of a large range of equipment, especially apparatus used in X-ray therapy, including X-ray measuring instruments), and Westinghouse.

Gradually, and by increments, the committee lowered the tolerance dose, and changed its significance: from a *maximum* level of exposure—that is, how much an individual could tolerate without becoming ill—to a *minimum* level, the smallest amount suspected to have lasting affect. It was not officially acknowledged that the amount of radiation an individual absorbed is cumulative—that the chances of damage increase with the quantity that hits the body—and that no amount of fresh air and fresh milk will dissipate it. Nor was it known that a superdose could wreak more havoc than the same quantity doled out in installments. Yet Donald Parker, whose radiologist father Carl Parker had allowed his adolescent son to have weekly X-rays taken for orthodonture (they were free, after all) suddenly developed a radiation scar four years into his dental adventure. Fifteen years later his professors at Harvard Medical School refused to allow him to specialize in radiology. "They told me I'd had enough radiation for a lifetime," he recalls.[24] And echoing that experience, Betty Parker, his wife, remembers that as a nursing student in Chicago in 1940, her whole class had been cautioned against sticking their feet in fluoroscopes, a good twenty years before the machines were removed from shoe stores.[25]

Among those most eager to establish standards of radiation exposure were manufacturers, especially those who produced better, more expensive equipment and found it hard to compete with dealers who sold less-shielded apparatus. They looked to the advisory committee to announce safety levels that would force competitors who were selling cheaper, less efficient instruments either to make safety improvements or get out of the market. Self-interest, in this instance, paralleled the public interest, but the advisory committee was reluctant to enter the commercial fray.

Manufacturers were also concerned about their employees, especially those with branches in countries with strong workers' compensation laws. A study of workers in X-ray factories under the auspices of the Philips company in Holland at this time concluded that a daily dose of .01 roentgens of soft rays appeared to be safe, but it also concluded that wearing film badges that clouded slowly with accumulated exposure to radiation should be required of all X-ray workers.

The economic turmoil of the Depression had drawn attention to public health, especially preventive medicine. Literally millions of people had their chests X-rayed, and because stories about X-rays made headlines, each X-ray draftee, so to speak, was a possible litigant. Few suits materialized, but the spread of preventive medical care to the have-nots was not welcomed by everyone in American medicine. Malpractice suits notwithstanding, free chest screenings struck some doctors as the foot-in-the-door of "socialized medicine."

In the disarray of the Depression, the American College of Radiology, which had begun as an honorary group in 1923, took on the responsibility of defending the economic interests of its members. Hospitals continued to grow during the Depression, supported in part by payments from the newly organized Blue Cross and other insurers. But hospitals were budget-wary. They wanted to employ radiologists as though they were just another hospital service, or worse, change the radiologist's traditional fee-for-service arrangement to a salary. California radiologists urged members of the American Roentgen Ray Society and the Radiological Society of North America to join with the American Radium Society and support an Intersociety Committee, which in turn collected a "war chest" to finance activities to negotiate radiologist-hospital relationships, that is, to protect their incomes against any kind of outside control. It argued that as the job of reading X-rays grew increasingly complex, radiologists deserved compensation commensurate with their status as experts.

By the mid-1930s, the RSNA had grown into a formidable organization that was sensitive to both the improvements in X-ray technology, and the needs of its members. By being on top of the issue of dangerous side effects, organized radiologists moved to control all radiation in medicine.

Only an Expert

With better machines, expert radiologists were getting remarkable images of parts of the gastrointestinal track, the neck, and even the brain, although X-rays of chests and broken bones still predominated. What laypeople, especially juries, were likely to find in these images was hard, and is still hard, to know. There had been sporadic complaints from the earliest years of radiology from doctors who insisted that only specialists could interpret radiographs. From time to time judges had agreed. But more often lawyers for both defense and prosecution found it useful to show X-rays directly to the jury—as the prosecution had done in Denver in 1896 when James Smith fell off a ladder and broke his leg.

After World War I no state in the Union refused X-ray evidence of medical miscalculations or evidence of a crime. Yet a minority voice within the medical profession persisted in questioning the use of radiographs by themselves. They argued that pictures alone did not tell the story, especially when the provenance of the pictures was not always clear. (Why, for instance, accept that the radiograph of shattered bones displayed to the jury were actually images of the supposedly injured plaintiff?) Even if authenticated, they insisted, the X-rays were not necessarily taken from a useful angle.

Many people, including physicians, simply could not tell what they were looking at in a radiograph or through a fluoroscope. When H. S. Ward published *Practical Radiography* in 1896, he included a frontispiece captioned "The Human Heart *in situ*." And so it was, but it was upside down! And so it remained, unnoticed, through twenty years of reprints.

In October 1897, Harvey R. Reed read a paper to the Fourth Annual

Meeting of the American Academy of Railway Surgeons in which he held up the X-ray to medicolegal scrutiny. There is a "halo of uncertainty" surrounding X-rays, he warned, and he proceeded to recount personal experiences where radiographs had not found bullets or foreign bodies known to be in a brain or abdominal cavity, but which were found by him, surgically. "Here is a case, which if circumstances had brought it into court, and the X-ray had been admitted as testimony, the evidence would have been far from being the truth, the whole truth and nothing but the truth."[26] He elaborated on this theme, referring to instances in which radiographs had been distorted by magnification, elongation, and shadows.

Seven years later in Britain, Halls Dally likened a radiograph to a painting by Turner. "Without intuition or previous study the one is almost as incomprehensible as the other, but as we gaze the wealth of detail rises before our vision until finally we are able to interpret the meaning of streaks and shadows that to the untrained eye are meaningless."[27]

Radiographers who testified in court in 1899 were warned to explain to the jury that they had to take into account not only the fact that the picture reverses the image from black to white, but also that the position of the tube and the photographic plate can distort the picture. Mihran Kassabian cautioned in his textbook in 1907 that there were always "numerous shadows . . . that defy all efforts of interpretation."[28]

There was a certain amount of understandable skepticism among physicians, like F. S. Shattuck, who noted at a medical meeting in 1903: "Frank Williams has just shown you some plates and tells you that the heart is here and the lung is here. Now I can't see a thing in these plates, and to be truthful, I don't think he can."[29]

These naysayers were left behind in the flood of enthusiasm from the converted who declared that now they understood that the naked eye sees only a small part of reality, while the X-ray exposes the *real*—what is underneath. They understood that the surface that the human eye sees is only a veil, perhaps even camouflage. And just as the myopic see a sharper world with glasses, even the sharp-eyed, without benefit of X-rays, see the world through only a small band of the electromagnetic spectrum. But, with the aid of X-rays, a world that had lain beyond the scope of human vision was, in theory, now exposed to everyone.

But theory was not reality. Anyone could line up at the Grand Central Palace fluoroscope and see his finger bones, but not everyone could look at a chest X-ray and diagnose tuberculosis, or at a dental plate and see an impacted molar. X-rays were never photographs, and the process of capturing an X-ray image can, and often does, distort that image in ways quite different from ordinary photographs.

While lawyers piggybacked X-ray images onto the legal precedent of photographic images, insisting that X-rays be accepted as evidence on the same grounds as photographs, radiologists, as they became more sophisticated about their profession, responded that X-rays did not reflect reality. Lawyers who opposed allowing X-rays into the courtroom without an expert to explain them argued that radiographs are *not* pictures of real objects at all but only *shadows* of objects which could never have been seen by the naked eye. Not photographs, they were images of shadows, and often distorted shadows to boot.[30]

It is probably safe to claim that Samantha A. Call was not considering setting any medical or legal precedent about X-ray evidence on October 14, 1934, when she decided to return some quilting frames to a Mrs. Matthews, but she did. Mrs. Call was driving along Third Street in the city of Burley, Idaho, at between ten and fifteen miles per hour when the car's front wheels suddenly dropped into a ditch where the city was laying a water pipe. Mrs. Call fell off her seat, injuring her back so badly that she was confined to bed for three months. She brought suit against the city to recover medical expenses.

Mrs. Call's lawyer introduced X-ray pictures of her pelvis and back. Recognizing that the pictures were not as clear as he might have wished, he told the jury: "X-ray pictures are not like the man that looks in a glass. . . . 'For he beholdeth himself, and goeth his way, and straightway forgetteth what manner of man he was.'" And the judge acknowledged that the *science* of X-rays was so well-founded that it was no longer necessary to prove that the pictures are reliable. However, this time the court said, "In the case at bar the X-ray picture that was introduced would be utterly useless as evidence without being explained, as it is clear, upon a view of the picture, that the average layman would get no information about the injury here complained of unless the alleged fracture is pointed out and explained to him. After examining this exhibit, we find ourselves in very much the same state of uncertainty about what the picture discloses."[31] The gist of the court's decision was that X-ray exhibits are only useful when they are interpreted and explained to a jury by competent X-ray experts. In other words, jurors in 1935 had to be told what to see. Radiologists were on the brink of victory.

Three years later, in San Francisco, L. H. Garland, a radiologist at San Francisco County Hospital, addressed a group of doctors and lawyers. Decrying the acceptance of X-ray films as if they were the same as "pictures," he argued that an X-ray is not a photograph. A photo is a representation of what the eye actually sees, he argued, and may be interpreted with reasonable ability by many laypersons. X-rays are different. He drew an analogy between the X-ray of an oil painting and the painting itself, between a photograph of an arm and an X-ray picture of that same arm. Under the X-ray, he pointed to the painting, the viewer sees brush strokes and lines but not the flesh tones of the final picture. Likewise, in the X-ray of the arm, there may be a hole in the arm that is normal, or it may represent a cancer. To know which kind of hole it is, you need an experienced person. Garland pleaded: "At first, there were no doctors qualified to interpret radiographs, but after years of development a group of specially trained doctors devoted themselves to this work. They are called radiologists." Radiologists, he went on, are not simply photographers. They are physicians, trained in radiology as a surgeon is trained in surgery. Quoting from a

1921 medical textbook, Garland argued that "roentgenology is not a picture process, but a medical procedure." Looking back to the warnings of Francis Williams, he quoted: "Radiographs should be read not only by a surgeon, but by a surgeon who is trained in reading them." As you wouldn't take a poisoning case to a jury without a chemist's expertise, so must X-rays have a professional to explain them. Garland concluded, "It would be much better if competent interpretation of the X-rays were presented to the jury rather than the misleading shadowgraphs themselves."

Garland understood that "there are several jurisdictions in this country where the courts rely entirely on expert interpretation, without demonstration of the films themselves, as the most desirable method of informing the jury. It is to be hoped that this custom will increase, and that written reports will replace *meaningless shadowgraphs.*"[32]

By 1940 the *Year Book of Radiology* had bought Garland's argument. "Obviously members of the average jury not only cannot understand and appreciate significant changes disclosed on an X-ray film, but also can be misled into entirely incorrect conclusions by their superficial examinations of the 'picture.'"

The *Year Book* went on, "Misleading X-ray appearances are common," and there are cases where money has been awarded by juries who could not possibly have understood "the imitation of fractures by growth . . . the fact that silicosis can be simulated by a variety of conditions, including blurred films, asthma, simple congestion and chronic bronchitis" and that even tuberculosis can be diagnosed when it isn't there.[33]

The X-ray image, hailed in 1896 as the equivalent of taking a photograph with a flashlight inside the body, had shifted in the mind of the law. A radiograph, far from being as clear as a photograph, now, along with fingerprints and ballistics, had to be interpreted through the trained eyes and testimony of an "expert." Yet, while legal and medical authorities argued that medical images were too obscure for ordinary folk to comprehend, popular culture thought otherwise. It had assimilated the X-ray images as a beam that exposed truth beneath opaque surfaces.

Something had changed between 1896 when Judge Owen Le Fevre in Denver had hailed the future in unveiling X-ray evidence to the jury and the 1935 Idaho jury. Part of the change came from improvements in X-ray apparatus that made possible spot-film snapshots of the intestine, tomographs of the lungs, and shots of the pelvis and spine—parts of the body that, unlike thigh bones, were simply unfamiliar to most people. Even today, highly intelligent laypeople find these radiographs hard to discern. Yet there is the possibility that the earlier pictures welcomed by judge and jury alike had been just as difficult to read, but were understood, or misunderstood, because the jurors believed they were clear.

Looking at the catalogue of radiographs collected during the first forty years is eye-opening to the late twentieth-century viewer. The earlier images are often remarkably clear when they show familiar bones, and utterly mysterious when they show internal organs. It is hard to avoid wondering what, if anything, had really been "seen" by doctors and jurors alike in the early years and if everyone had colluded in an emperor's-new-clothes scenario. Were the radiographs qualitatively different? Or had radiographers succeeded as part of their continued effort to exclude amateurs and ensure their incomes as certified experts whenever X-rays were used in court?

Although the answers require a combination of explanations, and the obvious self-interest of physicians cannot be overlooked, the truth lies in the changing nature of how both laypeople and physicians used their eyes. Despite the arguments of medical and legal experts, the majority of radiographs that came before juries showed fractured bones and foreign objects, not tubercular lungs or suspicious tumors. These were images that the ordinary juror, with a little explanation, could easily see and understand. Yet the experts had done their work well. Just as those physicians who could not see much in the blurred radiographs of the 1890s had caved in under pressure from their peers, a similar pressure affected the lay public forty years down the road, but in reverse. The aura of expertise projected by the purveyors of scientific medicine had convinced the public that they could not see the straightforward images of obvious irregularities or a scissor or safety pin dropped during surgery. They no longer believed that the only expertise needed was common sense. Jurists and jurors alike accepted the radiologists' claim that only they, the trained experts, could interpret images. They had a new visual understanding, a new preconception which differed from the untutored eye.

In 1940 a doctor's bag still contained a stethoscope, but if an X-ray tube would have fit in, it would have been on top. Most midcentury physicians would have agreed with their colleagues who had been convinced of the value of X-rays earlier in the century: "Sight is a much more satisfactory agent of information than hearing or touch."[34] Medicine was, a physician concluded as early as 1899, "gradually relegating hearing to a lower intellectual plane than sight."[35] The untutored eye could not interpret the X-rays, but most laypeople and general practitioners trusted the images to reveal evidence of injury or disease.

Five

Technological Innovation 1918–1940

Sharper, Clearer, Deeper

Just Air

Nineteen days after a trolley car tossed a forty-seven-year-old machinist headfirst onto the pavement in uptown Manhattan, medical history was made. It was November 24, 1912, when the man first arrived at Harlem Hospital disoriented, head swollen, blood oozing from a gash over his right eyebrow and his tongue slippery with bloody slime. Suspecting a fracture of the eye bone, H. M. Luckett, the surgeon on call, asked William Stewart, the radiologist, to take two plates. The pictures confirmed Luckett's suspicion: there was a circular fracture of the frontal bone. He would have operated immediately, he recalled later, had not the patient begun sitting up in bed, making what looked like a miraculous recovery. Luckett decided, instead, to wait and watch. Still watching some twelve days later, he was unhappy when, against his advice, the bored and restless patient checked himself out.

Yet Luckett was surprised the following week when the machinist returned, complaining of a terrible headache, vomiting, and lethargy. And then the man sneezed, releasing a cupful of clear liquid from his nose. Luckett immediately ordered a new set of X-rays, and this time he and Stewart stared in astonishment. The pictures had changed. There were now shadows where no one had ever reported seeing shadows before. Stewart concluded "that we were dealing with a case of fracture of the skull complicated by distended cerebral

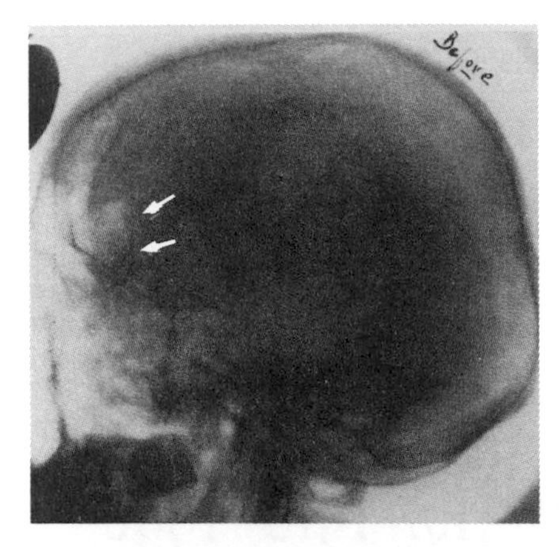

19. Air in the brain following skull fractures after a tram accident (1913). *Left,* on the initial radiograph, two small arrows indicate the fracture of the outer table of the right frontal sinus. Middle, lateral, and *(below)* posteroanterior plates made three weeks later by Dr. William Luckett show the same fracture and the cerebral ventricles distended with air. Courtesy of the American Roentgen Ray Society.

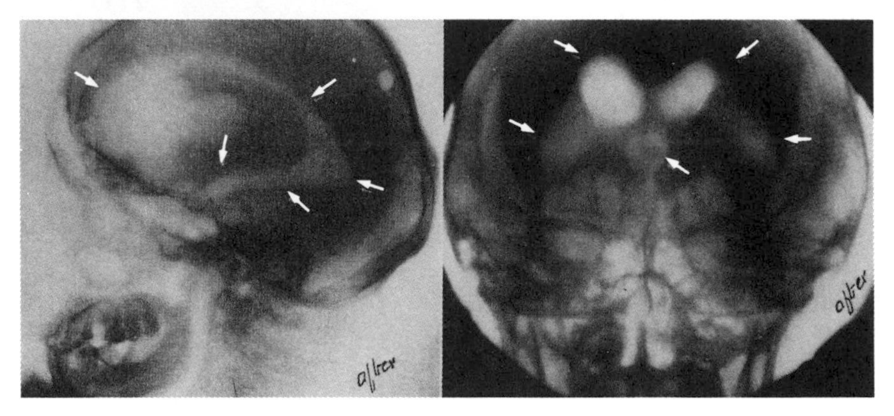

ventriculus [inflated] with air or gas."[1] He labeled the condition "spontaneous pneumoencephalography."

This time he operated and, with the skull opened, noticed some kind of gas bubbling out of the injured tissue. Three days later the machinist died, and the pathologist found a fracture in the wall of the frontal sinus. On submerging the brain in water during the autopsy, he noted air still bubbling out. Luckett deduced that the slime on the patient's tongue had been cerebral spinal fluid which had begun to leak out after the skull had cracked on impact with the pavement. Later, the force of sneezing or simply blowing his nose had forced more fluid out and allowed air to come in. And air, as had been pointed out by the prescient Francis Williams in his 1901 textbook, is a splendid contrast medium for X-rays. "Pneumocephalus," as Luckett dubbed the condition, once identified, was reported twenty-eight more times in the next few years, each time the result of an accident.

Luckett was on to something but did not fully understand the ramifications of his suspicion. Ever since the first years of X-rays, radiologists had realized that many parts of the body that could not be seen clearly with simple X-rays were beautifully clear when a contrast medium was present. Dyes of one sort or another were injected into cadavers and animal models, but the only contrast media known to be safe for human consumption were "meals" made out of bismuth and barium. Opaque to the rays, they outline the stomach and intestines without causing discomfort or poisoning, then pass completely out of the system. (Bismuth had been imported from Europe, so after 1914 American radiologists switched to barium sulfate.) Before World War I, the interior of the gastrointestinal track was the most familiar organ system known to medicine.

But the brain was still terra incognita in June 1915, when a thirty-eight-year-old woman arrived at a London hospital complaining of a terrible headache and a feeling that "her brain was splashing." Gilbert Scott, the radiologist on call that day, had never heard such a bizarre complaint. To humor her, he recorded, "I took hold of her head in both hands and shook it vigorously. The sensation imparted to my hands, together with the sound produced by this procedure, was most extraordinary, not to say alarming, and I instinctively let go. Free fluid in considerable quantity could be felt moving about in the cranium, coming up with a resounding smack against the frontal bone . . . as these signs indicated the presence of air and fluid . . . I expected to find interesting radiographic appearances. In this I was not disappointed."[2]

The air in the woman's brain provided an excellent picture of the orbit over her eye, from which a bony tumor had been removed nine years earlier. Scott speculated that during that surgery, a small opening had been made into the cranium, and over the years cerebral spinal fluid and air had leaked in. The patient seemed mentally healthy, and after the frontal bone was trephined (to allow the removal of liquid), she left the hospital and the public record. She would have been entirely forgotten, save that Scott decided to publish this case in 1917, a year after X-ray examinations on the battlefield in Flanders showed that gas from gangrene in head wounds was yet another example of air as a contrast medium.

These cases were noted as curiosities and apparently set aside. Ever since Edison's failure to get a picture of the brain, it had been treated as beyond the reach of X-rays. Even though Luckett and Stewart had been so impressed by their experience with the ill-starred machinist that between them they described the incident in three separate medical publications, they treated this incident, as did their readers, as anomalous.

By the end of World War I, X-rays were being routinely used for locating foreign objects in the rest of the body, observing broken or fractured bones, and for examining tubercular or otherwise infected lungs. They were, however, seldom used to examine the brain.

The brain had remained private longer than any other part of the body. At almost exactly the same time that explorers like Carl Akeley were closing in on the forests of Africa and southeast Asia, radiological map makers began to enter the cranal interior, what they called the last "dark continent" of the human body.

In the 1920s, doctors grew more adventurous. Success in manufacturing better X-ray equipment, specifically the Coolidge tube and the new grids, stimulated an urge to capture better images of every part of the body.

The possibility of seeing organs and tissue that had been invisible to earlier X-ray machines became a reality as physicians and surgeons introduced new contrast agents into previously unseen areas—especially the brain, the spinal column, the heart, and the arteries. The systematic search for new contrast agents was the first technological advance in the postwar period. The invention of machines to make new kinds of radiographs was the second great technological leap of the interwar years.

While new contrast agents were sought widely, the breakthroughs occurred sequentially, one leading to the next. But the development of new machines occurred almost simultaneously—a pattern that would continue—with credit for priority frequently left unresolved.

Out of Thin Air

The first "new" contrast agent was ordinary air, which Luckett had noted is an excellent contrast agent. But it took a major leap of imagination to shift perspective from marveling at incidents like those recorded in New York and London, to deliberately introducing air into the body, especially the brain, to enhance X-ray images. That leap was made by Walter Dandy, then a thirty-two-year-old resident in surgery at the Johns Hopkins Hospital. Whether or not Dandy was familiar with Luckett's article or with the scattered reports from the military medics about the use of air in the radiology of the brain is not clear. He said he got the idea himself while working under the celebrated surgeon William Halsted. (Halsted was famous for, among other things, overcoming his own cocaine addiction and developing radical mastectomies for cancer.) Dandy recalled Halsted mumbling to his residents, as he operated on intestines, that gases in the intestines were strong enough to perforate bone. Dandy put together the fact that there is an apparently harmless presence of gas in the abdominal cavity with the fact that gas (usually air) absorbs X-rays and so enhances radiographs. Dandy realized that harmless gas could be used to X-ray the part of the body of special interest to him—the brain.

Dandy was eager to perform surgery to treat hydrocephalus (water on the brain) in infants, as well as tumors and edemas in adults, and he had been searching for a way to look into the skull before operating. What he needed was a harmless substance he could introduce into a patient that would satisfy the absorption demands of the X-ray and still be comfortable. The living brain, as Luckett, Scott, and all neurologists knew from experience, is afloat in cerebrospinal fluid. In 1919 Dandy decided to substitute air for a portion of that fluid, to do deliberately what had happened accidentally to the unfortunate New York machinist and the London matron.

In his initial efforts, Dandy injected air directly through the skull into the brain's ventricles. This procedure, known as ventriculography, produced excellent X-ray pictures. But it was only useful for infants. With adults, Dandy had to drill a hole through the skull in order to insert the needle. The procedure was much easier with hydrocephalic infants: he injected the air through the soft fontanelle at the top of the skull where the bones had not yet knit together. These first patients, infants threatened with death or retardation, responded remarkably to shunts that removed the excess fluid after their hydrocephalus had been verified by X-ray.

Dandy had been using ventriculography successfully for about a year when he startled the medical world in 1919 with another revolutionary procedure, pneumoencephalography, which is the injection of air by lumbar puncture into the base of the spinal column. This technique involves placing two needles adjacent to each other so that as air is injected through one needle, fluid is removed through the other, taking care that the volume of air and the volume of fluid was the same. Dandy found that air injected into the space surrounding the spinal column rose until it filled the ventriculi—the spaces—in the brain as well as other, smaller, cavities. This process was, however, very painful. Dandy refined it by reducing the proportion of fluid removed so that patients could bear the pain without anesthesia and therefore remain awake to cooperate during the operation. The procedure made Dandy a celebrity, and his fame symbolized the glamour of the heroes of the new hospital-centered medicine.

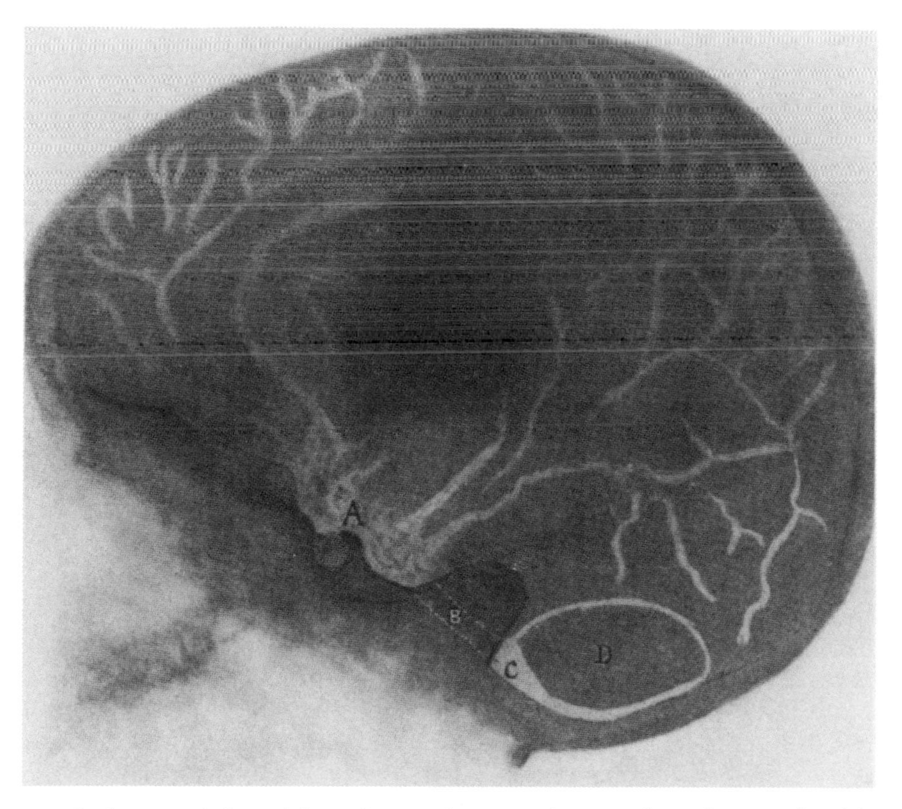

20. The first encephalograph by Walter Dandy (1919). This X-ray shows the ventricles of the brain after an injection of air. Courtesy of *Annals of Surgery,* Lippincott-Raven Publishers.

For all its impenetrability, the brain gave up its secrets without a struggle: once the surface was penetrated, the brain—unlike the lungs, the heart, and the intestines—has no large moving parts. (Newer forms of imaging can monitor blood flow and even neuronal connections, but they do not enter the story for another fifty years.) Ventriculography—the ability to see the cerebral ventricles outlined clearly—more than doubled the scope of what doctors could see inside the brain. By 1937, it had become the method of choice for examinations prior to brain surgery and it was the procedure performed in Beverly Hills, California, that July on the composer George Gershwin.

Gershwin, at thirty-eight, had been experiencing odd symptoms for several years, but most of them were subtle and camouflaged by the influence of the heavy-handed psychoanalysis that Gershwin was undergoing. The symptoms had become extreme earlier that year when Gershwin had lost consciousness for a fraction of a minute while playing his Concerto in F Major with the Los Angeles Philharmonic at the Hollywood Bowl. In trying to recall the episode, he mentioned smelling burning rubber before losing his place. Gershwin's medical history included more than a decade of constantly upset stomachs (dismissed by one doctor as "composer's stomach"), and increasingly frequent headaches associated with a scent of burning rubber that no one else could smell.[3] By July it was obvious that his problem was neurological, and he was brought to Cedars of Lebanon Hospital where a neurosurgeon, Carl Rand, saw at once what he was dealing with and asked to consult with Walter Dandy. The celebrated surgeon turned out to be sailing on Chesapeake Bay with the Maryland governor. Gershwin's family contacted the White House where a secretary called the navy. The navy, in turn, dispatched a coast guard cutter to bring Dandy ashore, where he was sped by police escort to the airport in Cumberland, Maryland, to fly to the West Coast. Rand had also sent for a locally prominent surgeon, Howard Nafziger, who was summoned back from Lake Tahoe. He telephoned Dandy at the Maryland airport and they agreed there was no time to wait. Gershwin was already semiparalyzed on his right side, and his eyes were swollen and protruding.

Ordinary X-rays revealed nothing, but by this time the neurologists suspected a tumor. Before operating, the surgical team opened Gershwin's skull and took X-ray images from several angles for two and a half hours, to get the best idea of the tumor's position. Then they performed ventriculography, and saw that both lateral ventricles were displaced because of the large tumor in the right temporal region. Nafziger performed a partial resection, but it was too late. Gershwin's glioblastoma—a fast-growing malignant tumor—had grown too large and he never recovered consciousness.

A few years earlier, in France, Maurice Ravel had begun to suffer headaches after a blow to his head in what had seemed a minor traffic accident in 1932. He began to have trouble moving his body and by the summer of 1933 could no longer swim. At the same time he had begun to make spelling errors, and by the end of the year was unable even to sign his name (a condition known as agraphia). While he could still play the piano, he had lost the ability to translate from one mental sensation to another. Ravel's disease, unlike Gershwin's, began to destroy his brain by making his life unbearable—he could hear new music inside his head but was unable to set it down on paper or play it on an instrument. Ravel's head was X-rayed, and his condition diagnosed as "shrinking of the brain." In a last-ditch effort to rescue his creative powers, Ravel agreed to admittedly desperate, experimental surgery in the winter of 1937. Some kind of fluid would be injected into his skull to nourish the receding tissues. Ravel died during the operation.[4]

Before the development of modern neurobiology, the study of the function and structure of the brain was the domain of psychologists and surgeons. It was not the domain of radiologists, so it is not surprising that both ventriculography and pneumoencephalography were developed by surgeons. Surgeons used radiology to guide them in their mission to alleviate particular kinds of life-threatening conditions, including hydrocephalus and tumors.

Oil

Jan Athanase Sicard, a French contemporary of Dandy, was looking for a way to relieve pain, not necessarily headaches, when he came upon a remarkable new contrast agent. Sicard had a reputation in Paris for his successful treatment of sciatica, and it was in connection with this painful back condition that he, ever on the lookout for pharmaceutical painkillers, happened across lipiodol. An iodine-based compound suspended in oil, lipiodol had been on pharmacy shelves since 1901 and was used as a painkiller in muscles. It had long been dismissed by radiologists because it tends to linger in the system and, like all iodine compounds, is radio-opaque. The presence of lipiodol interfered with routine X-ray examinations.

Legend has Sicard directing a student to inject the material into a patient's lumbar muscles, and has the student realizing in horror that he had, instead, accidentally punctured the cavity around the spinal cord. Rushing to confess his error to Sicard, the master is reported to have responded, "And the patient? How had this affected him?"[5] Apparently not at all, so Sicard investigated further by having the patient brought in on a table before a fluoroscope. There Sicard discovered that when he tipped the table that supported the supine man, he could watch on the fluoroscope as the oil moved along the nerve sheath and throughout the spinal region, highlighting tumors, bone spurs, and whatever other irregularities were causing pain or paralysis.

This was in 1921. Sicard and his associate Jacques Forestier then experimented on dogs, injecting them everywhere with lipiodol, under the skin, into the muscles and the peritoneum. Eventually radiologists all over Europe were using lipiodol to get X-ray images of the spine. It took another few years to catch on in the United States, because the particular iodized oil that was first tested in several hospitals was not quite the same as the French mixture, and it had killed an experimental animal.

Americans might have had to wait another decade for the benefits of lipiodol had not Ethel Russell, a radiologist at the Philadelphia General Hospital, decided to try it on a particularly frustrating case in February 1924. A young dental mechanic who had been paralyzed in both legs for over two years had been left a ward of the hospital, where his condition continued to deteriorate until he was incontinent. At this juncture Russell decided to reconsider her options. She knew that somewhere in the young man's lumbar region his spinal fluid was blocked. So far, the blockage had remained hidden. Desperate, she decided to try the new French technique of myelography (radiology of the spinal cord). She injected the lipiodol into the base of his spine and then took X-rays. The iodine enabled her to localize the blocked area so precisely that a surgeon could, and did, remove a large, but benign, tumor. The patient began walking again, and soon left the hospital and returned to work.

The next year Walter Dandy began using lipiodol where air diagnosis was not good enough, and loudly praised its efficacy. His surgical colleagues rushed to emulate him.

Meanwhile, Sicard and Forestier extended their use of lipiodol to other areas of the body, including the bronchial tubes, the uterus, Fallopian tubes, seminal vesicles, bladder, urinary system, and assorted joints, tissues, and organs. Lipiodol became the contrast agent of choice for the next twenty years. Injected into the bladder and urethra as well as the nervous system, lipiodol left no residue, allowing the most sensitive and heretofore radiologically opaque organs to be seen inside and out.

By 1925, air and lipiodol headed the roster of contrast agents, especially among physicians who wanted to see the recesses of the brain and spinal column. Lipiodol did not, however, lend itself to use in the last holdouts in the human body to give up their internal secrets to film—the blood vessels. Physicians and surgeons were very much aware that if they could find a way to get pictures of the inside of the veins and arteries, they would be able to diagnose and perhaps treat the most profound medical problems of the brain and heart. So far they had had little luck. They had only been able to see the delicately branching arterial tree in the radiographs of dead people—to whom an injection of dye held no threat.

Iodine

For imaging the blood stream, an oil-based agent like lipiodol was out of the question: oil could cause embolisms—fatal obstructions of gas bubbles. The possibility of introducing a nontoxic substance into the vascular system spurred the imagination of many doctors, but the first to make a breakthrough was Egaz Moniz at the medical school of the University of Lisbon. Moniz had studied medicine in Paris and then returned to Portugal where he first practiced ophthalmology and then moved deeper into the brain, which is to say he became a neurologist. Moniz came from such a prominent family that he was asked, as a young physician, to add diplomatic chores to his schedule. He had been appointed ambassador to Madrid during the first world war and then been selected to lead the Portuguese delegation to the Peace Conference at Versailles. While in Paris, he managed to fight a duel (by that time illegal in France), become a gourmand, publish a book on the history of playing cards, and begin work on a biography of John XXI, the only doctor ever to become Pope.

In 1927, at an international meeting of neurologists, Moniz startled his colleagues with his account of successful angiography. Moniz did for the cerebral arteries what Sicard had done for the spine. He had sought and discovered a contrast agent that enabled him to get clear pictures of tumors in the cerebrum.

The goal was clear: Moniz needed a nontoxic substance that would be eliminated from the body, but would not be diluted by the flow of blood before an X-ray could be taken. Nor could the contrast agent produce emboli or clots. Moniz looked to salts of iodine and bromine and settled on iodine because of its greater radiographic density.

A man of enormous imagination, ego, and ambition, Moniz suffered so acutely from gout in his hands that he could not use them and performed surgery with a partner, Almeida Lima. Together they operated to ensure that the sodium iodide was where he needed it to be when he was ready to take X-rays. They managed this by cutting into the internal carotid artery, injecting the iodine salt, then closing the artery and opening it again to release the iodine solution immediately before taking the X-ray to outline the arteries on the radiograph.

Moniz perfected what we now call an angiogram, changing contrast agents from time to time. He began experimenting with dogs, and then tried his technique with six patients, using a solution of 70 percent strontium bromide. Five of his subjects produced disappointing images. After the sixth died, he switched to a solution that was 25 percent sodium iodide, but the pictures they produced had poor contrast. Finally the ninth case, a twenty-year-old blind man complaining of severe headaches and vomiting, was revealed to have a pituitary tumor. The process, as far as Moniz was concerned, was a success.[6]

Moniz soon replaced sodium iodine with thorium dioxide, a radioactive compound. Marketed under the trade name Thorotrast, it was the first choice for many radiologists up through the early 1950s because the radioactivity enhanced the contrast in the image. Only then, after thirty years, did the penny drop. While the iodine in sodium iodide had been excreted almost immediately, the particles of Thorotrast are insoluble in water and they were trapped in the liver and spleen, irradiating the cells they rested in and slowly killing their hosts. When used for neuroradiology, the thorium often leaked into the brain, and the patients eventually developed brain tumors.[7]

That was in a future Moniz would not know. In the late 1920s, he moved on professionally, with Lima still acting as his "hands," to pioneer a technique of drilling holes through the skull and then removing part, or all, of the patient's frontal lobes in order to curb embarrassing or unconventional social behavior. This procedure, frontal lobotomy, won Moniz the Nobel Prize in physiology or medicine in 1949. His fame brought him to the United States, where he traveled from city to city, operating with his assistant on half a dozen patients in a single afternoon, "curing" by reducing the patients' ability to respond emotionally or intellectually. In hindsight, many critics consider Moniz's surgery as little more than authorized butchery. His admirers argue that Moniz was a great physician entitled to his laurels, not for lobotomy but for cerebral angiography.

It took only a few years more before the living heart, along with the brain, yielded to visual penetration. There had been early efforts to get an image of the heart, notably by Mihran Kassabian who, in 1907, reported on injecting infants with bismuth subnitrate. However, his and other episodic efforts to examine the heart never became routine procedures; the contrast agents were hard to control, and the moving heart is a difficult target for the X-ray camera.

But in the late 1920s a new method was introduced that would revolutionize the procedure. This was examination by catheterization—a technique in which, today, a needle pulling a slim tube is inserted into a vein and pushed through to the part of the body under consideration. The first experiment occurred in the summer of 1929 when, after practicing on cadavers, Werner Forssmann, an intern in Eberswalde, Germany, asked the head of surgery at his hospital if he could experiment on a patient. Flatly denied access, Forssmann suggested he try it on himself. This, too, was ruled out, but Forssmann was able to talk a nurse, Eva, into helping him on the pretext that she would be the volunteer. After he let her get him the equipment he needed, he tied Eva to a gurney and applied a local anesthetic to his own left elbow. Then he inserted a needle attached to a catheter thirty centimeters long into his own vein. At this point he released Eva and asked her to find the X-ray technician. Meanwhile, with the needle still in place, Forssmann walked downstairs to the basement radiology lab, looked in a mirror in front of a fluoroscope to check that he had done his work properly, and then took a radiograph documenting the experiment. He published the image of the catheter in his right atrium later that year (followed by a memoir entitled *Experiments on Myself*).[8]

Forssmann's impetuous behavior earned him dismissal from several hospitals, but he continued investigating the heart. Still using himself as a subject, he injected an iodine-based contrast material into his vein; the agent was harmless, but did not provide a clear X-ray image. At the time his work was hailed for its results, but his colleagues' condemnation of his behavior thwarted his surgical career.[9] Eventually, after World War II, his research was resurrected, and in 1956 he shared a Nobel Prize for his work on catheterization.[10]

Heart catheterization, like X-raying the lungs, remained more useful in fluoroscopy than in still images because the beating heart can blur the radiograph. Naturally, the ability to see inside the heart enabled cardiologists to diagnose conditions with much greater precision and to treat them, if possible. Today's open-heart surgery relies on a map of the heart provided by angiography. Equally dramatic has been the extension of catheterization techniques to the new radiological subspecialty of "interventional radiology." Contemporary Forssmanns not only push catheters through blood vessels to image the abnormal arteries on a screen, but they now treat those abnormal arteries with balloon angioplasty to widen the artery or by inserting stents, which place a small metal fence within the artery over which the artery heals.[11]

The introduction of new contrast agents into previously inaccessible regions of the body was complemented, during the 1920s and 1930s, by improvements in the X-ray apparatus itself. To the incremental improvements, such as machines with better electrical insulation, better shielding against excess radiation, and better focusing, more dramatic changes were added. New kinds of pictures became available as ways were discovered to fix images from fluoroscopes through the use of the spot-film device—a machine that recorded a fluoroscopic image instantaneously on X-ray film—better screens, and the first images of planes deep inside the body.

The years after World War I saw the widespread adoption into standard practice of technological innovations that had been invented before 1918. The old gas tubes were replaced with the new Coolidge apparatus as finances permitted. As engineers learned from physicists that X-rays varied within the spectrum much as colors vary in the spectrum of visible light, they learned ways of exploring this range of rays. It was common knowledge that high-voltage X-rays had shorter wavelengths, and that the shortest wavelengths, the gamma rays, had their own limitations and advantages. They called the not-quite gamma rays "hard" rays, and used them to penetrate deep into the body. At the same time they were able to regulate and send "soft" rays into tissue close to the surface of the skin.

As these innovations were brought to the marketplace, a new generation of physicians could penetrate the body more deeply and with more precision than ever before.

Steriography

Dandy's surgical colleague, J. W. Pierson, explained to an audience at the International Conference on Radiology in 1925 that of course ventriculography and pneumoencephalography were still dangerous and complicated procedures (and, he could have added, extremely painful), but whatever their shortcomings —as today's imagers would echo when describing their own new methods— they were a lot safer for the patient than the kind of exploratory brain surgery that had theretofore been the patient's only option.

From the very beginning of radiology in 1896, medical radiologists had been frustrated because what they wanted to see was often behind some other structure that blurred, distorted, or completely obstructed their view. Starting with stereoradiography, there had been a steady effort to place injuries, tumors, and especially foreign objects in three-dimensional space inside the body. The desire to see beneath or around other bones and internal organs was combined with the hope of seeing the body's interior in three dimensions.

The first successful efforts were those of radiographers like young Elizabeth Fleischmann in San Francisco during the Spanish-American War who earned praise from the surgeon general for her plates which, taken from different angles, triangulated the guilty piece of shrapnel or shot.

An Interior Slice

Ever since the Bucky-Potter grid, the device that kept scattered X-rays from blurring the edges of the image, improving the sharpness of the images, radiographers had known that when the X-ray tube and film moved in parallel planes opposite to each other, the blur caused by their movement removed the images of some of the structures that were in the way. As early as 1914 a Polish doctor, Carol Mayer, was able to get a reasonable image of the heart by blurring out the shadow of the ribs, leaving the image of a single plane, or slice. Techniques for producing these slices, which were soon called *tomographs*—*tomo* comes from a Greek term meaning a section or cut—were patented nine times with at least three different names in five different countries during the 1920s, but the first instrument was not built until 1931.

The promise of tomography was tantalizing. There are times when some new development is in the air: the need for the technique is obvious and the general technology is advanced enough to allow more than a single solution to the general problem. While it is beyond dispute that the discovery of X-rays was a complete surprise, once discovered, its practical applications were clear. Within days scientists and inventors in Europe and North America had proposed fluoroscopes—machines that did not make permanent pictures but instead provided an opportunity to watch what was going on inside the body in real time. By the end of 1896, a variety of experts were working on a few problems: they worked to improve the focus of the tube, to improve the stability of the tube, to protect the operator from excessive radiation, to get faster pictures, crisper pictures, and pictures of internal organs that were protected by bones that blocked the X-rays. In every one of these efforts—focus tubes, photographic plates, lead shielding—there were competing patents. The result was a slow, incremental improvement on the basic X-ray machine. The more dramatic changes took longer to reach the market because they demanded often expensive new equipment to manufacture them, and because they were too expensive for most self-employed physicians to buy. Like the fluoroscope and focus tubes, the idea of tomography occurred to several people at the same time in different parts of the world.

In 1921 alone, three Frenchmen applied for two patents: André Edmund Marie Bocage, a dermatologist who thought up the idea while in the army X-raying wounded soldiers, and F. Portes and M. Chausse, but no one actually constructed either instrument. The idea languished until 1930 when Alessandro Vallebona in Italy built a machine that got an image of a phantom, or artificial object representing an internal organ, inside a model of a patient. He called this method "stratigraphy." This was followed a year later by the "planigraph" of a body section inside a patient by a Dutch physician, Bernard

Ziedes des Plantes. Although these were working prototypes, neither went into production for many years.

Meanwhile in 1928 in the United States, Jean Kieffer, a French immigrant with little formal education, found a job in the X-ray department of a TB sanitarium in Connecticut. When he suffered a relapse of his own tuberculosis, he was conveniently put to bed at his work place. The doctors could not see the lesions, however, because they were in his mediastinum, a part of the lungs invisible to ordinary X-rays because of the bones surrounding it. Lying in bed and staring at the ceiling (all he could do in his condition), Kieffer pondered the problem of visualizing his own lungs.

He eventually worked out a system in which the X-ray tube and film were connected as if on a seesaw around the patient. The tube could be moved to focus on selected planes in the patient's body, and the film at the other end would then move with it. Kieffer's design was flexible; his instrument could move back and forth or up and down while the two important elements—the tube and the film—stayed in synchrony. Using the principle of delayed-exposure photography (albeit with the exposure only a few seconds), Kieffer had the focus stay on the target area as the X-ray tube and camera moved around it. The result was a clear image of the plane of interest, with the area around it blurred out. The thickness of the "slice" could be adjusted at will, as could the size of the focus area. To top it off, Kieffer's device was designed to work with a Potter-Bucky grid so that the image was especially sharp. Delighted with his solution, Kieffer applied for a patent in 1929. Like his predecessors in France, Italy, and Germany, however, he could not get anyone to build it.

The various X-ray companies he approached declined the opportunity to buy the patent on the grounds that it probably wouldn't work, or if it did, it would be useless and certainly not marketable. One manufacturer snubbed him: if the idea were worthwhile, one of his own engineers would have designed it already.[12] Kieffer is unique in the history of imaging devices, because he made his discovery without a formal education, as a patient and not a doctor.

Kieffer, Ziedes des Plantes, and Vallebona shared the distinction of not getting their devices manufactured. But in 1936 the early patent of André Bocage was taken up by the French firm of Massiot. At this point European and North American efforts parted.

In the United States that year, at the annual meeting of the American Roentgen Ray Society in Cleveland, a press release touted a new X-ray machine which did "body section roentgenography," that is to say, it got X-ray pictures of slices of the head or organs heretofore obscured by other tissue. At a demonstration by its inventors—Dr. Robert Andrews and Robert Stava from the Cleveland University Hospital—an "unassuming, unpretentious, and somewhat reticent chap" came up to say that he considered himself the inventor of their machine.[13] It was Jean Kieffer. But when they met later, privately, Andrews and Stava explained that he was only one among many claimants.

Andrews, who was a doctoral candidate in physics as well as a physician, had examined the European literature and then collaborated with Stava, who worked at the Picker X-Ray Corporation in Cleveland. Together they had built the model. They told Kieffer that, while the press release had brought people to the exhibition—including Kieffer—no one was buying the machine. The pictures produced by what they called their "planigraph" looked very raw and fuzzy to radiologists accustomed to ordinary X-rays.

Fortunately, however, the head of the Mallinckrodt Institute of Radiology at Washington University in St. Louis grasped the implications of the new machine and talked with all three men—the Cleveland doctor and engineer, and the Connecticut inventor. He arranged for Kieffer's version of the tomograph to be built in St. Louis. It was from St. Louis in 1937 that Kieffer wrote excitedly to his wife in New England, "I am so tickled at the machine and what it does that I would like to dance a jig!"[14] He had gotten a picture of an abdominal aneurism that was not only supposedly impossible to get, but that verified a questioned diagnosis. By the fall of 1939, more than a thousand patients had had what they were calling "laminagraphs" in St. Louis. Soon a commercial model, known as the Kieffer laminagraph, was in production.

The tomographs that were finally manufactured in the 1930s were based on Kieffer's design, which moved the X-ray tube and film while the focal plane remained stationary. The result was a clear image of that single slice. By moving the focus from one plane to the next and the next, the operator could build up a sequence of images. This series could then be arranged to give a good facsimile of the patient's interior space. A single tomograph could get around the problem of interference. A series of tomographic slices gave the impression of volume.

There were many variations and improvements on tomographs between 1939 and 1960 as the technique was applied to different parts of the body. In the early years tomography was used mostly for chest and gastrointestinal examinations, but in the 1940s and 1950s the technology was applied to skeletal problems, ear, sinus, and nose difficulties, and kidney and urethral complications. Tomography gave physicians their best pictures of organs hidden deep inside the body until computerized tomography took over in the 1970s.

Physics, Film, and Fluoroscopes

By the 1920s, double emulsion film (which was able to produce a picture in half the time with half the radiation) had all but replaced glass plates. Pathé in Europe had been selling nonflammable film for years but it did not produce as sharp a picture as Eastman Kodak's flammable cellulose nitrate product. Consequently, fires broke out so regularly in American doctors' offices that it was standard for fire departments to be alerted to the dangers from X-ray libraries. There was no apparent effort to make the American film safer until 1929 when an inferno that began in the X-ray storage area at the Cleveland Clinic killed 124 people. In response, the Picker X-Ray Corporation immediately ordered safety film from France, and within a year Kodak had perfected its own safety film. Soon Du Pont had one, too, with a blue tint that made the film easier to read and soon became standard for all X-ray pictures. The history of flammable film is a reminder that safety improvements, like the ill-fated lead-lined radiologists suit, were not developed when the market showed no interest in paying something extra for safety. Only the threat of being locked out of the particular market pushed American film manufacturers to match the French competition.

Kodak announced another innovation in X-ray film with great fanfare at the Century of Progress Exhibition in Chicago in 1934. Its great achievement was the first full-length, full-size, one-piece X-ray picture of a complete human being. (Before this all whole-body pictures had been composites.) *Time* magazine's story on the life-size X-ray describes the model, a woman, as "pretty," 20 years old, 115 pounds, with a size 13 dress, a size 21 hat, soft brown eyes, and a cupid-bow mouth (none of these attributes, of course, was apparent in the X-ray photograph).[15] Kodak suggested that such full-length films would be useful for getting a picture of all broken bones at once at an accident scene with minimal discomfort, or to show all secondary cancers, or the full extent of rickets. This large-size film never caught on commercially, however, and whole-body scans only became practical with the introduction of nuclear medicine in the 1980s.

But new methods for using ordinary size film were a different story. The first major advance was the spot-film device. The device entered North America via the port of Boston in 1932. It had been ordered sight unseen by Joseph Pratt, physician-in-chief at the venerable Boston Dispensary (the first public clinic in the United States, founded in 1796). Pratt had done postdoctoral work in Germany and had remained in touch with colleagues there. They wrote to him about the remarkable invention of Hans Berg, a gastrointestinal specialist in Berlin.

The device revolutionized X-ray studies of the gastrointestinal tract in two ways: it was able to capture successive fluoroscopic images of the stomach and duodenum during a barium exam, and, with an adjunct unit, it could show ulcers and monitor their treatment. Pratt wrote to Berg in Berlin, ordered a device and offered to pay the expenses of an assistant—a physician—who could bring it across the Atlantic, install it at the dispensary, and demonstrate its use.

That is how Alice Ettinger arrived in the United States in July 1932. (Pratt would have preferred a man, he had written to Berg, but soon appreciated the young woman who carried the bulky device in her suitcase.)[16] A veritable impresario of the gastrointestinal tract, Ettinger demonstrated the device throughout New England, published papers about its subtleties, and after the election of Hitler as Chancellor in Germany in 1933, accepted Pratt's offer to join the faculty at the Tufts University School of Medicine where, in 1939, she became the chief of radiology at the Boston Dispensary. Before America joined World War II against Germany, Pratt made a point of hiring other displaced German Jewish physicians, all of whom remained in Boston at the New England Medical Center, an association of the Dispensary and of the medical and dental schools of Tufts University.

Before the introduction of the spot-film device, fluoroscopy and radiography were entirely separate procedures. Fluoroscopy, where the image of the patient appears immediately on a screen, was especially useful for examining an internal organ in action. The new device enabled the physician to see a process in real time, as it was happening, on the fluoroscope and then, with the spot-film, freeze and record the particular image needed for diagnosis. It was like a still from a movie, except that there was no moving-picture film. The spot-film device enabled radiologists to select an opportune moment—during peristalsis, for example—to get a picture, which could then be compared with other images.

The fluoroscopic image had always been more difficult to read than an image on film, and from the first decades of this century, fluoroscope manufacturers kept developing and marketing improved screens. They used different fluorescent chemicals, with distinctly different lifespans, to produce increasingly brighter images. But none of these increased the intensity of the light on the screen enough to make it bright enough for the goal of making film strips.

In 1941, however, Edward Chamberlain demonstrated to a formidable audience of radiologists that he could make excellent radiographs from film held against a fluoroscopic screen. The fluoroscopic image is weak, he explained, echoing Antoine Béclère, because of limitations of the human eye, not the machine. Chamberlain reasoned that fluoroscopes would be improved if their screens were bright enough for the human eye to see well. At that time fluoroscopic screens converted only about 30 percent of the X-ray's energy into visible light. One way to get a brighter image was to make a brighter screen. But even a brighter screen was not enough if it meant capturing more X-rays. What was needed was a way to amplify the light without increasing radiation.

This was solved by the invention of the intensifier, a device containing a screen coated with a phosphorescent material that glows when struck by electrons. The first intensifiers were recommended as early as 1896 by the English photographer Archibald Campbell Swinton, who coated his screens with calcium tungstate, enabling him to get a brighter image and reduce exposure time. But there was no real progress until World War II when the development of electronics led to the invention of image intensifiers. These work by letting radiation from an X-ray tube pass through a patient to impinge on a fluorescent screen that is in contact with a small window. As the screen generates light, a photoelectric layer on the inner surface of the window emits electrons. These electrons are then accelerated onto a second fluorescent screen producing an intense light. In 1953 Westinghouse marketed a commercial version which it called the Fluorex. Although the Fluorex's useful field was only about three inches in diameter, it liberated those radiologists who had access to it from the encumbrance of wearing red goggles because the fluoroscopic images were now clearly visible in ordinary light. More important, it allowed doctors to capture those fluoroscopic images permanently on film or videotape. This was only a start, since image intensifiers did not become standard equipment until the mid-1960s.[17]

The image intensifier worked with other fluoroscopic improvements, including the spot-film attachment, making it an even more reliable way to capture a needed image. Like the new tomography, these images were excellent for the specialist, yet incomprehensible to the lay viewer and to most ordinary physicians. The spot-film, a great advance for gastroenterologists, captured a special instant from real-time observations of the body in motion, but only the physician who ordered and read the particular picture understood what it was all about.

On a New Scale

Ettinger was not the only female radiologist. Although women have never crowded the field, there have been prominent women in the community of X-ray experts from the days of Elizabeth Fleischmann. As a branch of medicine, radiology was a good niche for a woman: the hours were more regular than those of other specialties, and contractual relationships with hospitals allowed women to chose between being hospital employees or fee-for-service specialists. Many female radiologists were single, like Ettinger; others were married to physicians, or to scientists, like Sigrid Lauritsen.

Lauritsen, who had been educated in Denmark, studied medicine at the University of Southern California, a "mature" student who got her medical degree the same year her son received his bachelor's from the California Institute of Technology. During her student years she brought her radiology colleagues from Los Angeles Memorial Hospital to Friday evening meetings of Caltech's physicists' "light conversation and heavy drinking association" in Pasadena.[18]

Sigrid and her husband, Charles Christian Lauritsen, had come to California in 1928, after Charles Lauritsen, who was working in St. Louis, met and was mesmerized by Robert Millikan, the Nobel laureate who headed the California Institute of Technology. The Lauritsens followed Millikan to Pasadena, where Charles earned his Ph.D. the next year working with Robert Oppenheimer on the practical side of constructing a giant million-volt transformer.

Millikan's personal commitment to basic science did not blind him to the advantages of funding science through technology. Rather than wait for science to produce technological spin-offs—which had been the case with the study of electromagnetism—Millikan was happy to let technology provide the electrical power he hoped would produce scientific spin-offs. This, indeed, was the gist of the plan he had worked out with the Southern California Edison Company, which had provided Caltech with a high-voltage laboratory in 1920, and with the newly formed Metropolitan Water District. The Water District and the Edison Company were interested in long-distance electrical power transmission. Millikan, following his own research ambitions, wanted to produce voltage high enough to study, among other things, the nature of high-energy X-rays. Physicists of the day, Lauritsen among them, used the same technology to produce high-energy charged particles for the purpose of pursuing their interests in nuclear physics. Lauritsen met the challenge by erecting an enormous tube—a variation of the Coolidge tube—on a fourteen-foot-high redwood scaffolding in Pasadena. Lauritsen explained in the 1930 patent application that his tube, which could operate at a million volts, was "the full equivalent of a gram of radium in the treatment of disease."[19]

Lauritsen, in collaboration with a local physician, Seeley Mudd, and encouraged by his wife's clinical interests, developed high-voltage X-ray machines for radiation therapy. Millikan and Lauritsen then invited Albert Soiland, who ran a tumor clinic in Los Angeles, to use their 750,000 volt X-ray tube on patients. Starting in 1930, Soiland used what was, for the Depression, exceedingly expensive technology on several hundred patients suffering from inoperable cancers. Soiland established a precedent that would become enormously important in the years after World War II—the collaboration of basic science research and medical radiology.

The gap between research in the physical and in the biological sciences was enormous. While biologists and physicians were just beginning to understand the effects of ionizing radiation on human tissue—its dangers and its therapeutic uses—physicists were exploring the fundamental phenomena of matter including quantum mechanics, cosmic rays, subnuclear particles, and radiation. Chemists eagerly filled in gaps in the periodic table of the elements, explored the alchemical goal of changing one element into another, and searched for isotopes of elements like hydrogen. When in 1934 Irène Curie and her husband Frédéric Joliot bombarded the nuclei of nonradioactive elements with atomic particles, they produced new radioactive isotopes, for which, it will be remembered, they shared a Nobel Prize in 1934.

At this time, however, almost as soon as physicians and scientists from the former Allied nations had ended the often vicious and certainly self-destructive ostracism of their German and Austrian colleagues, the rise of Nazism in Germany changed the field on which the players met. One-time associates fell into two camps—pro- and anti-fascist. Soon the United States found itself accepting Jewish physicians like Alice Ettinger who were being forced out of the job market in Germany.

Preparedness, Again

The American military began seriously preparing its medical support system as Europe went to war in 1939. Westinghouse had developed the idea of recording X-rays on 35 millimeter film, which they sold to the military when the draft began. Both the army and the navy were determined to have a pre-induction health record of all recruits so as not to be caught, as they had been a generation earlier, by veterans who insisted that they had contracted tuberculosis in service and expected the military to pay for treatment. The navy liked Westinghouse's plan for rapid processing of inductees, and it worked out a routine whereby chest X-rays could be snapped as fast as the men had shots for typhoid fever. The navy got what it considered to be a complete diagnostic record in less than a minute.[20] (By 1944 the Public Health Service extended the X-ray part of the routine to people working in war industries and war agencies.)

The United States entered World War II with a large stock of new portable X-ray equipment redesigned by the Picker Company which had produced over 10,000 units by 1945 (and returned three million dollars to the U.S. treasury after VJ Day, refusing to profit from war). They also had a new portable X-ray field table, faster and smaller film radiographs, and the ability to establish X-ray facilities on every front. The improvements in X-ray technology during the war were limited to refinements on portability and speed, because few other changes were necessary for wartime medicine. Radiology was already an integral part of every military hospital and, as in the previous war, additional radiology officers and technicians were trained to meet the new patient load.

The war effort focused on producing large quantities of easily portable apparatus. It was not a time for basic research in radiology. Yet basic research continued in other sciences related to defense, including radar, submarine detection, and the development of nuclear weapons. In the quarter century after 1945 these strictly military projects would lead to the development of new ways to make clinically useful images of the body's interior. The contrast agents and tomographic machines developed between the wars prepared the way for the wave of new flesh-penetrating imagers that revolutionized medicine in the second half of the twentieth century and altered anew the way people understood the human body.

Six

X-Rays in the Imagination

The Avant-Garde through Surrealism

From the day that Bertha Roentgen's living bones appeared in newspapers around the world, those who saw them understood their bodies in a different way. Looking at a radiograph, patients, as well as physicians, could see the unmistakable line of a broken bone, or the presence of a machine-made object like a bullet or a needle. In making the interior of the body visible, X-rays shifted an assumption that had guided human behavior throughout recorded history. Visual penetration of one living person by another had been blocked by the skin. That barrier had dissolved. The X-ray unilaterally altered ages of societal accord by making public what was once private.

Conservatives flinched at that vision, including a reporter for the London *Pall Mall Gazette,* who commented early in 1896 "on the revolting indecency" of looking at other people's bones. He suggested that "the best thing would be for all civilized nations to combine to burn all works on the roentgen rays, to execute all the discoverers, and to corner all the tungstate in the world and whelm it in the middle of the ocean. Let the fish contemplate each other's bones if they like, but not us."[1]

Writers of fiction were the first to recognize the impact of X-rays on the collective psyche. They immediately began to posit scenarios of how the power to see through opaque objects might affect individuals and whole societies. A decade later painters began to offer graphic musings of what the new "insight" meant to their own vision. The X-ray was also the ideal metaphor for the geopolitical upheavals that characterized the next thirty years as it "exposed" the promises of new ideologues and offered a "new vision" of the world.

The X-Rays in Story

Fascinated by the possibilities of invisibility, H. G. Wells was the first well-known writer to explore the effects of X-rays from the point of view of the X-rayed subject. His portrait of an amoral scientist in *The Invisible Man* (1897) has haunted the twentieth-century imagination, both through the original novel and a series of movies. Wells conflates the idea of an exposed inner image with the mysterious power of invisible rays. If X-rays can make solid flesh disappear on a photographic plate, Wells reasoned, why not another scientific leap that would make a body itself totally transparent? His hero discovers rays akin to "roentgen rays," which make his body invisible, but the invisible man is visually vulnerable after eating because his meals remain visible in his stomach and intestines until they are absorbed. Wells knew some science, having apprenticed as a pharmacist before entering the London School of Science in 1884, but he had no medical training. So although he was credible when elaborating on the physical properties that make invisibility possible, his imagination did not extend to making predictions about the possible medical advantages of transparency. His narrative ploy seems likely to have been drawn from accounts of the barium meal that patients were already swallowing in 1897 for fluoroscopic examinations.

Nonetheless, he devotes an entire chapter to providing the reader with a thinly disguised physics lesson, summing up what the late Victorian man in the street could be expected to know about science.

> Just think of all the things that are transparent and seem not to be so. Paper, for instance, is made up of transparent fibers, and it is white and opaque only for the same reason that a powder of glass is white and opaque. Oil white paper, fill up the interstices between the particles with oil so that there is no longer refraction or reflection except at the surfaces, and it becomes as transparent as glass. And not only paper, but cotton fibre, line fibre, woody fibre, and *bone . . . flesh . . . hair . . . nails and nerves* . . . in fact the whole fabric of a man except the red of his blood and black pigment of hair, are all made up of transparent, colorless tissue.[2]

He has it all figured out, or at least enough to be convincing.

Looking at the X-rays in a happier light was A. A. Merrill, in *The Great Awakening: The Story of the Twenty-Second Century* (1899), who envisioned X-ray-like rays as a kind of super-antiseptic discovered by a biologist while "experimenting with etheric waves and their effect on microbes." Not surprisingly for 1899, these waves were fatal to the tuberculosis germ, and after a long course of study and twenty years of experiments, the hero-scientist is able to cure the disease.[3] Obviously familiar with tales of X-ray-induced burns, Merrill's "patient is subjected to the rays from this instrument for short periods of time until all the germs are killed; but the rays, being detrimental to the cellular tissues, have to be handled with great care, and the patient often has to undergo another treatment to overcome those bad effects."[4]

The first popular fiction to exploit the imaging potential of rays akin to, but specifically *not,* X-rays, was Jack London's short story "A Thousand Deaths," also published in 1899. In it a pair of scientists, father and son, attempt to conquer death through scientific gadgetry. One of the methods included "a glass vacuum, similar to but not exactly like a Crookes' tube," that, when placed in a magnetic field, emitted invisible rays similar to the X-ray. The father scientist photographed the apparently dead son and found an infinite number of blurred shadows indicating ongoing chemical motion—like that which is now distinguishable with MRI—and this activity was "proof that the rigor mortis in which I lay was not genuine; that is, those mysterious forces, those delicate bonds which held my soul to my body, were still in action."[5]

A more positive approach to the future of imaging was advanced a year later in 1900 by Jack Adams in his novel *Nequa; or, The Problem of the Ages.* This odd, feminist tale follows a woman, dressed as a man, into a subterranean civilization beneath the North Pole where she discovers an X-ray instrument that "secure[s] a photograph through wood and metal" and improves on it by attaching the eyepiece to an optical instrument that "casts the reflection on the retina of the eye." This makes it easy for doctors to "look into the bodies of their patients and examine the internal organs."[6]

Responding to William Randolph Hearst's desire to X-ray the brain, the time-traveling hero in the Reverend W. S. Harris's *Life in a Thousand Worlds* (1905) encounters "thought photography." Fulfilling the ambitions of later psychologists, philosophers, neurologists, and computer scientists, Harris's scientists were able "to follow the course of a thought in a living cerebrum after the brain has been made visible by a light more potent than the X-ray."[7] These early futurists, of whom Wells alone reached a broad public, were, apparently, the only visible literary figures inspired by X-rays before World War I.

In the interwar years storytellers in the new field of pulp science fiction usually used X-rays positively. They were still described as antiseptic rays that revealed "naked truth." Fluoroscopes and X-rays are useful tools for distinguishing friend from foe. In Lawrence Manning's "The Man Who Awoke" (1933), time travelers prove their antiquity as Homo sapiens to a future generation of humans by fluoroscoping their appendixes, organs that had evolved out of existence over the thousands of intervening years since the time travelers' own era.[8] Three years later, John Campbell's "The Brain Stealers of Mars" turn out to be giant bacteria that have disguised themselves as humans. X-rays reveal their nonskeletal interiors, saving humanity from certain extinction.[9]

Erotic and Eugenic Rays

The X-rays "unmasked" aliens disguised as humans, but they also penetrated the flesh of human women, unveiling their age-old secrets, or so it seemed. Since much of the "unveiling" was done by men, it can be construed as a kind of visual deflowering. Nineteenth-century American physicians (unlike their colleagues in France) did not examine their female patients with the relatively newly invented vaginal speculum because it was held to be "unjustifiable on the grounds of propriety and morality" for a physician to look at a woman's genitalia. Female patients stood behind velvet curtains, extending only a hand for the doctor to examine, as can be seen in Winthrop Chandler's nineteenth-century portrait of Dr. William Clysson examining a woman.[10] Male physicians could, in fact, proceed further than touching a hand to examine female patients, even going so far as breaking the hymen with a finger, as long as they did not look. As an insightful historian of medicine has observed, "In the United States in the late nineteenth century the gaze was a far more potent cultural symbol of eroticism than the touch."[11]

Much of this protection of female modesty was provided by men who were protecting their "property rights." For women, the new ability to see through their bodies was a path to freedom. Those who needed evidence found that the X-ray images supported their demands to free themselves from the unhealthy constraints of corsets; ardent feminists saw the rays as dissolving the barriers of all obstructive clothing. The American dancers Isadora Duncan and Loïe Fuller were convinced that new technologies like X-rays would interact with the arts. Duncan swirled in robes reminiscent of ancient Greek translucent fabrics, and Fuller designed colored lights so that as she whirled on her own axis, countless yards of veil-like materials gave the impression that she appeared and disappeared as she spun, a body seen through a fluoroscope.[12]

Before World War I, when X-rays were not yet routine, they evoked the mysteries that surrounded translucent garments and strange sparks of light. They were part of the package of scientific mysticism. If X-rays revealed the inner secrets of the living body, and radioactivity revealed the secrets of the atom, perhaps other hidden realms—the soul and sexuality—could be opened up as well. The possibility tantalized some scientists and much of the lay public.

The very idea of radioactivity, with its proof of the fabled transmutation of elements, and suggestion of a fourth dimension, attracted people who had rejected traditional religion and were grasping for validation of their intuitive sense of a deeper reality. The mysterious glow of X-rays and radium evoked the spirit world (magicians and mediums had long exploited the phenomenon of phosphorescence) to produce ghostly effects. William Crookes, the chemist whose tube had been the starting point of Roentgen's research, believed his interest in psychic matters was integral to his investigations into the nature of matter. And in 1911 the physicist Ernest Rutherford speculated that matter, under the influence of radiation, might somehow evolve—much as animals did—so that lower elements became more complex ones.

If famous scientists could play with such ideas, they were fair game for science popularizers. The report that radium, when held close to the optic nerve of a blind girl, had given her sensations of light prompted a newspaper editor to wonder if radium might not only revive a dead nerve, but a body as well.[13] The self-promoting French writer Gustave Le Bon floated the possibility that radioactivity was the secret to vitality, to life! These ideas evaporated in the scientific discourse of the 1920s, but not before leaving a profound impression on the general public. Similarly, it was an easy step from speculation about the nature of time and the fourth dimension (stimulated by the innovative formulas of Riemannian mathematics) to the mysterious X-rays that seemed to create visual auras that might be a signal from a higher dimension, a parallel universe. The link between X-rays as an optical phenomenon and the world of the supernatural—between the transparent and the invisible—would remain throughout the century.

Even before the bloody trenches had divided forever the seemingly placid prewar world from the social turmoil that followed, artists and poets, the elite of the avant-garde, were inspired by the X-ray's dissolution of opacity. The X-ray heralded future art movements by exposing the interior of bodies, and, by extension, exposing subtexts and the subconscious.

World War I introduced X-rays into the lives of middle- and working class patients. But scientific medicine in the form of X-ray diagnosis notwithstanding, the years after World War I were still filled with the sense that the invisible rays were supernatural. The difference between the prewar and postwar expressions of mysticism is that, after 1920, devotees used a new, scientized vocabulary.

Their embrace of X-rays in the postwar era was in some ways more critical than the naive embrace of their predecessors. The original description of the fourth dimension had been stated in mathematical terms that were inaccessible to almost everyone. After 1919 the General Theory of Relativity became the icon of inscrutable science. The mathematics of relativity was beyond the ken of most people, but the *idea* entranced them. Articles connecting relativity and radiation filled popular science periodicals. Compared with relativity—which was said to be understood by only a handful of people in the entire world—X-rays and radiation were familiar and accessible.

With demobilized veterans everywhere, most people had either been X-rayed themselves or knew someone who had been. The transparency of the flesh had become commonplace. At a deeper level, too, ordinary people now had a different understanding of their own bodies, structurally and sexually. From almost the day of their discovery, X-rays had been connected facetiously, frivolously, sensuously, pruriently, and seriously with sexuality, everywhere from cartoons and doggerel in popular publications to the apocryphal effort by a New Jersey assemblyman to outlaw X-ray opera glasses.[14]

This was fertile territory for Sigmund Freud, who wrote frankly about sex dominating the unconscious mind, which he had recently mapped using new words such as the *id* and *ego.* Women figured largely in Freud's published case studies, and the mystery of women was one of the uncharted territories he sought to define. But as he generalized from the claustrophobic lives of a handful of bourgeois women trapped in what seems to have been particularly authoritarian homes, another kind of woman attracted attention in the postwar world.

Marie Curie and her daughter, Irène, personified the blend of scientific innovator with womanly virtues. Together the Curies whistle-stopped across the

United States in May of 1921, supported by the federation of American Women's Clubs whose members greeted them at every station. The Curies brought the newly discovered structure of the atom (now understood as itself divisible and uncertain) down to earth with the familial terminology of "daughter" and "parent" atoms.

The popularity of the Curies was one indication of the change of the role of women in the 1920s, part of what we now recognize as the effort of women in the twentieth century to free themselves from many constraints, including what some saw as the bondage of housewifery, corsets, and veils, but also the bondage of privacy. The veils and walls that had protected their limbs and faces from the eyes of strangers had defined women as the possessions of men. Any display of their own bodies—"flaunting" as it was commonly called—was an assertion that women could do as they would with something that was theirs to expose. In fashion, as women gathered a sense of personal power, skirts crept to heights unseen before in adults. At the same time women flattened their breasts, the telltale secondary sexual trait that belied their efforts to prove they were identical to men.

Women had no model for behavior in the light of new explanations of sexuality. The sexually regenerative power of X-rays is the core of Gertrude Atherton's 1923 novel, *Black Oxen,* whose characters equate sexuality with youth. In *Black Oxen* the mysterious Countess Zattiany, née Mary Ogden, returns to her native New York City after an absence of thirty-four years, so unchanged by the passage of time that her high society friends assume she is her own (illegitimate) daughter. She explains that X-ray treatments on her "lower ovaries" in Vienna in 1919 cured not only her psychological depression, but also her whole body of the degenerative signs of age.

The society women are initially shocked: "How horrible!" "Did you feel as if you were being electrocuted?" " Are you scarred?" They do not expect the Countess's account of "an interior drama, not to put too fine a point on it, a drama of one's insides, and especially one that dealt with the raising from the dead of that section which refined women ceased to discuss after they had got rid of it." Once the secret of her regeneration is revealed, the heroine is asked, very delicately, if sexual desire has also returned. When she affirms that this has happened, despite the reaction of the chorus of naysayers, the author is obviously delighted, as are, presumably, her readers.[15]

In 1924 Thomas Mann made X-rays an evocative image of mortality and sexual desire. His hero in *The Magic Mountain* enters the X-ray laboratory's anteroom where he sees a gallery of "various members: hands, feet, knee-pans, thigh and leg bones, arms and pelvises. But he notes that the round living form of these portions of the human body was vague and shadowy, like a pale and misty envelope, within which stood out the clear, sharp nucleus—the skeleton." The technician comments: "Useful object-lesson for the young. There is a female arm, you can tell by its delicacy. That's what they put around you when they make love, you know."[16]

To Mann's hero, the sight of X-rays of his beloved's bones within her living body was sexually stimulating. They served as a preview and an analogy to the sex act, one of life's few opportunities of being inside another person. Similarly, the hero of the 1994 novel *They Whisper,* by the Pulitzer Prize winner Robert Butler, recalls a visit to his uncle's shoe store, the last shoe store in Wabash, Illinois, to install a fluoroscope. He is standing beside a friend, a little girl who is examining her new Mary Janes inside the machine: "There have been few moments in my life as intimate as the sight of Karen Granger's actual bones, her actual articulated bones with their shape visible to me, the shape that had been secret even when she stood barefoot in the grass of her front yard. . . . She wriggled her toes in the green glow of the X-ray and she let me keep my arm around her."[17]

The confidence and authority of doctors and surgeons expanded as the X-ray allowed them to see the internal structures of the organs they treated. And for a while the medical status of internal organs grew in proportion to their depth in the body and to the tenacity with which they held their secrets.

As the 1920s advanced, neuroradiologists, who were beginning to see the interior of the living brain, competed with Freud and his psychoanalytical colleagues to make their own maps of the seats of "sexual repression" and "sexual desire."[18] Women's hemlines fell with the stock market in 1929, but simply covering their legs once again could not recover the veiled attitudes of the nineteenth century. Sexuality, revealed, would not again be easily hidden, and social scientists followed physicians in using the X-ray to penetrate its secrets.

They were late into the game. During the 1930s, over 100,000 people worldwide were X-rayed every day, prompting the British biologist J.B.S. Haldane to predict that someday there would be neighborhood radiologist's shops. The X-ray was a fine excuse for medical voyeurism; at about this time one male X-ray technician told his psychiatrist that he chose his profession out of a deep-seated longing to see inside his mother's body. Male doctors seemed to take a special interest in irradiating female organs, as evidenced by the fact that gynecological experiments led the way in both X-ray and radium therapy as male doctors experimented by "poking X-ray projectors and radioactive substances into every part of their patient's bodies . . . with a special interest in irradiating the vagina and the uterus."[19]

By the mid-1930s, some of this "unveiling" had reached into the area of investigating sexual proclivities. In the spring of 1935 a group of homosexuals and lesbians in New York City who had helped establish the Committee for the Study of Sex Variants, headed by George Henry, a psychiatrist associated with the Payne Whitney Clinic, volunteered to participate in a study of homosexual behavior. The participants wanted primarily to understand themselves, and secondarily to show they were not dangerous. Their objective was betrayed, however, as the final document explained that the study was promoted by fear among the city's leaders that the homosexual population of the city was expanding and by the hope that "this research would go toward preventing the spread of sex variance through the 'general population.'"

The initiator of the project, a lesbian who called herself "Jan Gay," rounded up eighty homosexual volunteers between twenty and forty years of age, an equal number of men and women. They took written tests composed by Lewis Terman of IQ-testing fame.[20] And they submitted to physical examinations, including X-rays designed to measure the cranial densities of their skulls, and, for the women, the "carrying angles" of their pelvises. The angles were supposed to reveal masculine or feminine bone structure, that is, a skeletal explanation for what the committee termed "variant" sexual behavior.[21]

Among the remarkable aspects of the project is the fact that so many women, in particular, agreed to having their sexual organs pried, measured, and sketched (the report contains remarkably detailed, quasi-pornographic illustrations). Whatever else it uncovered, the study reveals an enormous relaxation of the boundaries of privacy, a process that had been accelerated by X-ray penetration.

Unlike the many other New Yorkers who were voluntarily X-rayed to treat acne (and who often developed cases of skin cancer years later), the volunteers in the sexual deviancy study suffered from no organic disease for which X-rays might conceivably be useful. The study manifests a remarkable lack of worry about the reproductive health of the lesbian volunteers. For the sake of collecting "scientific" data their reproductive organs were exposed to X-rays, and it is hard to believe the directors of the study were ignorant of the sterilizing effects of radiation. It was well known in the medical literature. The researchers apparently either assumed that lesbians would not want to reproduce, or even, perhaps, that it would be better for all concerned if they did not.[22] That point of view—very much in line with contemporary eugenic beliefs—was echoed in the Michigan law passed in 1939 that legalized sterilization by X-ray for certain miscreants.

In Nazi Germany the demonstrable ability of X-rays to render people sterile, without ever touching them, was seen as a distinct advantage of the technology. In 1941 Viktor Brack, head of the German euthanasia program, introduced a plan to secretly irradiate Jewish men with 500 to 600 roentgens, and Jewish women with 300 to 350 roentgens, amounts that the physicians had discovered would destroy the reproductive capabilities of the testicles or ovaries. Brack suggested this be done by having individuals stand in front of a counter where, under the pretext that they were filling out forms, they would be sterilized. Although the pass-through rate, estimated at 4,000 people a day, seems to have been rejected as too slow, the efficacy of radiation for sterilization was no secret.[23]

Brack was familiar with the lethal powers of radiation. In 1938 the radiological community had dedicated a monument to martyrs of radiology—mostly physicians and technicians—in Hamburg. As a rule, however, most people felt safe from radiation-induced diseases. With thousands of deaths from other occupational hazards, those relatively few traceable to X radiation, or radium, were insignificant by comparison.[24] Well before the start of World War II, X-rays, now quantified and labeled "tolerable" at specific dosages, were part of the standard medical package. X-ray machines had been improved incrementally throughout the decade, radiation leakage had been minimized, and cheaper film and faster processing had made chest X-rays part of the health "check-up"—itself a new procedure that rapidly became routine within the middle class.[25]

The X-ray was associated with good health, with fitting shoes and being told you did not have tuberculosis. It was enough of a by-word by 1934 that millions of Americans smiled when Dizzy Dean, who had been pitching for St. Louis during the World Series and got bopped in the head in the course of stopping a double play, soothed Cardinal fans the next day by reporting, "They X-rayed my head and found nothing."[26]

Radiation was considered benign in 1939 when Street and Smith Publications endowed Superman, their comic book hero from another planet, with both extraordinary strength and X-ray vision.[27] Superman's X-ray vision, like real X-rays, was blocked by lead. Like ordinary X-rays, his eyes could see through walls and, one supposes, clothing. But this hero's X-ray vision was never associated with anything so prurient as peering beneath a woman's skirt.[28] Nor, for that matter, did he ever frighten the good citizens of Metropolis with the ionizing radiation to which his X-ray vision must have exposed those forces of evil against which he fought. At the outbreak of World War II, X-rays were still the magic rays of turn-of-the-century fiction: Luddites and Cassandras decried them, but their voices were few and the general public seemed still to see them as mysterious, selectively penetrating, and, on the whole, innocent.

The Avant-Garde Offers a New Slant on Things

Artists in the counterculture that arose in Europe in the first decades of the twentieth century found the X-ray a formidable tool for shattering the cultural restraints that the guardians of society were trying desperately to maintain on manners and morals. In their manifestoes and canvases, "truth" took on new meaning, and so did the term "superficial." Peering through and beyond became the watchwords of the twentieth-century rebels, activists obsessed with the visual and at the same time skeptical about what they saw.

The razzle-dazzle that greeted X-rays in tabloids and journals throughout 1896 was echoed in comic strips of the day, but not in the paintings of serious artists like Degas or Renoir. It took over a decade for painters within the French establishment (even those in revolt from it) to incorporate the lessons of X-rays into their work. The first to portray the transparency and simultaneity of seeing through the body were the cubists, especially Picasso and Braque. Cubism repudiated the classical rules of depicting reality with natural light and one-point perspective, replacing them with multi-perspectives as seen by the artists.[29] Although the cubists did not mention the X-ray specifically as an inspiration, they adopted monochrome palettes—a deliberate abandonment of color—and depicted objects broken into surfaces with light coming from a variety of angles. They showed a limb simultaneously from top and bottom, much as X-ray technologists like Elizabeth Fleischmann had done with stereoptical cameras. Her pictures of the patient from different angles achieved a multiplicity of planes and a volumetric view of the patient's interior. Picasso, likewise, used many different perspectives of his models in his *Les Demoiselles d'Avignon* (1907). Here a seated woman turns her back to the viewer, but at the same time she shows her face and we can see the interior planes of her body.

Excitement about new scientific discoveries spread rapidly all over Europe, but France was a special magnet for people on the so-called cutting edge. In Paris in the years before World War I an intimate cosmopolitan culture flourished. Politics, patriotism, and national origins mattered little in their shared fervor for new art forms. Picasso came from Spain, Francis Picabia from Cuba,

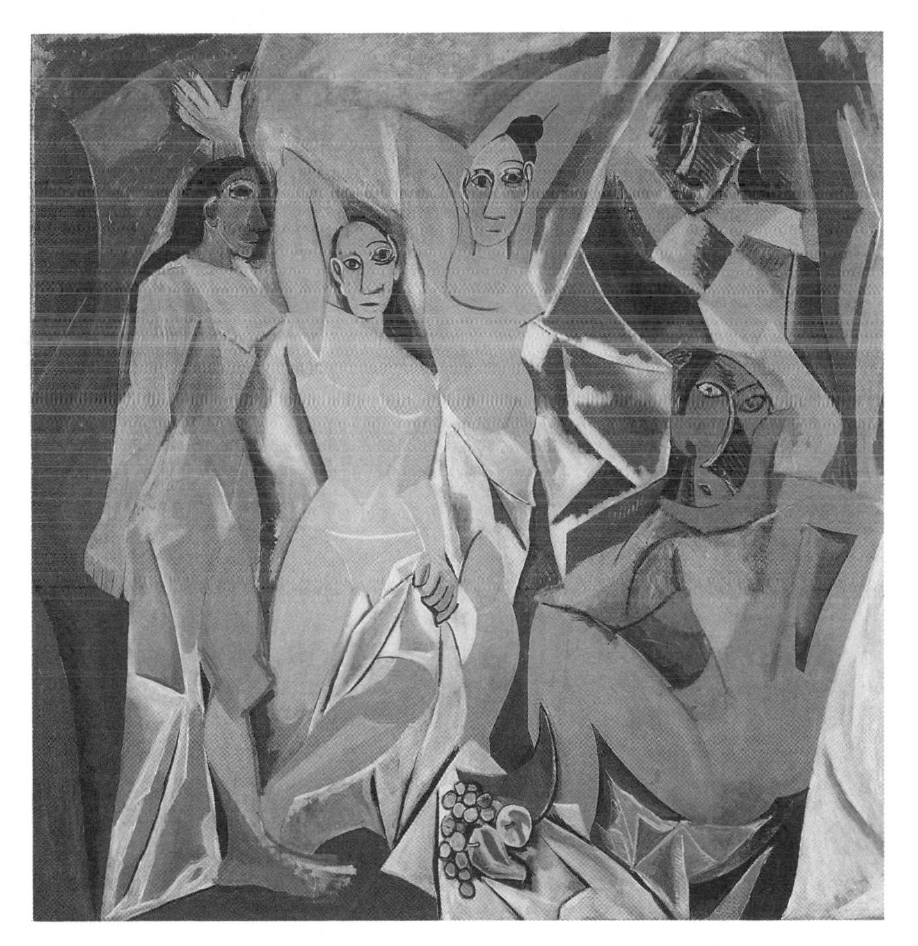

21. Pablo Picasso, *Les Demoiselles d'Avignon,* Paris (June/July 1907). Oil on canvas, 8' x 7'8" (243.9 cm x 233.7 cm). Copyright © 1997 Succession Picasso/Artists Rights Society (ARS), New York. Courtesy of the Museum of Modern Art, New York. Acquired through the Lillie P. Bliss bequest.

Frantizek Kupka from Prague. The Duchamp brothers, Marcel and Raymond Duchamp-Villon, and Gabrielle Buffet were French.[30] The artistic rebels who called themselves the "avant-garde" studied art and optics, painting and medicine, and moved easily from studio to laboratory and back again.

The cafés were abuzz in 1912 with news about X-ray crystallography, the passage of X-ray beams through crystals that left an impression of the arrangement of its atoms on film. With the atomic world visually available, at least in projected shadows, and the human body partially translucent, if not transparent, painters were understandably restless with what they saw as stale in the illustrative art around them. Yet where the impressive new technology of X-rays gave science and medicine new assurance, the ability to see through surfaces only undermined the artists' confidence. They had been taught to see one way, but they could no longer depend on their all-too-human eyes.

They read the work of the new physicists—much of it still written without intensive mathematics—and followed experiments as they were reported in medical journals as well as in the popular press. If the world beyond the fluoroscope revealed bones and ligaments, then what they saw with the naked eye was somehow false. This new sight devalued the visual world they had always assumed was the whole world. In short, many artists felt that they could no longer trust their eyes now that they knew that another level of reality underlay the superficial. If the X-ray had dissolved one layer of opacity, what remained? What structures awaited yet a newer way to breach a still deeper opacity? Cubists regarded the photograph and now the radiograph as receptors more sensitive than the human eye. If film could record studies of movements and sights hidden from ordinary vision, it seemed logical that film might also be able to capture hidden spirits and bodily emanations.

The avant-garde dived into this rich sea of new ideas. Art was their passion, but they could not ignore the implications of science. An earlier generation's study of the optics of color and perception had produced impressionism. But the heady discoveries in physics and chemistry made the impressionists' preoccupation with visible light (and the optical spectrum) seem suddenly narrow and antiquated. The avant-garde held fast to the impressionists' scientific approach but they rejected the science upon which impressionism was founded. They knew, along with everyone else, that matter could be penetrated, and revealed, by X-ray light. In the romantic view, artists possessed unusually keen sensibilities needed to reveal the real world. Now it was up to the new generation of artists to adapt the X-rays to reveal a different reality. To this end Marcel Duchamp studied non-Euclidian geometry, science, and technology while one of his brothers, Raymond Duchamp-Villons, a doctor, bubbled with excitement about X-rays and radium and what they meant to a new vision of the body and the whole natural world.

It was into this atmosphere that Frantizek Kupka arrived from Prague in 1905 to study optics and perception at the Sorbonne. As a painter, he tried to reflect the impression of transparency as captured on X-rays in his paintings. In *The Dream* (1906–1909) he makes his purpose explicit in his description of the artist's mind: "an ultrasensitive film, capable of seeing even the unknown worlds of which the rhythms would seem incomprehensible to us."[31]

Raymond Duchamp-Villon's connection with the medical world had an impact on his own art and on the work of his formidable brother, Marcel. Duchamp's 1910 painting of his brothers playing chess is, perhaps, the most emblematic of all X-ray influenced work because in it Duchamp shows the interiors of the men's heads, where we see ideographs of the chess pieces they are concentrating on. The next year Duchamp took up the challenge of revealing in paint the images captured by the physiologist-photographer Etienne-Jules Marey, whose sequential images broke down movements such as walking as taken by fast film, or as seen fluidly on a fluoroscope. Duchamp suggests different layers of space, contrasting internal versus external space in *Yvonne and Madeleine Torn in Tatters* (1911). The explicit influence of X-rays is evident in his rendition of Madeleine's nose. Because noses are made of cartilage, not bone, an X-ray of the skull leaves a triangular gap for the nose on the glass plate, and so he left a dark shadow in his portrait.[32] The most literal depiction of the everyday fear that X-rays stripped the body bare (a frequent theme in ribald rhymes and cartoons) was captured in *Dulcinea*: Duchamp overlaps images in a series reminiscent of Marey's chronophotographs, except that his subject loses her clothing as she progresses, ending up with only a hat. In his better known *Nude Descending a Staircase* (1912), the subject also loses, as she would before an X ray, all of her flesh. The idea that art could make an intellectual contribution to society lay at the heart of Duchamp's ambitions. Hoping to catch up with advances in science and perception, he declared that he wanted to "put painting once again at the service of the mind."[33]

From the first months of X-ray photography, the possibility of seeing into the workings of the mind preoccupied a few people to the point of obsession. Francis Picabia, self-appointed evangelist of the avant-garde, decided to accompany Duchamp's masterpieces, as well as Picasso's, Braque's, and a few of his own works to New York in 1913. With his wife, the painter Gabrielle Buffet, he sailed in style aboard the steamship *Lorraine* in January 1913. They would represent Paris at the opening of the Armory Show, America's first chance to look at what we have come to know as the great art of the early twentieth century.

Out of this whirlwind experience Picabia produced two X-ray-inspired works. One is a sketch titled *Mechanical Expression as seen through our own Mechanical Expression,* a very personal portrait of another passenger on the *Lorraine,* a ballet dancer by the name of Udnie Napierkowska.[34] She rehearsed daily aboard ship and developed a close friendship with the Picabias. During the weeks after their arrival, the Picabias were embraced by America's innovative artists, and Napierkowska danced for all of them until her performances were declared lewd and she was deported. As immortalized by Picabia, her actions are anything but. His drawing shows a spinning X-ray tube (not

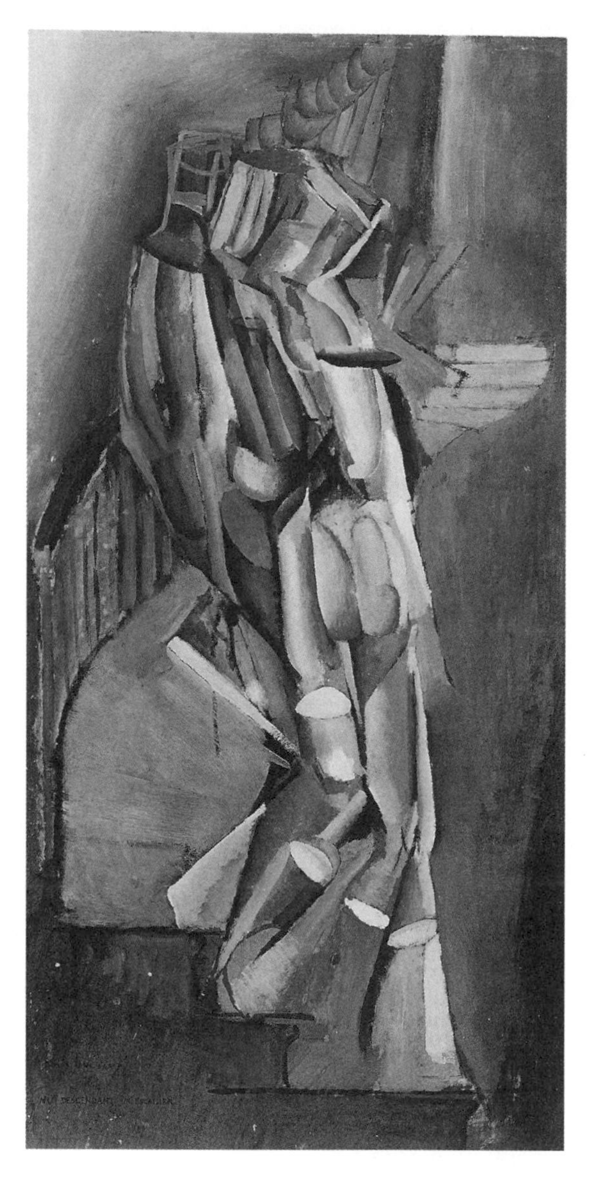

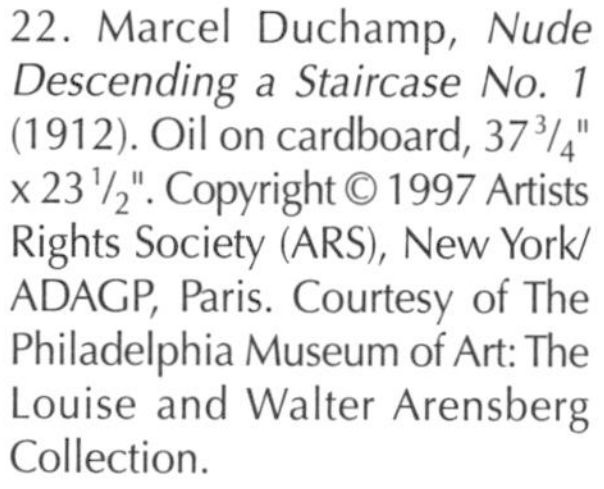

22. Marcel Duchamp, *Nude Descending a Staircase No. 1* (1912). Oil on cardboard, 37 3/4" x 23 1/2". Copyright © 1997 Artists Rights Society (ARS), New York/ ADAGP, Paris. Courtesy of The Philadelphia Museum of Art: The Louise and Walter Arensberg Collection.

simply a cathode-ray tube, but specifically an X-ray tube, as evidenced by the small funnel on the side which was a product of tube improvements in the first decade of the century). It sparks, as the old gas tubes often did, but the spark serves as a sexual metaphor for the comely Udnie. The tube is also an analogy for the grace of the dancer as she spins naked, open to the scrutiny of an X-ray's penetrating light.

Picabia's second picture, a watercolor, is very different. He signed *New York through an X-Ray* on all four sides to show that it can be seen from any angle. It is abstract except for the borders which have skyscrapers, the emblem of New

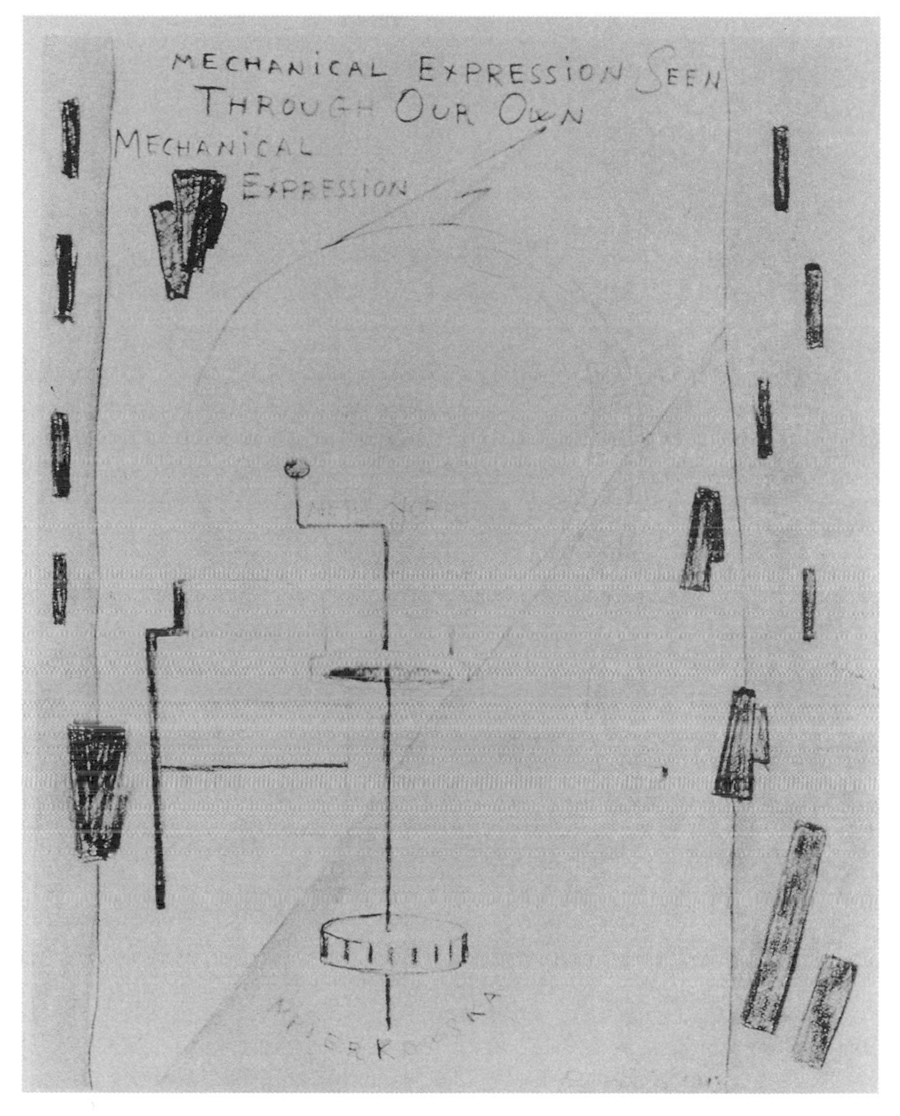

23. Francis Picabia, *Mechanical Expression as seen through our own Mechanical Expression* (1913). Watercolor and pencil on paper. Copyright © 1997 Artists Rights Society (ARS), New York/ADAGP/SPADEM, Paris. Courtesy of Pascal Sernet Fine Art.

York. New York delighted him, and on another visit two years later he remarked that "upon coming to America it flashed on me that the genius of the modern world is in machinery and that through machinery art ought to find a most vivid expression . . . . I mean simply to work on and on until I attain the pinnacle of mechanical symbolism."[35]

The Armory Show was hailed by sophisticated critics as a wake-up call. Christian Brinton, writing in the April 1913 issue of *The International Studio,* used his review to suggest that American painters seek inspiration in their own experience, as the better Europeans have, and to avoid pedantry. He advised:

> There is no phase of activity or facet of nature which should be forbidden the creative artist. The X-ray may as legitimately claim his attention as the rainbow, and if he so desire he is equally entitled to renounce the still and devote his energies to the kinetoscopic. . . . There is scant reason why those [discoveries] of von Roentgen or Edison along other lines should be ignored by Expressionist and Futurist. . . . The point is that they will add nothing thereto, unless they keep alive that primal wonder and curiosity concerning the universe, both visible and invisible . . . which has proved the mainstay of art throughout successive centuries.[36]

Outside of France and the United States, artists explained their break with the pictorial past in words that echo the impact of their new ability to see through objects that were only recently opaque. In Italy a group announced themselves as *futurists* in 1910 and described their artistic goal as the capture of the ephemeral in two dimensions. They spelled out their intention of incorporating X-ray imagery in the *Technical Manifesto of Futurist Painting,* explaining, "Our bodies penetrate the sofas upon which we sit, and the sofas penetrate our bodies." Their spokesman, Umberto Boccioni, asked, "Who can still believe in the opacity of bodies . . . when our sharpened and multiplied sensibility allows us to perceive the obscure disclosures of mediumistic phenomena? Why should we continue to create without taking into account our perceptive powers which can give results analogous to those of X-rays?"[37]

In Munich another group issued a manifesto, calling themselves *Rayonnists.* Their pictures featured the penetration of objects by now-visible rays that were a spin-off of the ubiquitous X-rays. Raising the ray to emblematic status, they illustrated the whole electromagnetic spectrum, visible and invisible energy, as if all energy were rays of light emanating from an organic source.

X-rays influenced a group of Russian painters, especially Mikhail Larionov and Malevich. Larionov's paintings were characterized by the contemporary poet Mayakovsky as "a Cubist interpretation of Impressionism."[38] His 1912 *Woman Walking on the Boulevard* captures motion by showing multiple legs in the walking woman, as seen through her transparent clothing. Malevich picked up on the possibility of "seeing through," writing in 1915 that "objects have vanished like smoke."[39] What he meant was twofold: that objects as the subjects of painting had become irrelevant, and that the new optics, including X-rays, dissolved whatever had been tangible about things, reducing them to the familiar smokiness of the space inside a radiograph. The Russian avant-garde was fascinated by the idea of seeing through as a precursor to seeing beyond. Speaking for them as a group, Pavel Florensky wrote in 1921 that the aim of art was to "overcome sensual visuality."[40] This translated into an art that was enthusiastic about representing transparency, sometimes in paint and sometimes through transparent media like the newly invented plastics.

After the war, artists from the old avant-garde continued, with renewed enthusiasm, to rebel against the now discredited aesthetics of the prewar establishment. They still used the X-ray as a guide to the figure beyond nudity by removing the skin to show the skeleton beneath.[41] Many of these artists had had intimate experiences with X-rays either as soldiers who had been wounded and treated at field hospitals, or as medics. The future surrealists André Breton and Louis Aragon, and the filmmaker and artist Jean Cocteau, had all joined ambulance units, which on both sides in the First World War were well supplied with portable X-ray machines.

The war changed the way artists interpreted X-rays. They were now familiar with them as a battlefront medical accessory, and they saw them in their medical role as messengers of life and death. The grim experience of battle with its legacy of dead tree trunks and blackened fields erased the delight in the glory of color that had so moved prewar painters. The truth of war, like the radiograph, appeared monochrome.

One of the artists to emerge energized from the fray was Naum Gabo. He had left St. Petersburg in 1910 under the name Naum Pevsner to study medicine in Munich. While there he took at least one course with Roentgen, gave up medicine for art, and changed his surname. The constructions and drawings he made on his return to Russia at the outbreak of war incorporated the vision of Roentgen's rays. His sculptures rely on translucent and transparent materials, and they draw on the sophisticated X-ray crystallographic research done by one of Roentgen's protégés at the State X-ray and Radiological Institute in the newly renamed city of Petrograd. In 1920 Gabo managed to publish his *Realist Manifesto.* Recalling perhaps Roentgen's lectures, and engaged by the upheaval of war, Gabo declared his own rules of art. Just as X-rays are shaded from black to white, so are the layers of tissue they reveal. That gray scale is reality. The *real,* Gabo announced, is what is beneath, not what is superficially apparent. "We do not turn away from nature, but, on the contrary, we penetrate her more profoundly than naturalistic art ever was able to do." He went on to reject what the X-ray does not reveal. "We renounce colour as a pictorial element, colour is the idealistic optical surface of objects; an exterior and superficial impression of them and has nothing in common with the innermost essence of a thing. . . . We affirm *depth* as the only pictorial and plastic form in space."[42] Gabo would continue to explore the lessons of X-rays and experiment with the problems of translucence over the next five decades.

In practice this led him to a rediscovery of glass as an artistic medium and to a delight in plastics that were just being developed. Now, as an artist, he was able to create with transparencies, emulating in abstract forms and in figurative sculpture what he had seen with X-rays. This is an aesthetic of looking through, not looking at.

With his brother Anton Pevsner, Gabo designed the sets for Diaghilev's 1927 production of *La Chatte,* a ballet in which a young man falls in love with a cat and beseeches Venus to transform it into a woman. To illustrate this Aesopian fable about the instability and unreality of outward appearances, the brothers designed a circular, revolving stage studded with constructions of mica and celluloid. Like a series of stereoscopic lenses, the assemblages reminded the audience that they were constantly looking through to spaces beyond their changing perspective.

The Soviet Union would enjoy another decade of unbridled artistic creativity in the 1920s, including the work of Pavel Mansurov, an abstract artist who briefly headed the Experimental Section of the State Institute of Artistic Culture in Petrograd. He was especially interested in connecting art and nature and saw the X-ray as a tool linking the creative process with the exact sciences. He had access to laboratories and studios and was able to "investigate the various forms of organic structures including man," and "analyze the expediency of decorations affecting vision, touch, smell, hearing, taste, and sex." And he accepted the X-ray as "an important weapon in the campaign to link the creative process with the exact sciences, especially with engineering, physics and mathematics."[43] The X-ray was *the* tool of transparency, an aesthetic of looking beneath surfaces that was discouraged by the Soviets. In 1927, before going into exile, Gabo explained: "The only thing I maintain is that the artists cannot go on forever painting the view from their window and pretending that this is all there is in the world, because it is not. There are many specters in the world, unseen, unfelt and unexperienced which have to be conveyed and we have the right to do this."[44] The X-ray, as the specific instrument for literally seeing through the body, became a metaphor for theories such as Freud's hidden motivations that guide external behavior, as well as assertions that supposedly solid objects were made of atomic and subatomic particles.

Gabo's earlier 1920 manifesto was one of a string of artistic declarations announcing a new aesthetic. He was succeeded by the surrealists and preceded by dada. Each group felt obliged to explain their artistic credos to each other as well as to the general public. Gabo's usurpation of transparency as a realist goal was also adapted as part of the aesthetic of German artists at the Bauhaus School in 1925. There, at the Weimar Republic's most enduring legacy of innovative art, the architect Mies Van Der Rohe interpreted this new aesthetic of transparency—displaying the underlying units of structure—into a building in which the skeleton was covered only by a "skin" of glass, as transparent as a body is when seen through an X-ray.[45]

For all the familiarity of X-rays to the well-educated artists of the avant-garde, the radiographs themselves were still costly objects that were usually kept by the doctors or hospitals that had made them. They were not easy for nonphysicians to acquire. When Marcel Duchamp moved from painting to making collages of artifacts and simple "found" pieces before the war, he did not incorporate radiographs. Neither did the artists who embraced dada (an artistic reaction that had evolved during World War I as a nihilistic response to the violence of war in which all art styles that had preceded the war, especially those that enshrined "beauty," were rejected) and deliberately made art from junk. X-ray plates were still too fragile to be regarded as flotsam and jetsam. Instead, the radiographs inspired artists to imitate and recreate the effects of X-rays, and science, to reveal heretofore hidden kinds of space.

X-rays were an obvious metaphoric device for the surrealists, whose name itself conjures up views through a fluoroscope—sur-real, above the real, or "super" real. Inspired by Freud, the surrealists looked to the unconscious to find a different kind of reality, one with layers of psychological possibilities, as exemplified in Salvador Dali's 1928 dream seascape where the viewer sees transparent images through the body of *The Spectral Cow.*

At about the same time Picasso, who had never joined any postwar artistic movement, began almost routinely to include those internal organs once hidden inside the body in his figurative renditions. His *Girl Before a Mirror* (1932) presented the model with her uterus and ovaries exposed to view—as

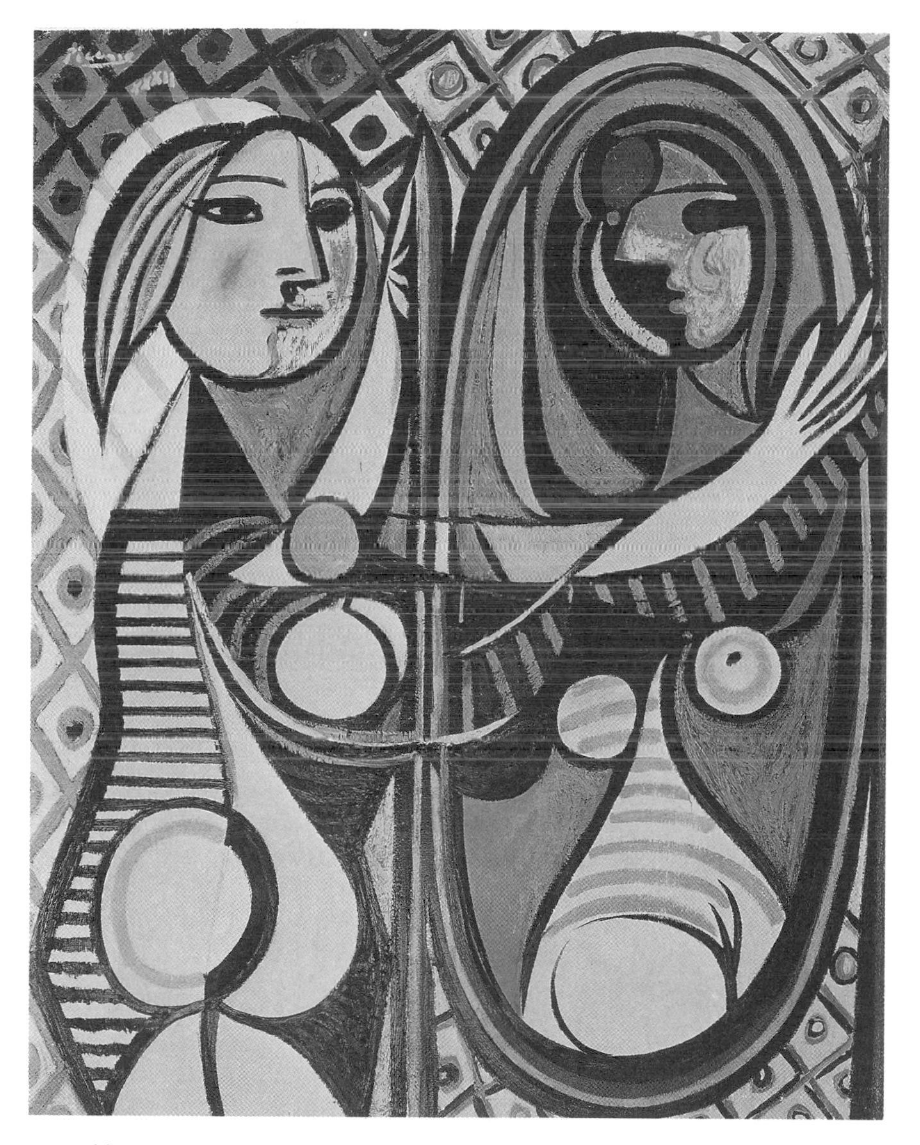

24. Pablo Picasso, *Girl Before a Mirror* (Boisgeloup, March 1932). Oil on canvas, 64" x 51 1/4" (162.3 cm x 130.2 cm). Copyright © 1997 Succession Picasso/Artists Rights Society (ARS), New York. Courtesy of The Museum of Modern Art, New York, Gift of Mrs. Simon Guggenheim. Photo copyright © 1996 The Museum of Modern Art.

in a tomograph—along with her external sexual traits, her breasts and rounded buttocks. Picasso's artistic vocabulary had expanded to routinely include internal body parts that had been made familiarly visible through X-rays.

The technology affected male and female artists differently. The rays simultaneously de-eroticized the body—breast bones without breasts are essentially asexual—while they accentuated the differences in the pelvic girdle and exposed uterus and ovaries. One artist who used the message of transparency was Frida Kahlo, a formidable Mexican painter born in 1907 who had studied anatomy as a premedical student before changing professions. She used X-ray-like images to portray the transparent body, singling out the reproductive organs, in a series of surrealistic, autobiographical canvases.

Kahlo was familiar with the inside of the living body from her studies, and more intimately by looking into her own body as a patient. When she was nineteen the car she was in collided with a tram: her pelvis and part of her spine were shattered, leaving her in constant pain, and transforming her body into a source of artistic inspiration. While she never incorporated radiographs, as such, into her work, she painted the insides of her body frequently, isolating internal organs but keeping them connected to her and to each other. In *The Broken Column* (1944), she depicts her spine as a fractured ionic pillar inside her flayed torso which is held together by a surgical brace. She deliberately overturned the conventions of anatomical surface and layers: an exoskeletal corset holds together the exposed substructure—an X-ray in reverse.[46] Kahlo's use of self-portraiture to describe the experience of her damaged body differs from the work of her husband, the muralist Diego Rivera who used an X-ray-like image of a woman in *Mechanized Maternity* (1933). Rivera displayed the model's open abdomen as if she were a machine, an analogy in the spirit of Picabia, emphasizing the depersonalizing effects of machines in capitalist society. Kahlo's exposed female interior was neither Luddite nor Marxist but emotional and personal.

Artists of the late nineteenth century had had no trouble domesticating photographic technology, but in the twentieth century all servants—human and technological—presented problems to those dependent upon them. The not always malleable technology of X-rays was one of those unreliable servants. Granted that X-rays penetrated the surface of objects to deeper truths, those truths were often painful, like the diagnosis of disease. Not surprisingly, there were occasional rages against the machine which in this instance was the messenger.

On another level the X-ray was disparaged in parts of the medical community because it was a machine in an era that saw a rapid proliferation of machinery at the expense of the healing touch of the human hand. It seemed like another effort to reduce the human body to just a machine that could be penetrated visually by yet another machine.

Other artists, however, saw the X-ray as a counterweight to homogenizing mechanization. The X-ray penetrated the human interior and found what

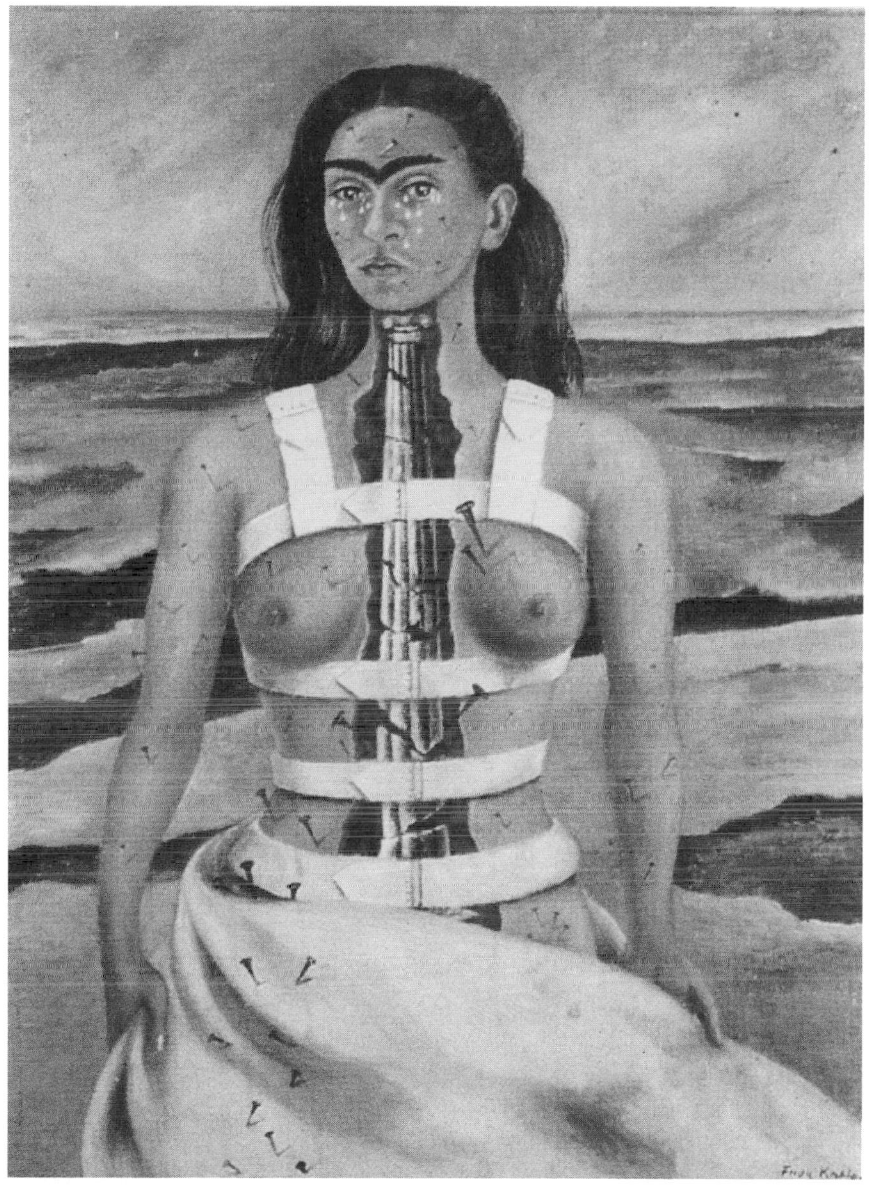

25. Frida Kahlo, *The Broken Column* (1944). Oil on masonite, $15\,^3/_4$" x $12\,^1/_4$". Courtesy of the Instituto Nacional de Bellas Artes y Literatura.

was unique inside each body. Artists diverged in their attitudes towards machines, including X-rays. They might reject them altogether in a back-to-basics return to hand-work, or satirize them as Picabia did in his sketch of a dancer-as-X-ray-tube, or embrace them completely, like Gabo, who saw the fruits of technology as tools for expressing truth. These last, at first a minority, were committed to the idea that looking deeper meant finding more.

See-Through Photography

X-rays closed one door in the art of photography and opened another. The rays tore up the unwritten contract between nineteenth-century painters and photographers that had allowed artists from Delacroix to Eakins to use the camera as a tool to help capture "reality." In those years the photograph represented a frozen instant in black and white which the painter controlled by first positioning, then framing, and then finally elaborating on in color. The photograph lent verisimilitude to those artists who saw their mission as capturing an image of reality. For them, a photograph acted as an armature for a painting.

Although a camera's lens is different from the human eye, the late nineteenth-century public accepted the photographic image not so much as different but as improved. Whereas the eye only glimpses a scene once, selecting whatever is especially interesting, a photograph captures everything and can be examined at leisure so that details passed over at first can be discovered at leisure. Photographs assumed the role of objective witness in popular culture. Emile Zola, a serious amateur photographer as well as journalist-novelist, declared: "We cannot claim to have really seen anything before having photographed it."[47]

The impact of seeing a captured instant of human misery inspired the reforms that followed the publication of Jacob Riis's photographs of the squalor of America's poor. Moreover, photographs do indeed pick up more than can be seen by the naked eye because the photographic plate is sensitive to wavelengths of light differently from the human retina. The photograph seemed to verify external reality until its power was suddenly undercut by its supposed companion technology, the X-ray. By revealing the skeleton beneath the skin, the X-ray destroyed not only faith in the judgment of the naked eye, but also faith in the total veracity of the photograph as a recorder of truth. The X-ray helped undermine not only the validity of the optical world but the idea that the artist's mission is to reflect that world.

Artists had to define a new mission. The armature of bone and muscle that the X-ray exposed was hard to ignore. Painters in these tumultuous years had to decide how to accept the new vision. Many found it a useful approach to the metaphorical world of the new psychoanalysis, others used it as satire, and still others found it a step on the road to abstraction.

There is no doubt that the X-ray inspired many painters to look through, around, and beyond the flesh. In the years before 1914, artists had reflected the impact of X-rays onto their perceptions of the world in pen and ink, paint and collage. By the 1920s, medical X-rays had become so familiar that artists and public alike expected to see X-ray impressions anywhere, and they accepted as normal those works of art that resembled X-ray images, and X-ray images that claimed to be works of art.

Imaginative photographers, however, saw opportunities in X-ray technologies to explore the photographic effects of other parts of the spectrum on a variety of surfaces, including film and chemically treated paper. Experimental photography now took on the look of X-rays as photographers tried to recreate using ordinary sunlight the translucent black-and-white appearance of X-rays. One approach was to expose paper coated with a photographic emulsion directly to a source of light. Among those who experimented with X-ray-like effects were a pair of Americans in Paris, Man Ray with his assistant Lee Miller.[48] Their "rayograms," as they called these images, like X-rays, are hazy and have the aesthetic of transparency. In his work as a fashion photographer Man Ray experimented with black and white portraits of people as well as objects, all apparently bathed in a halo of light.

Ordinary photographs had accustomed people to seeing the world in black, white, and shadows. X-rays increased the tendency to reject color as merely decorative or, even worse, as a misleading play of light. In the interwar years the German dadaists (who had rejected the "art" of the past as artifice and thus phoney) coined the term *photomontage* to describe the style of fitting photographs together to produce an artificial but realistic image. The term was supposed to signify that those who practiced it were engineers, not artists, for in German *montage* means assemble.[49] Chief among this group were Hannah Hoch and John Heartfield. Writing about her work, Hoch traces the roots of photomontage to postcards, war photography, and radiography.[50] Politically conscious, Hoch and Heartfield used the technique to express their political outrage and developed it into an art form that exposed hypocrisy by showing the evil within *as if* in X-ray images. Heartfield fine-tuned the superimposition of body parts on machine-made objects. A successful commercial photographer, Heartfield was a pacifist during World War I, changing his name from Herzfeld to symbolize his brotherhood with the British enemy. As a Communist in the 1930s, he was a fierce anti-Nazi. He used X-ray vision as metaphor in his pictures of Hitler—one showing Hitler's rib cage filled with coins where his heart should have been, and another showing a skeletal hand hovering over a busy populace.

Like the collage artists, photographers did not yet use X-ray prints, probably because they were hard to get because radiologists kept their patient's records. Although some professional photographers had access to X-ray equipment, they did not use it, perhaps out of an awareness of the dangers of exposure to radiation. Inevitably, however, some of the physicians who worked with X-rays used them to explore the beauty of organic structure. In the mid-1930s, Dain Tasker, a physician in Los Angeles, teamed up with the photographer Will Connell to make X-ray images of flowers. He echoes the artistic ideals of the realists: "When we eliminate color and fall back on outline and molded density as the basic beauty factors . . . we begin to realize nature's infinite variety of structural perfections." Tasker was proud that he didn't "pose" his flowers or "chemicalize" them in any manner. He treated them as he routinely treated human patients; he "experimented with weak iodine solutions in an effort to bring out the detail of the circulatory system of the stem and petals."[51] In this instance the physician and artist exploited an identical technology.

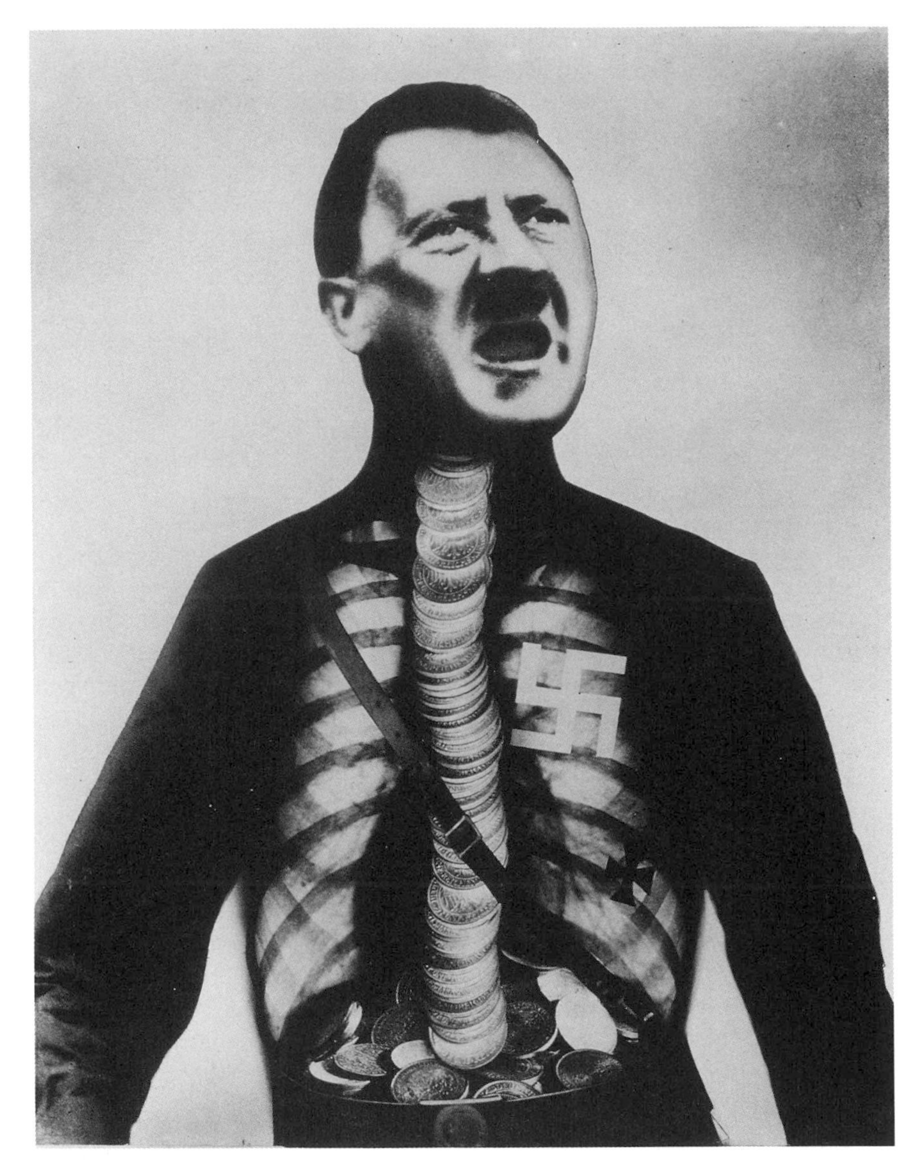

26. John Heartfield, *Hitler Swallows Gold and Spouts Junk.* Copyright © 1997 Artists Rights Society (ARS), New York/VG Bild-Kunst, Bonn.

Motion Pictures

In 1896 John MacIntyre at the Glasgow Royal Infirmary had the world's first totally electric medical laboratory. During that year of X-ray mania, MacIntyre experimented with two ways of making X-ray motion pictures, usually known as "cinemaradiology." He tried filming the fluoroscopic screen, and he tried passing film between the screen and the X-ray tube—the direct and indirect

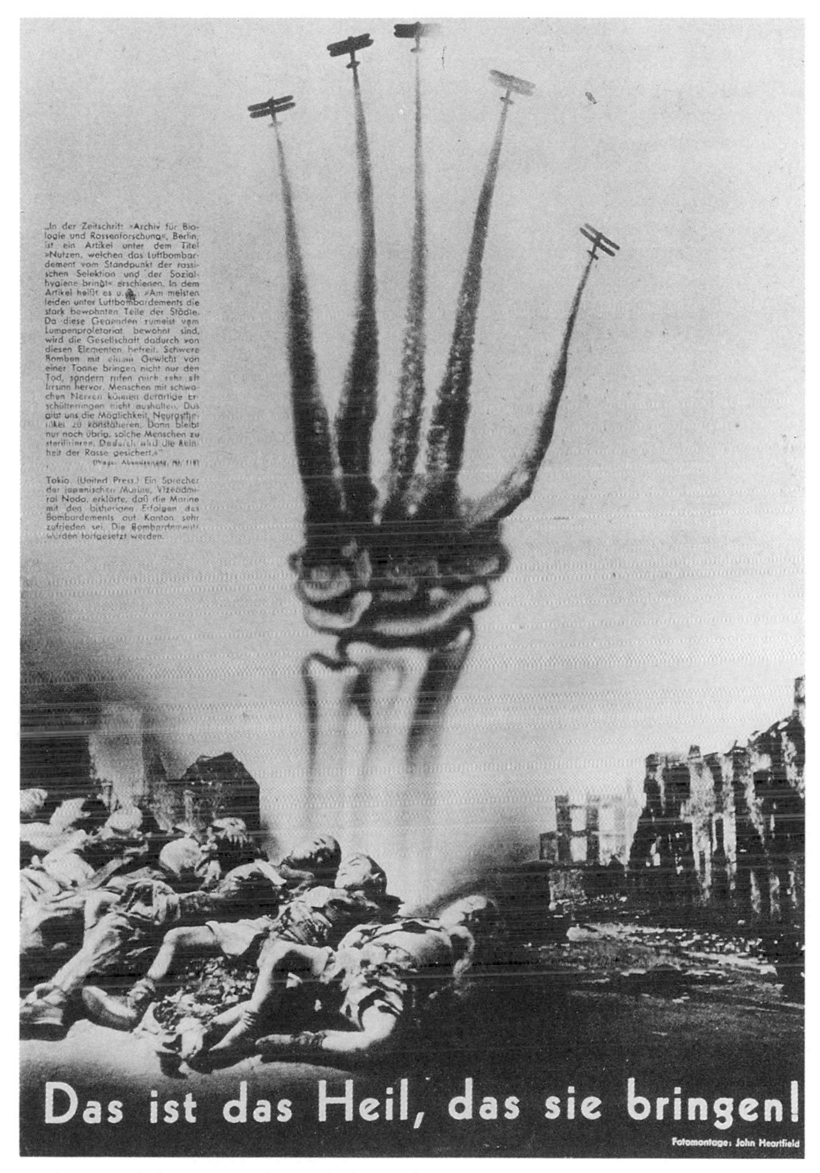

27. John Heartfield, *Das ist das Heil, das sie bringen!* Copyright © 1997 Artists Rights Society (ARS), New York/VG Bild-Kunst, Bonn.

method of making X-ray movies. But despite his efforts and the efforts of others during the next half century, no one would get very good moving pictures until after 1950.

Cinematography, the technology that the Lumière brothers had first presented to a Paris audience on December 28, 1895 (the same day Roentgen published his first communication about X-rays), seemed a natural venue for X-rays. There was the fluoroscope through which observers could watch a heart beating or track a piece of bread through the throat to the digestive tract. It seemed easy enough to transfer the technology to X-ray cinema. The trouble was, as radiologists knew too well, there was no way to capture a crisp moving image because the fluoroscopic image was dim. Movies, even at their most crude, have to move between ten and twenty images per second to give an illusion of movement, but an exposure time limited to a tenth or twentieth of a second was not long enough for early X-ray machines to get a decent picture.

Efforts to make X-ray movies waned until after World War I when a combination of entertainment cinema and a revived interest among physicians in studying the functioning of internal organs spurred new efforts to perfect cinemaradiology. When, in 1920, Kodak cooperated with American researchers, they found that they were unable to get a sharp image unless they exposed both patients and investigators to what they had begun to acknowledge was excessive radiation.

Then, in 1933, the German immigrant physician Hans Jarre reported that indirect methods, the filming of the fluoroscope, seemed promising because of the development of X-ray film that was six times as sensitive as ordinary film. Summing up the state of the art, Jarre pointed out that the direct approach—photographing from inside the fluoroscope—is complicated because X-rays are not refractable by ordinary lenses, and demanded considerable machinery; in addition, they took a long time, subjecting the patient to excessive exposure. With the indirect approach, however, a good motion picture could be made *if* the screens could be improved (intensified) and the film were faster. Jarre was right, but those improvements depended on technologies that would not become available for another twenty years.

Although medical X-ray cinema was at a standstill between the wars, movies featuring X-ray techniques were a feature of the new art of commercial cinema. Experimental two- and three-minute movies made by Man Ray in 1926 show images of feet atop and then through sidewalks, and fish photographed through water. The accidental occurrence of double exposures proved an excellent device for producing the impression of seeing through a fluoroscope. Man Ray took advantage of double exposure to give the impression of X-ray vision, and although there were no X-rays involved in the filming, their aesthetic influence is clear.

In 1930, X-ray images joined high culture in Jean Cocteau's full-length surrealist fantasy, *The Blood of the Poet.* In the opening scene a painter stands beside an easel, a cannon booming in the background. As he ducks behind his canvas, the canvas becomes a fluoroscope so we see the painter's bones in shadow, recalling the X-ray units on the front during the World War. As the story of a man imprisoned in a looking-glass world continues, a hollow head, like a hologram, spins slowly. Meanwhile, the hero moves to rid himself of a mouth that has transferred to his hand in a liquid-filled basin that looks just like a photographer's developing bath. The plot winds through complex, dreamlike scenes that come to a climax when a black angel becomes translucent, as if an X-ray image, and the indoors and outdoors become conflated just as the body's outside and inside were becoming equally familiar through the medium of X-rays.

As the decade advanced, Hollywood adapted Cocteau's illusory techniques. The first sound adaptation of the H. G. Wells novel *The Invisible Man* in 1933 portrays the dying protagonist as an empty plastercast in a hospital bed. His bones begin to show—as in an X-ray photograph—with muscles filling in on top of them. His *cloak* of invisibility disappears as his life seeps away. What is especially interesting in this interpretation of the saga of the invisible man is that the film audience has accepted transparency as the sign of life, and is not surprised that all they could see of the hero was his intestines absorbing food. Ironically, for the invisible man, his skin is only visible as he dies. The opaque curtain of skin becomes a shroud.

By 1940 X-ray machines were almost as ubiquitous as electric streetlights. X-rays were a routine procedure at the dentist, the draft board, and hospital emergency rooms. Their ordinariness may well have dampened the imaginations of serious artists and even diminished their interest in representing the body altogether (accelerating the movement towards nonobjective art). Other artists may have found inspiration in the blurred edges of the new tomographs for another kind of abstraction. However they were approached, radiographs, once understood as a clear gaze into the living body, were now redefined by radiology professors and medicolegal experts as too complicated for ordinary people to look at and understand.

But no matter who interpreted them, the presence of X-rays in everyday life raised few alarms. The dangers of ionizing radiation seemed to have been confined to occupational hazards, and those were being brought under control through safety precautions. The public appreciated that X-rays enabled doctors to diagnose disease or, in association with laboratories like Caltech's, to treat cancers. Only after 1945—fifty years after the publication of the image of Frau Roentgen's skeletal hand—did an X-ray image take center stage again, but this time it was the X-rayed silhouettes of the dead blasted into slabs of concrete in the ruins of Hiroshima.[52] Radiation filled newspaper headlines again, only now in the context of fallout (a new term) from nuclear weapons. In the same newspapers, however, the old optimism held firm in press releases from the Atomic Energy Commission about new nuclear-related medical promises.

Part II

Beyond the X-Ray

In 1937 the National Academy of Sciences ventured a prediction of the scientific breakthroughs that the future would bring. Although it was right about synthetic rubber, it missed the development of nuclear energy, computers, and the commercialization of television. These last two—television and computers—have together transformed the texture of almost every aspect of contemporary life, but nowhere so dramatically as in medical imaging

Television, which had been invented in the 1930s, entered America's living rooms in the 1950s. By reducing images to an array of tiny squares called *pixels* (for picture elements) which it showed on book-sized screens, television domesticated and personalized cinema. Television got people used to watching moving images that they could control.

In contrast to television, the computer—which evolved about a decade later but came onto the market at about the same time—symbolized the *impersonal.* The first computers were gigantic, room-sized monsters that seemed to reduce individual identities to mere holes in stacks of IBM cards. But the computer's ability to store and analyze huge quantities of complex information grew as the machines themselves shrunk, and by the 1980s the personal computer had begun making its way into offices and homes.

From their beginnings as mathematical problem solvers, computers evolved the capacity to reconstruct images from enormous amounts of mathematical data. After the Apollo missions sent back computer-reconstructed pictures of the moon, it did not stretch the imagination to propose that computers could reconstruct images of the interior of the human body which, like the pictures from space, could be manipulated in terms of color and displayed on a personal video monitor. Soon physicians and patients could explore the body's interior with CT (computerized tomography), MRI (magnetic resonance images), PET (positron emission tomographs), and ultrasound. The video monitor gives the impression that the images produced by these different machines are pretty much the same, but, in fact, they are very different from each other.

The first computerized image to enter the market, CT, used X-ray beams to accumulate information that it reconstructed into images of cross-sections, or slices, of the inside of the body. In contrast to the discovery of X-rays, which had startled a generation of scientists, engineers, and physicians into a flurry of experiments, computerized images had been anticipated by imagers for at least a decade. They did, however, startle and delight the ordinary citizen.

Potential patients were eager to have a glimpse inside heretofore hidden areas of their bodies, and gladly exchanged the benefits of diagnosis for the risk of exposure to ionizing radiation. The consumer trusted imaging science, so that when MRI entered the market, there was little anxiety about possible hazards from exposure to magnetic fields or, in the case of ultrasound, little worry about the dangers of being bombarded with sound waves. The advantages of seeing into the body overwhelmed the low probability of negative side effects.

As the technological juggernaut changed everyday life, the sight of computerized cross-sections of hearts, brains, and kidneys grew as familiar as pictures of the moon. But there was nothing inevitable about either lunar or anatomical images. In contrast to the X-ray with its single discoverer, each new technology owed its origin to more than one inventor. They, in turn, either cooperated or competed with each other—depending on the technology—and according to individual temperaments and the size of the anticipated prize. Looking over their shoulders from time to time, medical imagers recalled the perils of X-rays and, wary of possible side effects, took what precautions they could. As in the past, lawyers and artists quickly learned how to exploit these new ways of seeing into the body. And more swiftly than the first time around, they used the insights of these new medical imagers to question and reinterpret what it means to be human.

Seven

The Perfect Slice

The Story of CT Scanning

Ronald Reagan had been president of the United States for just over two months when he left the White House at 1:45 P.M. on March 30, 1981, to talk to the AFL-CIO's Building and Construction Workers Union. He was only going up the road to the Washington Hilton, but he went in full presidential style: a three-car motorcade including the White House physician and the press secretary, James S. Brady.

At 2:20 the president finished speaking to the generally unresponsive audience and stepped outside with his bodyguard. He was still wearing his trademark grin when the television cameras caught a change of expression. Seconds later he disappeared from view as he was pushed into a waiting limousine, which sped off.

Left behind, James Brady collapsed, his head bloodied. He had caught the first of six exploding "devastator" bullets that twenty-six-year-old John W. Hinckley, Jr., had just fired. The second bullet went astray; a third and fourth hit a D.C. police officer in the back, a fifth struck the chest and liver of a Secret Service agent, and the last ricocheted off the limousine and caught the president under his left armpit.

Unlike his predecessors, Garfield and McKinley, Reagan survived the assassin's attack, and the public was confident that his doctors could see exactly where the bullet was. There was plenty of X-ray apparatus in the emergency room at the George Washington Medical Center where the president had been rushed. Once they had located the bullet near the heart, the surgeon, Benjamin Aaron, operated and retrieved the dime-shaped fragment, which he displayed to the press. In the days that followed, no one marveled at the daily X-rays. They were as integral to his care as the antibiotics that saved him from the infections that had killed his predecessors.

James Brady's shattered brain was a different matter. Traditional X-rays were not much better at probing the brain in 1981 than they were in 1896, but the CT scanner in the emergency room was, and its use in 1981 signaled the acceptance of a new kind of image—a new way of seeing—into popular consciousness. This new instrument used X-ray beams to capture cross-sectional images beneath the skull and a computer to construct an image from the data. Like the tomographs of the 1930s, CT obtained images of slices inside the body, but unlike the old tomographs, the CT slice was not blurred by the intermediary bones. CT produces crisp, detailed pictures of bones and cartilage, and, most importantly, incredibly precise images of the brain itself.

When Brady arrived at the trauma unit minutes after Reagan, and lay bleeding on a gurney only a curtain away from his boss, Arthur Kobrine, the neurosurgeon on duty, saw immediately that the bullet had wreaked enormous damage as it blasted through. Wasting no time, he ordered a CT scan.[1]

In 1981 there were more than thirteen hundred CT scanners in the United States. The National Institutes of Health would soon pronounce them "safe, powerful and cost-effective."[2] CT was then called "CAT," the "A" standing for either "assisted" or "axial," depending on who was doing the explaining. It was shortened to CT by the end of the 1980s in medical circles, though it is still called CAT by much of the public. At the time of the shootings, scanners had been on the market for nine years and emergency room physicians had come to depend on the black and white cross-sectional slices of the interior of the body. David Davis, chief of neuroradiology, showed Kobrine the CT image of Brady's brain, with a huge blood clot. Recalling the scan as "fantastically useful," Davis says it showed exactly where Kobrine had to operate in order to pop the clot immediately. Without the CT scan they would not have seen the clot in time and Brady would have died.[3]

The entire operation—clearing away pieces of bone and tissue and parts of the shattered bullet—took almost seven hours. Kobrine could not predict the extent of the damage or the success of his repairs and was relieved on April 1 to see Brady tossing cotton balls with his wife and hear him pronounce her name and count from one to ten. Though Brady was never able to resume work, his humor and personality survived the assault. He was able to appreciate the role of the new CT scanner as well as his wife's campaign for gun control in a bill bearing his name.

In the nine years that CT machines had been available, they had become clinical fixtures, and "scan" had joined international medical terminology. The verb, which had once meant a superficial once-over, became a way of describing the meticulous gathering of data from computer-controlled sensors and its display on a screen.

From the crude instrument first demonstrated in London in 1971, CT scanners had evolved through four generations into a streamlined, swift, efficient machine. This was in large part the result of American medicine's response with open checkbooks—the machines started out at about half a million dollars apiece, including installation. Not every hospital could afford one, but every major research hospital could as well as large trauma centers. The CT scan enabled almost every kind of doctor, from brain specialist to pediatrician, to look deep within the patient without inflicting pain. It helped make "exploratory surgery" an increasingly rare event. Not only could CT spot tumors, but the scans enabled surgeons to save lives through rapid diagnoses of organ trauma, fractures, internal bleeding, masses, and swelling.

In 1981 Americans were used to watching computerized reconstructed images from NASA's planetary probes and did not question the provenance of the images on their doctor's computer screen. Most people knew that CT scans were produced by X-rays, but few understood that the X rays in CT scanners do not make any initial picture, much less an image on film. Instead, CT scanners send collimated beams of X-rays through the body to an array of detectors that send signals to a computer for processing. The computer's program turns the signals into pixels on the video monitor. The image can then be "enhanced," colored, or made larger or smaller by the computer. The system works in two ways: it can reveal an anatomical slice by mathematically reconstructing the data the computer has received, and it can take a weak image and clean it up—the equivalent of retouching a photograph.

This new machine, like the ancestral, noncomputerized versions manufactured in the 1930s, was conceived at almost the same time by a handful of people in different areas of science and in different parts of the world. Each had the impression that he was alone in stating the problem and suggesting the solution. That problem had arisen more than once in the history of science—how to make a two- or three-dimensional image of an *interior* slice of an object by reconstructing data from a large number of projections *through* the object. The theoretical problem suggested many approaches, but the amount of mathematical processing needed to solve it was daunting, even with the computers that were just becoming available. Computers in the early 1970s had limited data storage capacity which restricted the scope of problems they could solve and the resolution of the images they could project from the CT scan. Engineers had to take into consideration these limits. As computers became faster and added memory, the range of what the new scanners could do also expanded. What followed were a series of multiple, almost coincidental, discoveries—each of which could have led to the construction of a CT machine—had only other apparently necessary factors been in place.

The problem took concrete form in 1955 when Ronald Bracewell, an Australian astronomer and polymath who had just immigrated to Stanford University, needed to map sunspots—areas of intense microwave emission—with radiotelescopes. Because he could not focus the giant radio antenna dishes on localized points on the sun's "surface," he approached imaging as an engineering challenge. He was able to reconstruct the solar image by getting his data in narrow strips, like a bandage. Then using a series of these one-dimensional strips, he was able to reconstruct a two-dimensional map. In a paper published in 1956, Bracewell described how he had used a mathematical device called Fourier transforms to do this.[4]

A decade later in 1967, while using radio waves to construct a similar sort of map of the moon's brightness, Bracewell showed that he could reconstruct these lunar images without having to use Fourier transforms. Fourier transforms, he points out, are interesting mathematically but computationally wasteful, and this was especially true in the 1960s when computer memory was limited. Not only were they "wasteful," Bracewell adds, but Fourier transforms, which ought theoretically to have been ideal for reconstructing images, in practice produced "contaminated" pictures filled with "artifacts," things that aren't there, distortions that usually result from mathematical errors.[5] Bracewell's new mathematical solution appealed to scientists outside of astronomy, but not immediately. The mathematics, which would eventually be used in medical scanners, appeared only in an Australian physics journal, a publication light-years away from the libraries of physicians.[6]

While Bracewell looked at astronomical bodies, researchers in Cambridge, England, were looking at the extraordinarily small world of viruses through an electron microscope, and finding a similar problem. They needed to reconstruct a three-dimensional image of a virus from two-dimensional data of an electron micrograph, and they, too, succeeded by using a formula similar to Bracewell's.[7]

Those working on reconstructing images of the human body had a handier subject than the astronomers and virologists, but one that is far more complicated. The living human body presents two problems: it contains tissues with a large range of densities and it is susceptible to injury from excess radiation. The solution to both was arrived at in the late 1950s: a technique known as "back projections." Extremely narrow beams of X-rays which carry minute quantities of radiation are shot through the body. The energy of both the entering X-ray or gamma ray and of the same beam as it exits can be measured, and then, by subtracting the second number from the first, the computer finds the amount of energy absorbed by the tissue in a particular plane. An image is built up by sending thousands of beams from slightly separate angles through the body to intersect in that particular plane. Then the data from the transmitted beams is gathered and fed into a computer.

Unfortunately for William Oldendorf, another pioneer in modern CT technology, computers were not very powerful or available when he completed his residency in neurology at the University of Minnesota Hospitals in 1955. Oldendorf, who had grown up in Schenectady, New York, in the shadow of General Electric's research laboratory, was a precocious student, who had already built a telescope when he was twelve, three years before he graduated from high school. At Union College, he studied astronomy and worked as an announcer on the local radio station—developing the resonant voice which would contribute to his fame as a lecturer. Under contracts from GE's research laboratory, he ground two twelve-and-a-half-inch paraboloid mirrors for testing air flow on its new jet engine. After medical school, Oldendorf was board-certified in psychiatry and then in neurology, where he learned to perform angiography and pneumoencephalography, the latter still much as it had been done by Dandy in the 1920s—injecting air through the lumbar region into the brain. Struck by the inadequacy of brain imaging for the patient (it was extremely painful) and the doctor (it only revealed a limited area of the brain), he began looking for a better approach. He was still pondering the problem when he moved to Los Angeles and a joint appointment at UCLA's medical school and the Veterans Administration hospital.[8]

Convinced that there was a better way to get an image of the brain, he removed a donated brain from its skull and took ordinary X-rays. Even without the bone barrier, he demonstrated, radiographs show very little of what is going on inside. Inspiration came to him in 1958 from discussions with an engineer (Oldendorf himself was a member of IEEE, the Institute of Electrical and Electronics Engineers) who had been asked by a major orange growers cooperative to devise an apparatus that could sort out frostbitten oranges from good ones. The engineer described the problem: bad oranges looked good from the outside, but dehydrated orange segments hid beneath healthy skins. The dehydrated segments reminded Oldendorf of a human skull shielding its own bad segment, such as a tumor.

The orange-inspired engineer had toyed with using some kind of X-ray, but it was expensive and the machine was never built. Oldendorf, however, liked the idea. He reasoned that he could measure the radiodensity of an interior point within a complex object—one that is not homogeneous—by sending a beam of X-rays or gamma rays through the object and by having the emergent beams strike a detector on the opposite side. If the beam source and the detector were both rotated about the same axis within a plane, the X-ray beam would pass through the object from many angles, pinpointing a singular spot. By also moving the object along the path of a line, eventually he would be able to measure the density along a single line through the complex object and reconstruct density relationships and their positions.

The thought was father to the deed, and Oldendorf went to the electronics hobby room in his Los Angeles home where, with forty-one identical iron nails, one aluminum nail, and a plastic block (with holes for the nails) seated on an HO-gauge train flatcar and track (borrowed from his sons), he built himself a model in 1959–1960. This model machine scanned all points in the plane using rotational—isolating a point—and translational—moving the point along a line—motions. (Translate/rotate would become the catchwords of early CT scanning.) Mounted on a 16 rpm phonograph turntable, the machine moved the point of intersection of the axis and the beam through the model at 80 mm/hr. Oldendorf used a gamma-ray source within a lead shield, rather than X-rays, in this experiment, because it was easier to control. It sent a collimated beam of high-energy particles through a plane in the phantom (or model) head. The

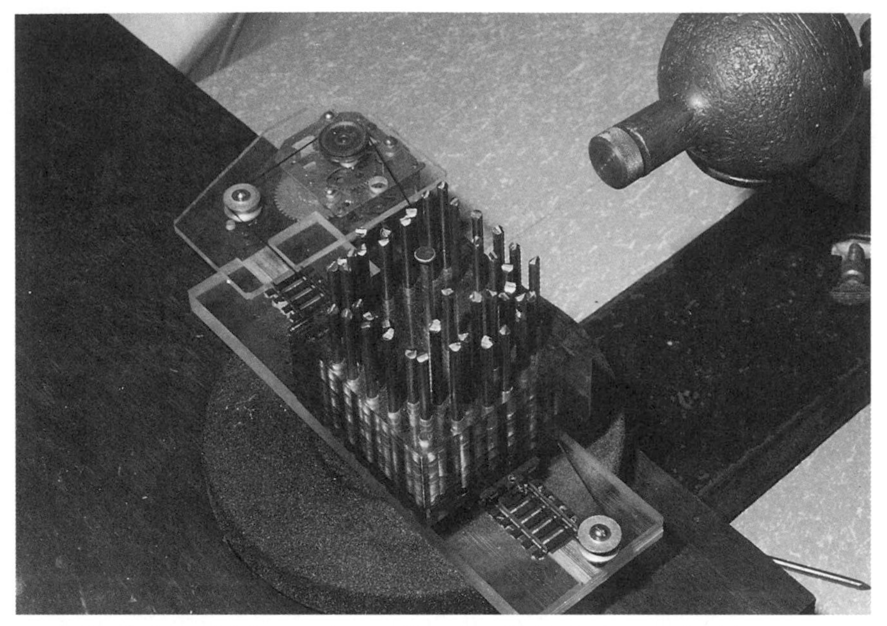

28. Oldendorf's model CT scanning machine (June 1960). A photograph of the arrangement known as Oldendorf's experiment. The gamma-ray source is to the upper right of the picture and the nail phantom is shown on its truck on the railway track. The clock mechanism is to the lower part of the picture. The whole arrangement is mounted on a rotating turntable. Courtesy of Stella Z. Oldendorf.

aim was to locate both the one iron and the one aluminum nail inserted in the center of the block when the other forty iron nails were ringed around them during and without rotation and with linear displacement. The particles emerged, struck a photon detector, were counted, and a recognizable dual pattern was displayed as a two-dimensional image. Oldendorf processed the signal using an electronic filter to separate the information he needed about the point he was aiming at from unwanted information about the density of the surrounding structure.

He explained how his machine, and all CT scans, work: "An observer standing stationary in a forest might have a difficult time viewing a distant person because that person might be blocked by trees in between. But if the observer begins to move through the forest, while at the same time looking in the direction of the distant person, then the trees in the foreground would seem to move past, while the distant individual would seem to stay still." Using this analogy, Oldendorf explained: "The distant person represents the nails in the center of his model, and the trees the line of nails obscuring it. The observer's line of sight is like the gamma ray beam that is continuously pointed through the surrounding ring of nails at the interior nail. As the gamma source circles, the nails in front and behind the central nail momentarily absorb gamma rays, deleting them from the beam, creating the equivalent of the blurring motion of trees in the forest. The interior nail itself, located at the center of motion of the gamma ray source, absorbs gamma rays continuously."[9]

Despite its apparent simplicity, Oldendorf's model incorporated the fundamental concepts of all later computerized tomographic scanners—except for the modern digital computer. At one point Oldendorf conferred with a physicist colleague at the University of Chicago who recalls that, in those precomputer days, he reckoned Oldendorf would need 28,000 simultaneous equations, and told him to forget it.[10]

Oldendorf did not have the computational tools to interpret the quantity of data he would need. But he had demonstrated that to measure the radiodensity—the ability to absorb radiation—of a point, he had to uncouple the effects of all the other points on the same plane. He had worked out back projections to reconstruct a two-dimensional display of images and the beginnings of the machine. Encouraged by the success of his jerry-built model, Oldendorf felt it was simply a matter of "scaling up the dimensions and sensitivity of this crude apparatus before [he] could similarly scan the head."[11]

With this in mind, and aware that with living patients his method might work with X-rays instead of gamma rays, Oldendorf applied for a patent in 1960 and published the results of his experiment in 1961 in *Bio-Medical Electronics*. When he received the patent in 1963, he approached X-ray manufacturers everywhere, and was roundly dismissed. One major corporation responded: "Even if it could be made to work as you suggest, we cannot imagine a significant market for such an expensive apparatus which would do nothing but make radiographic cross-sections of the head."[12]

A dynamic physician of extraordinary energy, Oldendorf gave his CT patent a metaphorical shrug, and turned his attention to exploring, and finding, bridges across the blood-brain barrier.

Allan Cormack, who is a nuclear physicist and the third pioneer in the exploration of CT, was initially well equipped mathematically but not medically for the problem that was to become an obsession for him from 1956 on through the next ten years. Still living in his native South Africa, his obsession began with a call from Cape Town's Groote Schuur Hospital (the site of the first heart transplant operation). The hospital was legally mandated, he learned, to have a physicist on hand to monitor radiation therapy. Its physicist had suddenly quit, and he was asked to fill in. Cormack, then a lecturer at the University of Cape Town, suspects he was the only person in Cape Town, and probably in all of South Africa at the time, who knew how to handle radioactive isotopes. So he took the day-and-a-half per week job for three months.

With a desk in the radiology department, he recalls, he could not help but notice the haphazard way radiotherapy treatments were designed. "I was horrified by what I saw, even though it was as good as anything in the world, because all planning was based on the absorption of radiation by homogenous matter approximating human tissue, and no account was taken of the differences in absorption between, say, bone, muscle, and lung tissue. It struck me that what was needed was a set of maps of absorption coefficients for many sections of the body."[13]

He was thinking about therapy, worried by the obvious unnecessary overexposure to radiation because it was applied in such a scattershot fashion. The situation led him to ponder the whole notion of body maps, although, he admits, he had no idea then how very interesting this line of thought would turn out to be.

Cormack embarked on a search for a way to map the body using X-rays. He was not consciously thinking in terms of images and had not yet even heard the word *tomograph.* The images, which were the logical by-product of his quest, did not interest him at this point nearly as much as solving the mathematical problem of measuring the X-ray absorption along lines through heterogeneous tissues of the body. It was what he called his "line-integral" problem. This was a problem, he was sure, that must have been solved by some nineteenth-century mathematician, but who or where he could not guess.

This line-integral problem continued to haunt Cormack. In the next year, 1957, he tried an experiment using a gamma-ray source on a circular phantom to test the theory he was developing. What happened next was a technician's error that he was quick to profit from. He had asked the university machinists to make a symmetrical phantom out of a uniform disk of aluminum surrounded by a wooden ring. He got an image, but found an anomaly in the data near the center. He questioned the machinists and discovered that the phantom was not uniform; the machinists had put a peg of slightly different density at the center of the disk. This "error" on the machinist's part revealed that Cormack was on the right track. His scanner had actually detected the small density difference. This unexpected bit of detection kept him working on the line-integral problem and formed the kernel of the paper he published in 1963.

At this point Cormack's attention shifted to his private life, his marriage to an American physicist and their move to Boston. There, as a nuclear physicist, he joined an experimental program at the Harvard cyclotron and soon joined the physics department at Tufts University. He relegated the line-integral problem to a kind of mental attic space where he continued to mull over it. He had come to think of it proprietorially as *his* problem—although he continued to sense that someone must have solved it already, and he wrote inquiries to mathematicians on three continents. Years later he learned that he had tried the wrong mathematicians. "His" problem had, indeed, been solved, and more than once, not by a Victorian Englishman as he had suspected, but by a Dutch physicist in 1905 and later by the Austrian mathematician, Johann Radon, in 1917.

In Boston he continued to work on the line-integral problem and in 1963 he was ready to experiment with another phantom, one that he designed deliberately with irregular symmetry. This time he had the help of a Tufts undergraduate, David Hennage, who was studying the new computer language FORTRAN and wanted to learn how to apply it. He helped Cormack build an experimental scanner that used a computer to reconstruct images of asymmetrical phantoms.

Cormack published the results of the experiment in 1963. Meanwhile, as a nuclear physicist, Cormack shared access to the Harvard cyclotron with doctors from Massachusetts General Hospital. They were busy using the radioisotopes produced by the cyclotron in nuclear medicine, especially with exploring the difference between the way normal and malignant tissue absorbed these isotopes. Cormack believed his solution could be adapted to help them find theirs, and so he approached them with the suggestion that his mathematics had applications for emission scanning, obtaining an image of the body's interior from an internal radioactive source. The doctors dismissed his suggestion, perhaps because he was an outsider, or perhaps because they could see no connection between sending X-rays through a body, and measuring radiation emitted from a body. Whichever, they ignored his approach only to take it up in nuclear scans a decade later.

Like Oldendorf in California, Cormack tried to drum up outside support. Unlike Oldendorf, he did not approach manufacturers but instead spoke to colleagues at NASA.[14] The single inquiry he received from his publication was from the University of Neuchâtel where a representative of the Swiss Avalanche Research Center wondered if Cormack's approach could predict the depth of snow.[15] At this point Cormack became the chairman of the physics department at Tufts, and had less time to ponder the line-integral problem which was moving on its own momentum toward a new field of physics, and a new kind of radiographic image.

Meanwhile, at the University of Pennsylvania, David Kuhl, a radiologist whose precocious interest in radioactive materials had begun while he was still a high school student in 1946, had by 1965 completed his compulsory military service in the navy. Tangential to his interest in nuclear medicine, he was doing a project for the navy at the Willow Grove Naval Air Station outside of Philadelphia. The navy had its own astronaut program then, and at this station had an assembly the size of half a freight car with a gondola inside. They used it to test volunteers who they strapped into the gondola, which they then spun like a giant centrifuge. They wanted to simulate the effect of large gravitational forces on the blood in the astronaut's lungs. According to Kuhl, "We made a system where the volunteers could self-inject themselves with a technetium compound [a mildly radioactive material which is not dangerous], a substance which had just come out at that time." Then they were rushed by ambulance to the university to see where the radioactivity was in their lungs, to get a snapshot of what had happened when they were under stress. "We developed the cross-sectional image to see where the radioactivity was."[16] Slowly, incrementally, the ingredients for a CT scanner were falling into place. Later that year Kuhl made an image of a subject's thorax without any internal source of radiation. Instead he coupled a radioactive source to a detector, not unlike Oldendorf's design.

This image was published with a paper describing the process in *Radiology,* a medical journal, in August 1966. It is the first cross-sectional image ever made by sending radioactive beams through a living subject to detectors on the other side.

Kuhl's machine was very sophisticated. It had a built-in computer, a processor, and a small interactive CRT monitor display. The Pennsylvania team made no effort to patent their approach, or to take it further. The Picker Corporation, which expressed some interest in it, thought of transmission imaging as an adjunct to planning radiation therapy, not as an imaging technology that could be refined into a better picture.

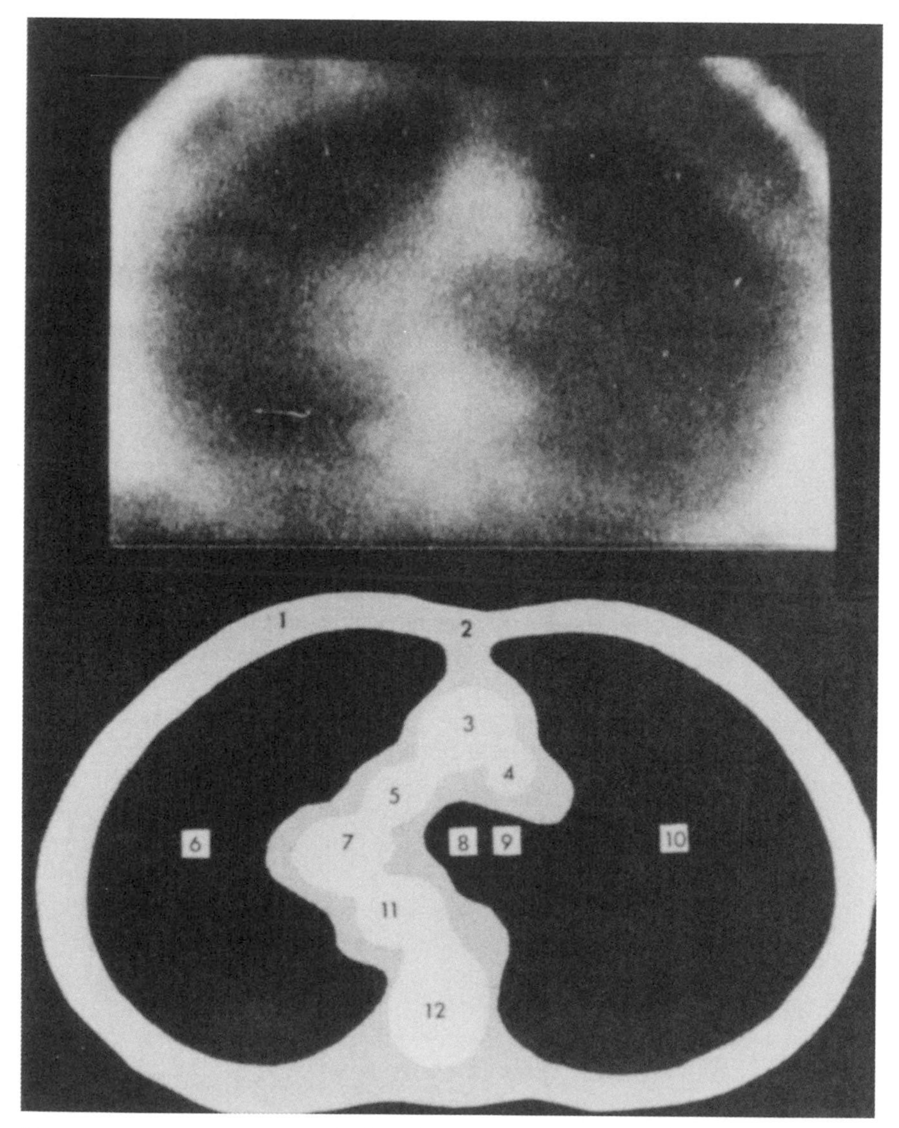

29. First transmission section scan of a living human thorax by David Kuhl (1965). ("Transmission Scanning," *Radiology* 87 [1966]: 278–284.) Courtesy of the Radiological Society of North America.

Kuhl had the technical capacity to expand his cross-sectional imaging machine into a computerized scanner, but he had his eye on another goal. He did not pursue *transmission* imaging because his real interest was *emission* imaging, reconstructing a picture of an internal organ, like the lungs, from an internal source of radiation. In retrospect, he realizes that he had all the ingredients in hand, including the mathematics, very like those that appeared a few years later in the first commercial CT machine.[17] All he would have had to do was replace his gamma-ray beam with the more penetrating X-rays, and he would have had a CT scanner. This is a perfect example of the Burke rule: "A way of seeing is also a way of not seeing—a focus upon Object A involves a neglect of Object B."[18]

EMI: The CT Scan on the Market

The commercial atmosphere changed abruptly in the early 1970s. The medical world crackled with excitement when London-based EMI, Electrical and Musical Industries Limited, patented and demonstrated a computerized tomographic scanner.

The precise details of the development of the commercially viable EMI scanner are hard to track because they occurred in the laboratory of a private corporation which sought patent protection immediately and for whose operations secrecy was key. There is no doubt that the man behind the patents was Godfrey Newbold Hounsfield. From his own account, his insight into a practical application of back projection came from his experience developing a computer for EMI, and a long-standing interest in pattern recognition. He may or may not at some point have been familiar with the efforts of Oldendorf and Kuhl as he moved toward a working machine. There is evidence that representatives from EMI were familiar with some of the work of each of them. Cormack and Kuhl recall either being contacted directly by EMI representatives, or having people they corresponded with contacted by them. Kuhl regrets that Hounsfield referenced none of his papers, since a year earlier, he had received a letter saying, "We at EMI have been following very closely your work and there is obviously some similarity."[19]

EMI was part of a business culture whose mores were orthogonal to those of academic science. The industry wanted to surprise the market with a finished product that would reap immediate profits, whereas in academia where priority is crucial, researchers usually make their discoveries public incrementally as they occur. Academic science takes a longer view, and while profit is not ignored, prestige and credit are also prizes, along with a sense of satisfaction in having made a contribution to a growing body of knowledge. Within the academy, attribution is paramount, along with the sense of sharing information and cross-pollinating ideas.[20] While universally admiring Hounsfield and the creation of the commercial scanner, almost every academic scientist who recalls any contact with EMI at this time marvels at its penchant for secrecy, which they saw demonstrated in the protective guard EMI deployed around its resident genius.

However much information Hounsfield actually garnered from earlier scientific publications, the idea of computed tomography was "in the air," and the solution he worked out idiosyncratically became the first commercial scanner. Manufactured by EMI, it was the product of cooperation between the company and the Medical Research Council (MRC) of Britain's Department of Health and Social Security (DHSS), which is analogous on a small scale to the National Institutes of Health (NIH) in the United States. The CT scanner made its debut at Atkinson Morley's Hospital in Wimbledon in 1971.

Godfrey Hounsfield, the link between theory and practical application, was born in Newark, Nottinghamshire, in 1919 and grew up on a farm in nearby Sutton-on-Trent. He is a mild-mannered genius who attributes his successes to a penchant for easily growing bored combined with an unquenchable curiosity. The youngest of five children of a steelworker-turned-farmer, Hounsfield recalls an idyllic boyhood spent exploring the soaring qualities of hang gliders (by leaping with them from the tops of haystacks), and rigging up a projector for the village cinema. He attended a local grammar school, but, a weak student, he did not follow his sister to Oxford or, for that matter, attend any university. Instead he went to work for a local builder and joined the air force reserves. With the outbreak of war in 1939, he was called up by the RAF and assigned to communications.

Here Hounsfield flourished, doing so well on his exam that he was assigned to teach the course, rather than take it, and was sent to the top-secret RDF (later called RADAR) school. He so excelled in radar research that on leaving the army in 1946, he won a government grant for further training. He undertook this at Faraday House in London, one of Britain's first polytechnics. After graduation in 1951, he joined EMI. He has spent his whole career there, free to follow his own bent, as long as the possible payoff dovetails with the company's interests.

EMI had been founded in 1898 as the Gramophone Company (a deliberate inversion of *phonogram,* Edison's term for a recording.[21] Over the years EMI bought patents for records made of shellac with up-and-down (instead of side-to-side) grooves. It had also acquired a painting by an English artist, Francis Barraud, of a dog seated listening to the horn of a phonograph, which became the British trademark of the HMV record label and the American trademark of RCA. By 1931, the original Gramophone Company had merged with two other large recording companies to become EMI. The new company supported an excellent research and development program which assisted in the development of television before 1939. After the war, in 1945, EMI worked briefly with the California-based Varian Associates, a company then manufacturing microwave tubes and components, equipment which would also play a role in the development of computerized imaging.

In the 1950s, EMI encouraged research in transistors and early computers, but never lost sight of its signature product—music recordings. EMI sold classic and popular music in whatever form was popular: hi-fi, stereo, and tapes. In the 1960s the success of its Beatles recordings accounted for over half of the company's considerable earnings; electronics accounted for less than a quarter of sales and medical instruments were virtually nonexistent.

This is the scene Hounsfield entered. His first assignment was to streamline the EMIDEC 1100, the first British computer. Hounsfield successfully redesigned it to work on transistors, but EMI needed cash for its rapidly diversifying record business and sold the computer facility (which was lucky, Hounsfield recalls, as transistors soon gave way to chips). EMI then sent Hounsfield to the central research laboratory where the director asked him what he wanted to do next.

Hounsfield looked at the list of offerings and opted for exploring pattern recognition, a problem he had been toying with that related to EMI's primary mission of recording and playing back information. Information theory is a highly theoretical, mathematical science which might have put off a less intrepid inventor. But Hounsfield was attracted by the puzzle and clearly not frightened by its complexity. He believes that "most of these problems are just generally reasoning around the problem and using common sense, and then proving it by maths afterwards. I think in general it does turn out that way whatever you're doing: you've just got to use the absolute minimum of maths but have a tremendous lot of intuition."[22]

Hounsfield's frame of reference included two very different experiences: work on storing image information on linear TV scans, and work positioning radar where the topographical features of the landscape are displayed on a cathode-ray tube screen by a spiral scan. Hounsfield recalls that he was thinking over these problems on "a long country ramble" when the seeds of the CT scanner began to grow in his mind.[23] If many measurements were made through an object at various angles, the information provided could be used to reconstruct the image, but that would take thousands of mathematical equations to achieve. Hounsfield knew that this could be managed by the proper mathematics, and he was confident that the computers he had so recently worked with could handle the vast array of data.

Hounsfield's familiarity with computers also informed him that computers can store pictures, bits that can be presented as sets of pixels. He knew, as Cormack had seen in the Groote Schuur Hospital, that ordinary X-ray filming is inefficient for two reasons: the random scatter of X-rays contributes no information to the film, and the superimposition of all sorts of images—bones and soft tissue, for instance—makes the image difficult to read. He was also aware of classical tomography and realized that it gave patients an unhealthily heavy dose of radiation.

A CT scan, as he envisaged it, would provide more information than an ordinary X-ray picture. Each scan would look like a cross-sectional cut; a series made close together could be built up into what looks like a three-dimensional image. The major question to be answered was whether he could get a fine enough image—free of noise—without administering an overdose of radiation. He wanted to try, and so presented his ideas in a report that became the basis for EMI's 1968 British patent: "A method of and apparatus for examination of a body by radiation such as x or gamma radiations."

At this point, Hounsfield's solution used much of the same reasoning as those of the Australian, South African, and American inventors, of whom only Oldendorf had filed a patent. The decision to put more than Hounsfield's time into the project seems to have been tipped by Hounsfield's boss, Len Broadway, the director of research. While not expert with computers, Broadway had worked with X-ray analysis of crystals and radiology. He asked EMI for the leeway to build a model to see if it would get a powerful enough signal-to-noise ratio to produce an image.

Hounsfield was eager to try. The mathematics that had obsessed Cormack did not worry him; he knew there were algorithms around, including Fourier transforms and Bracewell's published work, for reconstructing data from projections. As it turned out he rejected them all in favor of a simple "iterative" algebraic technique because he found it personally satisfying, even if the method is disparaged by mathematicians as both cumbersome and repetitive. This was fine for making the first scans, but was exceedingly slow and did not take advantage of the computer's potential. At this stage, however, Hounsfield was mostly interested in proving that he could do what he had promised. There would be time in the future to streamline the process, he recalls, and for the moment he was enjoying having hands-on control.[24]

EMI, however, hesitated and refused to provide more money for the instrument without some evidence of a market. Broadway realized that they needed a partner that could supply both development money and a clinic where they could test the machine.

His solution was at the Department of Health and Social Security (DHSS) in London. Hounsfield explained to the DHSS health officer that his proposed device would be useful for detecting tiny tumors. When the suggestion of mass screening for such growths did not excite the health officer, Hounsfield took a different tack. He presented his proposed machine as an opportunity to see inside the brain! Not only did this offer an economic bonus (most brain problems necessitated exploratory surgery) but throughout the seventy-five-year history of X-rays, the prospect of seeing into the brain had stirred the medical and popular imagination.

The DHSS put EMI, including Hounsfield, in touch with James Bull, a distinguished neuroradiologist who, recognizing the potential of the invention in 1967, in his turn put Hounsfield in touch with the neurosurgeon James Ambrose. Ambrose had been exploring other methods of imaging the brain and was impressed by the promise of Hounsfield's approach. Through 1968 and 1969 Hounsfield worked on models with phantom subjects, using gamma rays—as Kuhl and Oldendorf had—instead of X-rays. It took nine days to scan the subject and another two-and-a-half hours to process the data on a computer. This was obviously too long, so he replaced the gamma rays with X-rays, cutting the scan time to nine hours. As he continued to refine the system, he proceeded from artificial phantoms to using a pig's head (once leaving it wrapped neatly on the London Underground in a hurry not to miss his stop), and, eventually, to human organs provided by the Royal Marsden Hospital.

EMI and the Medical Research Council people who funded the DHSS had decided to develop an instrument to help neuroradiologists, and designed a machine that would scan just the head. Hounsfield was not part of this deal-making, and recalls a little regretfully (and perhaps unrealistically) that he could have as easily built a whole-body machine at the onset, only the medical people seemed set on a machine just for the brain.

With funds raised and the project headed for realization, secrecy became a priority, and it is difficult to discover how much was known, by whom, at what time. But on October 1, 1971, Ambrose and Hounsfield scanned their first patient, a forty-one-year-old woman who had symptoms suggesting a brain tumor somewhere in the frontal lobe.

She lay with a rubber cap on her head to one side of a plastic water-filled box. The water was necessary then because the density of water is closer to the density of bone than is the density of air. By excluding air, they reduced the range of information that would have to be processed and the calculations the computer would have to make. They sent a collimated beam of X-rays through her head, which was picked up by two scintillator detectors on the other side. Both the X-ray source and the detectors scanned the patient's head. Then the instruments were rotated one degree and the machines took another scan. This continued, rotating degree by degree, for 180 degrees, giving each

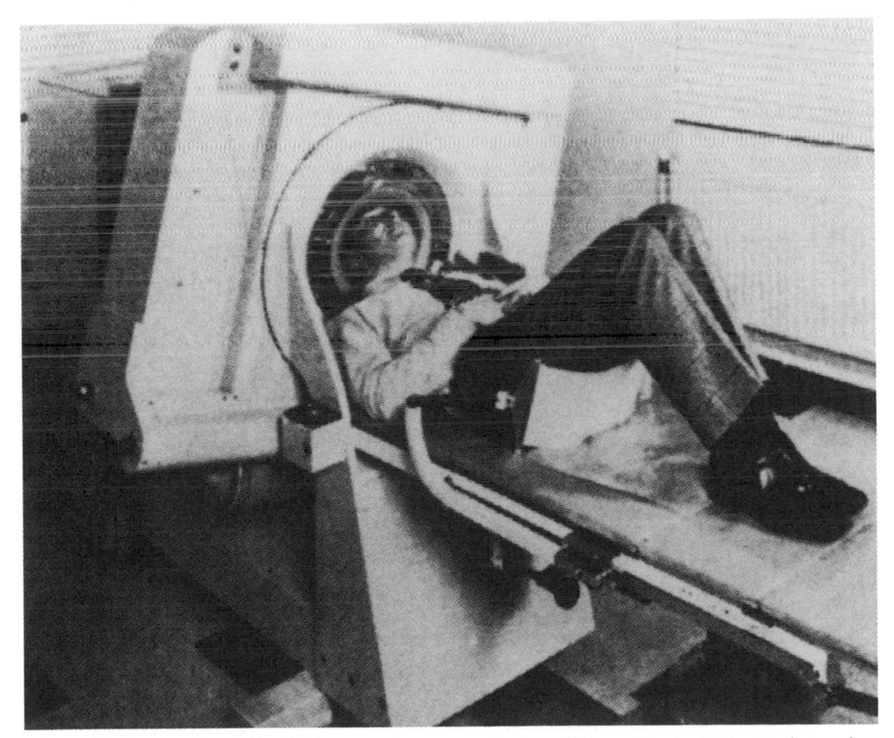

30. First clinical prototype EMI brain scanner, installed at Atkinson Morley's Hospital, London (1972). Note the water bag surrounding the patient's head. (G. N. Hounsfield, "Computed Medical Imaging," Nobel Lecture, *Journal of Computed Assisted Tomography* 4 [1980]: 665–674.) Courtesy of *Journal of Computed Assisted Tomography*, Lippincott-Raven Publishers.

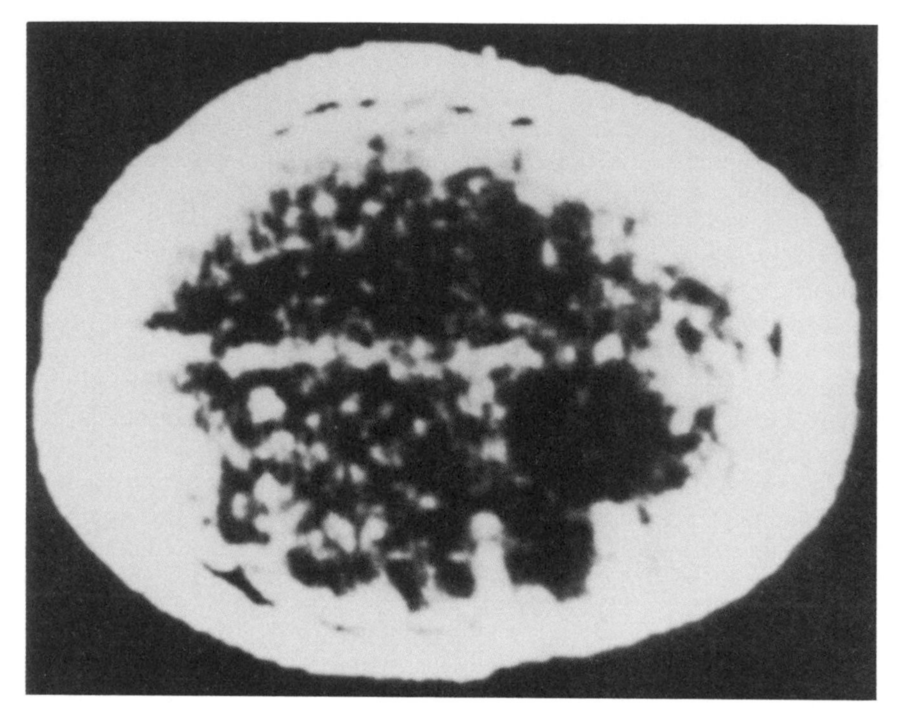

31. First clinical CT image obtained from EMI prototype unit (1972). In a woman with a suspected brain lesion, the scan clearly shows a dark circular cyst. (G. N. Hounsfield, "Computed Medical Imaging," Nobel Lecture, *Journal of Computed Assisted Tomography* 4 [1980]: 665–674.) Courtesy of *Journal of Computed Assisted Tomography,* Lippincott-Raven Publishers.

detector 28,000 readings, which were recorded on magnetic tape. Through it all the patient remained still, her head against the water-filled box for the entire fifteen hours it took to complete the task.

Ambrose then sent the data tape across London to a computer where it was processed. This was in turn processed by another computer that produced a cross-sectional image which was photographed from the monitor's screen after what now seems an intolerable wait. The photograph was finally carried back to Ambrose. He easily saw a tumor in the patient's left frontal lobe, which he soon excised.

Souped Up CT Evolution

In 1972 the British demonstrated their EMI scanner to the world and immediately got contracts to build five more machines. Of the original six prototypes, one remained in Wimbledon, one went to London, a third to Glasgow and the fourth to Manchester (both cities historically steeped in radiology). The Mayo Clinic in Rochester, Minnesota, and the Massachusetts General Hospital in Boston bought the two remaining machines for about $300,000 each.

At this same time—1971—David Davis, the neuroradiologist from George Washington University Medical Center who was to attend James Brady, was at a meeting in Europe and, hearing about the excitement over the machine, flew to London to see it for himself. Davis realized, even though the scanner was in its early stage, that brain imaging would never be the same, and he "went after the thing," convincing EMI to establish its American headquarters in nearby Reston, Virginia (the home of the American College of Radiology).[25] The pictures, crude by today's standards, astounded neuroradiologists and all other radiologists as well. Davis bought the next scanner to be delivered in the United States. It took four minutes per slice and still used a water bag. But as soon as it arrived, patients came from all over and gurneys lined the hallways. EMI scanners worked round the clock, proving beyond the wildest vision of its creators that hospitals would pay what would soon be half a million dollars for a machine that could see into the brain.

The only market EMI ever considered seriously was the United States. In November 1972, it presented, with great fanfare, the images from its clinical brain scanner to the annual RSNA gathering in Chicago, already the international showcase of innovations in imaging.

EMI dominated the exhibition.

In a description of the first scans in the *British Journal of Radiology*, Ambrose noted that doctors, like himself, could have the data in either numerical form or as an image.[26] When in 1974 the Hospital of the Good Samaritan in Los Angeles got the first scanner on the West Coast (and only the twenty-sixth in the world), they received their information in two versions: as computer printouts of numbers (enough for each scan to paper a small room) and as pictures. Although few, if any, radiologists ever looked at the numbers, they had not yet acknowledged their dependence on imagery.[27] Besides, in 1974 the CT's computer was so busy with scanning patients that radiologists had to wait for the doors to the clinic to close before using the scanner's image-producing mode.[28] As late as 1976 a scientist at the Mayo Clinic wondered if, in opting for an image over numbers, they were losing valuable information about the nature of the tissues.

EMI's images changed the way radiologists looked into the body. Robert Stanley, chairman of the Department of Radiology at the University of Alabama School of Medicine, in Birmingham, recalls a meeting in Puerto Rico in 1976, three and a half years after the introduction of the brain CT scanner, when he was still on the faculty at the Mallinckrodt Institute of Radiology at Washington University in St. Louis. About half a dozen people, mostly from the Mayo Clinic and the Mallinckrodt Institute, with experience in body CT banded together to insist that CT images be presented in the scientific literature as if the patient is being viewed from below, rather than viewed from above, as the brain CT images were presented. All textbook pictures of cross-sectional anatomy since the 1920s depicted the body as if seen from above. But imaging the body of a living person with a CT scanner reversed this convention. Stanley says that body CT took this approach so that the patient's left side of a CT image, presented on film or in a textbook, is to the viewer's right, in much the same way as conventional chest and abdominal radiographs are viewed. Soon the "brain folks followed suit." When Lee, Sagel, and Stanley's textbook with body CT images appeared in 1983, all earlier images of cross-sectional anatomy from the 1920s became obsolete.[29]

But salespeople at EMI had no doubts about the importance of images as they made marketing decisions. Broadway advised granting patent licenses to American companies. He reasoned that EMI did not have the resources, or more important, the familiarity with the medical market, to be able to compete with established medical firms. EMI had already been contacted by every big medical equipment manufacturer, with the exception of Siemens, about cooperative ventures. EMI, however, flush with its recording bonanza (although company officials denied that the Beatles' billions had anything to do with their decision), opted to go it alone.

Hounsfield was demonstrably not alone in conceiving the CT scanner, but it is hard to imagine how the instrument would have gone into production without the support of a company like EMI. We know others tried. The combination of the Beatles' success with the British system of research subsidies and the genius of one engineer broke the cash barrier and changed the face of modern medicine.

The first CT scanner, like Roentgen's X-ray apparatus, triggered improvements so rapidly that within three years the prototype had passed through several generations and EMI, always an anomaly on the medical scene, had ceded place to the familiar industrial giants. But in the interim a few other "upstarts" had a run for the money, too.

With EMI's machine unveiled, Robert Ledley, a professor of biophysics and radiology at Georgetown University Medical School in Washington, flew to London, had a close look, and on his return announced that he could build a better scanner, cheaper, and big enough to image the entire body. His team at Georgetown had experience in pattern recognition as did Hounsfield, and in two years was able to build the ACTA (Automatic Computerized Transverse Axial) scanner, still using what is known as "first-generation" CT technology. Its trial subject (with bows to Oldendorf's UCLA colleague) was a navel orange inside a skull in a bowl of water.

The first CT images were a puzzle to the physicians and surgeons who would be expected to use them. Ledley recalls that he felt obliged in 1976 to publish his own atlas to teach radiologists how to see the images his ACTA produced.[30] Ledley patented ACTA, claiming that it was an entirely different instrument from EMI's, that it had roots in the American precedents of Oldendorf and Cormack, and he licensed it to Pfizer, a pharmaceutical company with a worldwide medical sales force.[31]

First-generation scanners, including ACTA, are defined as those having a single, or perhaps dual, source of X-rays and a single detector that moved slowly around the subject in planes. They took a long time to get an image because the technicians had to translate and rotate the tube for each plane.

These were overtaken by second-generation scanners that used either a fanlike X-ray beam or multiple beams and multiple detectors, and a gantry that moved in larger steps, collecting more information in less time. The first of this second generation of scanners was also a whole-body scanner, invented by a research group at the Cleveland Clinic in Ohio. It was especially good at imaging the body below the neck. Patented as the Delta scanner, it was marketed in 1975 by Ohio Nuclear, and later sold to Technicare.

At almost the same time third-generation machines came on the market boasting a fan-shaped beam of X-rays broad enough to encompass the entire body. The beam rotated in sync with a bank of detectors, reducing single scan time from minutes to seconds. Yet there were still problems to sort out. The circular motion of the rotating tubes and detectors tended to distort the image, introducing circles, and producing artifacts, images of things that aren't there.

The solution to this last problem seemed to lie with the computer algorithm, not the hardware. When in 1974 the National Cancer Institutes let out a bid for an American company to develop a faster and more accurate scanner, American Science and Engineering, a small company then located on the MIT campus in Cambridge, won the contract.

American Science and Engineering was then staffed by some of the best young radioastronomers in the world (one of them, Riccardo Giacconi, later became head of the European Space Telescope). Because radioastronomers, like Bracewell, were familiar with imaging challenges, AS&E had entered the scanning market. It began when the U.S. Postal Service started X-raying the mail for firearms.[32] By the early 1970s, after a series of airplane hijackings, AS&E had produced an X-ray machine that would reveal what was inside hand luggage without fogging camera film. Now the same high-powered team went to work on CT.

Jay Stein, a leader of the team, attributes their success to his collaboration with Larry Shepp, a mathematician at Bell Laboratories in New Jersey. Shepp had been spending a lot of time in 1972 at Columbia University's Presbyterian Hospital where his young son had been diagnosed with a brain tumor.[33] He was in New York that day in April when Hounsfield made his first American presentation of EMI at Presbyterian Hospital, and his son's physicians asked him to attend the demonstration. They hoped his expertise in mathematics would help them evaluate EMI's machine.[34]

When Hounsfield finished speaking, Shepp asked how he was reconstructing the image—with a single formula, or with a procedure that required a long series of steps to arrive at a data point. When Hounsfield explained that he was using an iterative procedure—what Shepp describes as a clumsy trial-and-error approach—Shepp went home and worked on the problem for several months. Where Hounsfield had had to work on the first machine with a real patient, Shepp had the luxury of making simulations of images on the computer. He could ask, in effect, what formula can best produce this kind of image. Knowing that the system worked, Shepp emphasizes, he had the leeway to demonstrate the

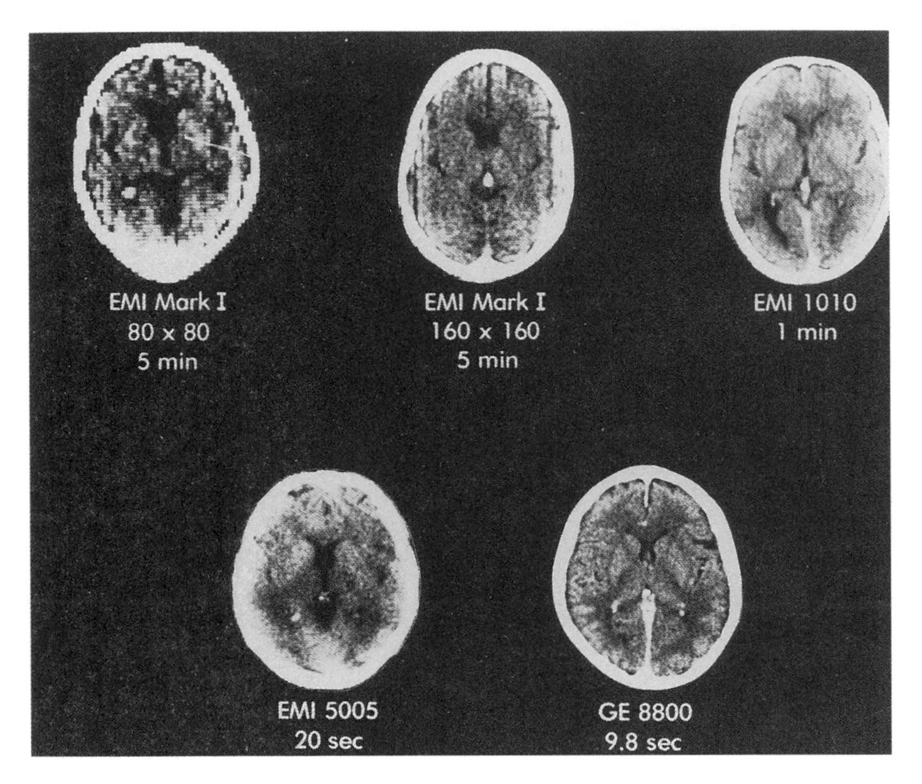

32. Five CT brain scans, 1974–1980. Images of the same midbrain in five different patients record the evolution of CT technology. *Top left,* 1974; *top middle,* 1976; *top right,* 1977; *bottom left,* 1978; *bottom right,* 1980. The difference in quality is apparent. (A. R. Margulis, "Radiologic Imaging: Changing Costs, Greater Benefits," *American Journal of Roentgenology* 136 [1987]: 657–665.) Courtesy of the American Roentgen Ray Society.

considerable advantage of using formulas over iterative procedures. Inspired by his son's illness, he stuck with the problem. When he met Jay Stein two years later at a mathematics meeting in San Francisco and discovered that they were both interested in the problems of scanning, they teamed up with the neurosurgical team at Columbia University to produce a new scanner design: the fourth-generation CT.[35] These fourth-generation machines included a ring of detectors so that only the X-ray tube had to move, avoiding the creation of the circles that plagued third-generation designs.[36] Most of the smaller companies could not tune their detectors to avoid these artifacts, but GE succeeded so that today its third-generation design dominates the market.

In the rush to upgrade CT scanners, the machines were fine-tuned, but the prices did not drop. EMI faced increasing competition. It had brought out its own second- and third-generation models and by 1975 had enlarged the computer display from 80 x 80 pixels, to 160 x 160. EMI, still a major manufacturer with machines all over the United States and Europe, fought to protect its lead by introducing a maze of lawsuits to obstruct the competition. Alan Cormack, who was asked to testify as an expert witness, describes EMI's legal manipulations as skilled brinkmanship in which they initiated many cases but stopped short each time before reaching open court, sealing the record as part of the out-of-court settlement.[37]

EMI successfully held off competitors by changing the rules in an old game. A representative from GE, testifying at a congressional committee, explained:

> Before CT, few X-ray companies bothered with patents, since all the X-ray companies recognized that no one company had a monopoly on the patents, each would have to license from the other to stay in business—the result being "why bother with patents?" EMI, which was new to the X-ray business, patented their CT designs, and by the end of the decade was requiring substantial royalties from all the CT suppliers. As a defensive measure, the X-ray companies substantially changed their patent policies; for example, we went from having a part-time use of one patent attorney to having three full-time patent attorneys. This, I believe, was totally the result of EMI's changing the practice of an industry.[38]

If EMI had been committed to medical instrumentation, it would have been in its interest to keep costs down and cooperate with its competitors. But EMI both underestimated and misunderstood the medical market. After Hounsfield's Chicago success, it sold the remaining prototype machines for $310,000 and in the next few years improved the machine and raised the price to about $500,000. EMI never tried to diversify into other medical instruments but looked on CT as a single product in the X-ray market. It had a large lead and competed successfully against the ACTA and Delta scanners. But, with the entry of GE and Siemens into the market, EMI found that the medical imaging business demanded frequent redesigns and a team of field representatives to attend to broken or damaged units. Pasadena's Huntington Memorial Hospital was not the only one that, fed up with relying on this or that new company for maintaining its very expensive machine, returned for their next purchases to GE and Siemens, whose representatives they knew and trusted.

In Britain, after EMI's astonishing initial success, there was no long-term plan. The Medical Research Council (MRC) was at least as eager to recoup its investment as EMI. They could not tap markets in countries with state-controlled health budgets like their own until the scanners had proved their value and the kinks had been worked out in the free market of American medicine. British engineers today still complain bitterly that British ingenuity, as displayed in the development of the scanner, suffered from a lack of correlative business leadership.[39] But university-based British scientists are not complaining. The MRC continues to support basic research.

In London, management shake-ups at EMI put an end to its medical odyssey. The company withdrew from all related research to return wholly to music. They sold the CT scanner to Ohio-based Picker, which in turn was taken over by a British-based conglomerate, the General Electric Corporation (GEC as distinguished from GE, the older U.S. company). It had been a grand adventure. Hounsfield remains with the company and spends a day a week looking at blood flow at the Brompton Hospital. Still interested in computers in 1994, he had two he worked with at home, playing with neural networks and simulations of evolution. As for the scanner, "It was the most interesting part of my life."[40]

As CT images became more highly resolved, they have been especially useful in enhancing the range of interventional radiology. CT allows the radiologist to see increased tissue definition and differentiation, exposing the delineation of abnormal tissues such as infections and tumors. By seeing the tissue, the radiologist uses imaging to place needles and catheters into the abnormal areas. Infections can then be drained through the skin without subjecting the patient to surgery, and, guided by CT, tumors can be treated very effectively. Using a combination of imaging techniques and specialized instruments, the interventional radiologist crosses beyond diagnosis into what the layperson would see as surgery.[41]

In to the late 1980s CT innovators continued to spin off variations. Douglas Boyd, a physicist in San Francisco at the University of California Medical School who had worked with some of the earliest computers as a graduate student at Rutgers, and who at Stanford had helped develop a sophisticated radiotherapy device that could treat tumors in three dimensions, introduced "superfast" scanning as a diagnostic device in 1985. His "imatron" has no moving parts and can get a picture in 50 to 100 milliseconds. That is rapid enough to image the heart between beats, so it is especially useful for coronary checkups. It can also get images in seven planes at once, allowing for a variety of perspectives.

Then in 1989 the first spiral CT entered the market. Unlike imatron, which offers speed, spiral CT provides continuous data acquisition over a large volume of the body—the entire chest, for instance—instead of a series of separate, parallel slices. The adoption of slip-ring technology (used for years in radar) freed the scanner from the cables that literally chained conventional CT to the wall and limited the circular movement of the X-ray tube. For after each single slice was made, the machine had to be stopped to unwind the cables to the wall outlet. The slip-ring channels the power source through the action of two rings slipping against each other: an outer ring houses the X-ray tube and detectors, to which brushes are attached that contact a stationary inner ring made of a metallic conductor. The outer ring with the X-ray tube rotates while the inner tube is stationary, leaving no coil to unwind. The result is a spiral motion during which the patient is moved swiftly through as data is constantly acquired.

This volumetric data can be reconstructed by the computer into a variety of cross-sections of different thicknesses—as thin as four millimeters—without having to subject the patient to additional discomfort or exposure to ionizing radiation. It is usually used without any contrast media, saving both money and any possible allergic reaction on the part of the patient. Spiral CT would not have been possible without improved X-ray tubes which tolerate high temperatures and greater currents.[42] This kind of data enables radiologists to create three-dimensional images that can be turned around on the monitor so that a skull, for instance, can be viewed from a variety of perspectives.

Competition among CT manufacturers has produced high-speed machines that are especially valuable in treating children or trauma cases. Where CT exams once took between thirty minutes and an hour, spiral scanning cuts the time to five or ten minutes. In an emergency room, cases can be imaged in twenty seconds.[43] Speed is its major advantage; the trade-off is somewhat poorer resolution.

The Dollar Spiral

Besides meeting competition within their own ranks, CT manufacturers had to face the creature of their own success—a machine whose enormous price tag had no place in the way traditional radiology departments made their budgets. CT arrived on the American scene in the wake of Medicare. As the national medical budget soared, CT, the first of the big-ticket body-penetrating cross-sectional imaging machines, became the whipping boy of medical cost containment. Many times the price of any earlier medical tool, they were an easy symbol of fiduciary profligacy. Joseph Califano, the Secretary of Health, Education and Welfare in the Carter administration, is reputed to have declared in 1976 that every hospital no more needed a CT scanner than every garage needed a Cadillac.

One of the first legislative tools of cost containment was certificate-of-need (CON) laws, regulations that required institutions to prove that they were not simply duplicating equipment available nearby. The Federal Health Planning Act of 1976 required states to create health-planning mechanisms for hospitals, and applied equally to capital improvements and new services.[44] The rules varied, but they started by declaring that all devices that cost more than $400,000 had to be reviewed for community need at state and local levels. Some states meshed these demands with CON regulations. Each state created its own bureaucracy, of varying degrees of complexity. Most state programs applied only to hospitals, and this encouraged them to contract with something new—free-standing independent imaging centers.[45]

While the advantages of a CT scan seemed obvious to physicians treating victims of trauma, stroke, and a host of other medical crises in emergency rooms, the heightened dependency on technology disturbed some physicians outside the emergency room who had never stopped suspecting that machines were becoming ever more a wedge between doctor and patient.[46] It is likely that some unnecessary scans were ordered by physicians or hospitals eager to amortize their investment in the machine. Indeed, a great deal of effort has been spent verifying the rise in scans as a factor in rising medical budgets. But, surprisingly, almost no alarm has been raised about the coincidental rise in unnecessary exposure to radiation from an unnecessary scan. CT scans, though well shielded, use ionizing radiation. And even though the typical scan exposes patients to less radiation than an angiogram or gastrointestinal fluoroscopy, it is ten times that of a simple chest X-ray (but produces perhaps a hundredfold more information).[47] Head scans can be especially dangerous to the eyes, which are very sensitive to radiation, and as narrow CT "slices" might overlap, the same sensitive cells could be exposed to additional radiation.

Sales outside of the United States followed a different pattern. Almost all other industrialized nations provided some kind of national health care by this time; with it went centralized control over acquisition and distributions of costly medical instruments like CT scanners. When acquired through a central authority, scanners were distributed according to population and demand. Some countries, like Japan, negotiated prices as well as the quality of the image the machine could produce. Other countries, like France, which lagged in its initial acquisition of CT machines, made up for it a decade later by acquiring high-end spiral and superfast models.

In the United States, grants from the NIH (the parent of the National Cancer Institutes), NASA, and the Department of Defense did help in the development of CT scanning through small grants to universities. But in 1974 government officials wondered why it was a British company that was actually producing machines. After all, Oldendorf, Cormack, Bracewell, and Kuhl had seen the promise of such a machine, built models, or, like Kuhl, had actually taken transmission pictures. As dollars crossed the Atlantic, there was enough disquiet for a U.S. government representative to visit Ronald Bracewell at his Stanford laboratory. What, he asked, could the American government have done?[48]

Budgetary obstacles notwithstanding, American hospitals bought CT scanners, not necessarily out of need, but to woo patients. X-ray manufacturers who had turned deaf ears to Oldendorf's early patent now bought improved patents without having had to invest in basic research. They had missed out on EMI's glory, but not the dividends.

But the glory that went to EMI spilled over onto the daring and cautious alike. The award of the Nobel Prize for physiology or medicine in 1979 to Godfrey Hounsfield and Alan Cormack validated the decisions of the hospitals that had bought the scanners. The prizes acknowledged a fait accompli—a revolution in diagnostic medicine. The awards were greeted by cheers and, inevitably, disappointment. The news that an award would be made to the inventors of CT scanning had apparently leaked out, and a host of people seemed to have volunteered to nominate one, two, or three possible candidates.

Hounsfield had been an obvious choice, but, from the perspective of scientists, what Hounsfield had done was good engineering, not science. He had not derived any original algorithm or invented the collimated beams or receptors that furnished his raw data. Yet the fact remains that Hounsfield had designed a machine that worked even though both theory and experience suggested it was too complicated to succeed. Shepp speaks for a lot of people when he confesses: "If I had known what he knew when he started, I would have said it wouldn't work, and never tried."[49] The theory for the mathematics had been articulated by Alan Cormack, who shared the prize. That choice would most likely have pleased Roentgen, who, although an experimentalist himself, is remembered for having said: "The physicist in preparing for his work needs three things, mathematics, mathematics, and mathematics."[50]

Whatever the politics of the prizes, the fact stands out that the awards for physiology or medicine in 1979 were not granted to physicians or biologists, but to an engineer and a nuclear physicist for developing a commercial machine. It had, apparently, been a difficult decision. The Nobel committee's minutes remain sealed for fifty years; only in 2039 we may learn why it delayed its press conference for an hour before announcing its choices.

Oldendorf, frankly disappointed, remarked to students that he had paid the price for being twenty years ahead of his time, and went back to his laboratory. Kuhl continued his work and made major contributions to another imaging technology. Bracewell, who had never thought he was a contender, turned to medical image reconstruction and joined the editorial board of the new *Journal of Computed Axial Tomography* in 1977. An editorial in the journal's first issue compared the invention of CT scanning to Roentgen's discovery, pointing out that like the X-ray, CT met skepticism on the grounds of medical outcomes and cost.

The editorial may have been responding to an editorial comment in the venerable *New England Journal of Medicine* the year before: "CAT fever has reached epidemic proportions and continues to spread among physicians, manufacturers, entrepreneurs and regulatory agencies. A cursory review of any radiologic or neuroscience journal attests to the virulence of this new disease. Within the United States alone, the costs of this epidemic are staggering."[51]

A medical writer crowed in the *New York Times* that the Nobel committee had delivered a "major blow against the bureaucrats in Washington who would like to halt, or even to reverse, the current technological revolution in United States medicine."[52]

The CT in Court

The scanner that helped save James Brady's life also saved the life of the man who shot him. John Hinckley, though obviously disturbed, had never before used a gun to shoot anyone. Caught with the weapon in his hand, his defense team needed to prove he was not responsible for his actions. They turned to psychiatric experts, who sought evidence in a CT image.

First they had to establish that Hinckley had a disease with a label. This was achieved by psychiatrist David Bear who, on his first day of testimony, lectured the court on "schizophrenia spectrum disorder," a condition he described as a progressive illness that produces depressive episodes. It was exacerbated on the day of the shooting by Hinckley's ingestion of Valium. To prove Hinckley's impoverished ability to reason, Bear introduced a CT scan—the first time that a CT scan had been admitted as evidence in an American court.

Judge Barrington D. Parker wanted to know how this new kind of image could help the case. Bear responded that "there is overwhelming evidence that the brain's physiology related to a person's emotions and that an abnormal appearance of the brain relates to schizophrenia."[53] Bear was specifically referring to a study from St. Elizabeth's Hospital in Washington that showed that, in the brains of one-third of the schizophrenics autopsied, the sulci (the folds and ridges on the surface of the brain) are more shallow than in normal people. He had a radiologist show the court a scan of Hinckley's brain and pointed to the widened sulci. He was saying that Hinckley's diminished brain was part of "a statistical fact." He did not say that the widened sulci caused schizophrenia, but he said the image indicated a good chance that Hinckley was suffering from the disease.

A witness for the prosecution testified that the degeneration of some of Hinckley's brain tissue, as revealed "on a device known as a CAT-scan—was the same as that found in half the nation's adult population."[54] He did not add that most of the human brain had not been mapped and the causes of schizophrenia are unknown so that reading the scan was akin to reading the entrails of a slaughtered eagle.

The judge pondered the problem, rejected the admissibility of the CT scan evidence, and then, nine days later, reversed his decision, adding a new legal precedent to the already unusual trial. The jury seemed to accept the meaning of the scan as the defense portrayed it and declared Hinckley not guilty by virtue of insanity. He was sent to St. Elizabeth's Hospital for an indefinite length of time in June 1982. The CT scan began a career as a staple in insanity pleas.

CT scans were already part of the coroner's toolbox. Like skeletal and dental X-rays, CT images of the brain are an excellent way of identifying otherwise unidentifiable corpses. When fingerprints are hard to read, or when there are no fingers to print from (canny murderers often remove them), final identification can be made from the shape of the frontal sinuses, if there is a CT on file. Sinuses are as individual to humans as nose prints are to gorillas. No two are the same, not even in the case of identical twins.

CT scans were officially deemed part of the expected "medical standard of care" in an action against the federal government in January 1983, retroactive to 1976.[55] The plaintiff was Kenneth Swanson, who had been honorably discharged from the United States Army in 1974 after serving in Germany for three years. He was discharged after his odd behavior earned him a diagnosis of acute schizophrenia. As his behavior grew stranger, he sought help at the Veterans Administration hospital in Salt Lake City. Doctors there added multiple sclerosis to the original diagnosis but offered no help. Then in 1976, in a checkup at the Portland VA hospital, a neurologist noted that his symptoms, which now included weakness in the right arm and leg and loss of hearing on the right side, slurred speech, and double vision, supported "the possibility of a brain stem lesion." She recommended that Swanson have his head examined by a CT scan. Soon he was having headaches as well and difficulty swallowing, but no one followed through with the scan. His condition continued to deteriorate until 1980 when, after being flown to Boise, Idaho, another VA neurologist ordered a CT scan. This time he got it and his physician saw that Swanson had neither schizophrenia nor multiple sclerosis, but rather he had a massive tumor which had become so lodged in his brain stem that by this time it was impossible to remove completely.

Swanson, severely impaired, won a settlement to help defray his substantial living expenses. The court ruled in 1983 that CT scans were the standard that Swanson's condition entitled him to have received in 1976—what Califano had referred to as "Cadillac" treatment. The court could not recall a time when CT was *not* the routine diagnostic procedure for any brain-related problem.

In 1976—when, according to the Utah court, Swanson should have been having his CT scan on the West Coast—Judith Richardson Haimes was being scanned in Philadelphia, and she wasn't at all happy about it. She also went to court, but in her case blamed the CT scan for having ruined, rather than potentially saving, her life. Haimes had a history of recurrent brain tumors. Seeking an explanation for their growth, her doctor ordered a CT scan. Wary of dyes, which were used to enhance the image, Haines asked the neuroradiologist at Temple University Hospital not to use them. But the neuroradiologist injected dye into her arteries anyway and went ahead with the scan.

Not long afterwards, Haimes began vomiting and developed a fierce headache.

Ten years later, Haimes had her day in court. In her suit against Temple University, she explained that the CT scan had ended her career as a psychic and destroyed her family. Testifying in her behalf, Raymond Schellhammer, a special agent with the New Jersey Commission of Investigation, described how before 1976 Haimes had helped the police find the body of a missing woman and track down the woman's husband, who had killed her. Haines testified that she had been born with an ability to read the auras that surround everyone. From the auras, she could tell the future, "see" things that had occurred in the past, and give warnings. She said that the CT scan had robbed her of that talent, and her whole life had fallen apart. She had lost her source of income, and, even worse, her family had lost the advantage of the annual readings in which she had advised them what to look out for in the year ahead. She attributed the death of her twenty-year-old son to her inability to read his aura. "The truth of the matter is, my son was killed in an automobile accident that didn't have to take place."[56]

The jury, against the recommendations of the judge, awarded her $986,000. Did the public in 1986, as represented by the jury, regard the CT as a killing ray? The temper of those times may be more accurately reflected by the judge who reversed the decision, noting that a jury's verdict should not be overturned unless it "causes the trial judge to lose his breath, temporarily, and causes him to almost fall from the bench." He wrote: "Although this court did not manifest any of the aforementioned gyrations, we nonetheless find the verdict to be so grossly excessive as to shock the court's sense of justice."[57] Emanuel Kanal, a radiologist at the University of Pittsburgh, questions her claim on different grounds: "If she could see the future," he asks, "Why didn't she know about the scan, and refuse to take it?"[58]

That same year Woody Allen's fictional hero was having a hard time just getting along with his wife in the popular film *Hannah and Her Sisters,* when he was terrified by a physician who ordered a CT scan and misread it. The resulting colored pictures, which the audience sees, show a serious brain problem, suggesting that our hero's time to work out his family affairs is very short indeed.[59] By 1986 the texture of everyday life in the United States had expanded to include familiarity with the insides of the brain as revealed in CT. Computerized scanning had been embraced as the standard of care by physicians, the courts, and Hollywood.

The skull now conjured up a new image: no longer a barrier, it was more like a door opening and bringing light into a dark room. CT scans soon explored the interiors of Egyptian mummies, examined the stomach contents of a three-thousand-year-old man found frozen in the Alps, and reconstructed the head of a two-million-year-old hominid fossil. Nothing with bone could escape the scanner. But CT went beyond bone: in 1995 a group of Dutch radiologists used a spiral CT scanner to examine a gypsum bust of the late singer Elvis Presley, and made three-millimeter thick reconstructions every two minutes. The resulting image, *Elvis Revisited with 3-D Spiral CT,* places medical technology right in the center of pop culture, dissolving, so to speak, whatever space remained between them.

Eight

A Subtler Slice

Magnetic Resonance Imaging

The particles inside an atom's nucleus can be manipulated beyond what was the realm of fantasy a century ago. Then scientists held the atom to be both indestructible and homogeneous, and the word *nucleus* had no meaning beyond the central structure in a plant or animal cell. Within the single generation between the wars, physicists probed the atom, discovered its cloud of electrons surrounding a nucleus containing other particles, and posited the possibility of tapping the energy inside. The next generation would discover how to manipulate these particles to obtain remarkable images of interior spaces in a procedure now known as magnetic resonance imaging, or more commonly, MRI.[1]

CT images bone, cartilage, and calcium deposits extremely well, but has difficulty imaging soft tissue surrounded by bone or cartilage. MRI does to bones what X-rays do to skin: in an MRI, bones disappear from view. The skeleton, the symbol of X-rays, dissolves completely. Without the carapace of bone, soft tissues are visible in all their complexity. The black negative spaces on an MRI are comparable to the black space on an X-ray or CT scan—they denote the places where no signal is picked up. On an X-ray or CT image, the tissue that does not absorb radiation is black. But in MR, bones are black and everything else is revealed in detail. The act of visual penetration no longer carries the association of stark white skeletons, and death.

A decade after MR machines entered the clinic, their images would be accepted as evidence in court. MRI pictures provided dramatic corroboration

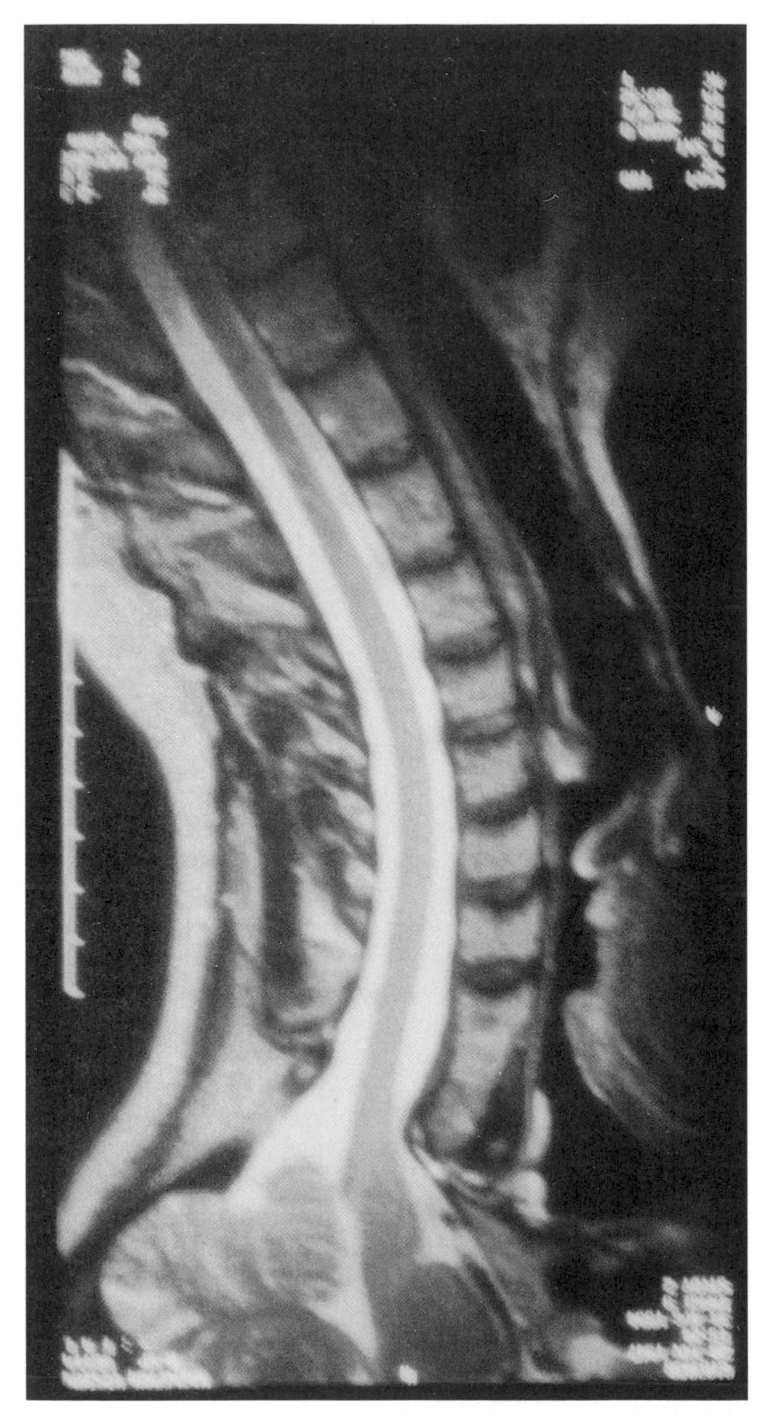

33. MRI of the normal anatomy of the spine. Most of the bone is not imaged so it appears as black, but intervertebral discs and glands are revealed in detail. (William G. Bradley, Jr., W. Ross Adey, Anton H. Hasso, *Magnetic Resonance Imaging of the Brain, Head, and Neck: A Text Atlas*, Rockville, Md.: Aspen Systems Corp., 1985.)

of the beating, fortuitously videotaped, of an African-American, Rodney G. King, by four white policemen in Los Angeles on March 3, 1991. The acquittal of those policemen on charges of police brutality sparked three days of riots the following May, but the images produced by magnetized hydrogen protons in King's bruised head convinced another jury in a civil trial to award King 3.8 million dollars in compensatory damages.

The second jury saw pictures akin to, yet qualitatively different from, the CT scans that the Hinckley jury had seen a decade earlier. Both images show slices of the interior of the targeted organ, but only MRI can produce an image of organic tissue wherever there is a trace of water, as there was in the swollen tissue inside Rodney King's scalp and right temporalis muscle. The MRI showed the jury where cerebral spinal fluid had leaked through multiple skull fractures (seen on accompanying CT images) into King's right maxillary sinus. Three years after the beating, physicians would attribute King's continued complaints of headaches, visual problems, numbness along the right side of his face, and memory loss to these injuries.[2]

When MRI images are used as evidence, they invariably appear as part of a triptych with the two earlier kinds of images X-ray and CT. King's victory in his civil suit was a victory for the use of MRI in court. MRI has had to overcome an obstacle that did not exist when X-rays were first accepted in the courtroom, and which CT avoided by being accepted as a version of X-ray radiographs. This obstacle was the Frye rule, a legal test of the scientific validity of a new technique.[3] King's lawyers had to convince the court that an MRI of the inside of his head was a scientifically accepted procedure that would show damage, otherwise invisible, that the police had inflicted that night.

Magnetic resonance imaging is inconceivable without computers. MRI benefited from the struggles CT developers had gone through a few years earlier to find the mathematics to reconstruct images. Although the nature of the signals differ, the human body remains the same, and the problem of reconstructing an image from a mass of data from within the body is essentially the same. In the few years separating the development of the two imaging technologies, the mathematics had been figured out. These algorithms were a major gift from CT.

In every other way, however, MRI has different scientific roots from CT—and its heroes began by exploring quite different problems. The two kinds of anatomical images meet often in the courtroom and on computer screens and today give the impression of being partners. But this was not always the case. Without CT's dramatic entry into the medical marketplace, it is hard to imagine how MRI would have gotten the kind of support it needed to trigger its own revolution, coming, as it happened, from a specialized area of particle physics.

Nuclear Magnetic Resonance (NMR)

The idea that the interior of the atom's nucleus could be manipulated grew from the suggestion of the Austrian physicist Wolfgang Pauli in 1924 that the protons or neutrons (or both) inside atomic nuclei would, under certain conditions, move with angular momentum, or "spin," and become magnetic.[4] Evidence of this nuclear magnetism was detected in frozen hydrogen by two Soviet scientists in 1937, the same year that the American physicist I. I. Rabi actually measured the magnetic moment (or spin) of the nucleus, for which he coined the phrase *nuclear magnetic resonance,* or NMR.

In the beginning there was only NMR, and it was the province of physicists. Rabi won the Nobel Prize in physics in 1944 for his method of measuring nuclear magnetic resonance. Eight years later NMR research earned the Nobel Prize in physics again when Edward Purcell and Felix Bloch shared the award for their independent but almost simultaneous announcements that they had measured NMR in bulk matter.

Echoing a pattern of much scientific discovery, the articles appeared within a month of each other in 1946, when Purcell at Harvard and Bloch at Stanford both published papers in the *Physical Review.* Both men knew that nuclei with odd numbers of protons, neutrons, or both, align themselves like little compasses when exposed to a strong magnetic field. Then, when an alternating magnetic induction is turned on at the radio frequency of the particular atom—its resonance frequency—the protons in the nuclei resonate with it. In laboratory NMR, and later in medical imaging, the nucleus imaged is usually hydrogen. As the major constituent of water it is the most prevalent element in the human body.

When the magnetic field is altered, the protons produce an alternating magnetic signal that can be picked up by a receiver. When the signal is turned off, the protons relax, which is to say they return to their original state. NMR records two signals: T_1 and T_2. T_1 and T_2 are both relaxation times, that is, they are measures of the times in which the components of the net magnetization of the excited nuclei return to equilibrium. T_1 is the relaxation time for the component in the direction of the external field; T_2 is the relaxation time for the component perpendicular to that field. T_2 can never exceed T_1. The difference between T_1 and T_2 from point to point reveals subtle differences in adjacent tissues. These are the basic data that NMR experiments always produce.

Eventually, when NMR was adapted to sophisticated imaging systems, it became possible to derive additional images from sophisticated manipulations of the radio signals. This was done by pulsing them (turning the frequency on and off rapidly), and by taking advantage of other qualities of the spinning nuclei.

This demonstration of the peculiar behavior of certain nuclei in certain conditions initiated the new scientific subdiscipline of NMR, a specialty that was almost immediately adopted by chemists who saw it as an excellent tool for chemical analysis. In the first decades after World War II, NMR was the interdisciplinary offspring of physics and chemistry. At this time NMR explored small, test-tube sized samples of homogeneous inorganic substances. Like Roentgen's discovery, it had absolutely nothing to do with medicine. But unlike the discovery of X-rays, where the medical advantages were immediately obvious, it would be twenty-five years before the medical applications of NMR would be realized.

NMR soon became the special province of chemists who used it to identify and determine the structures of molecules. The first NMR machines were cumbersome devices that utilized magnets, transmitters, and receivers connected to a unit that recorded spectra. During the early years, the Varian company in Palo Alto, California, the first commercial manufacturer of NMR spectrometers, had a virtual monopoly on the devices. Varian had the advantage both of holding the patent and having as a consultant the Swiss-born American physicist Felix Bloch, who was on the faculty at neighboring Stanford University.

Varian had marketed its machines exclusively to the chemical and petroleum industries until 1955, when the chemistry department at the California Institute of Technology (Caltech) ordered one and brought it into the realm of basic research. This first laboratory-size unit was set up on the third floor of the chemistry building, where it challenged the building's structural stability. The magnet alone weighed two thousand pounds. Among its array of pilot lamps, dials, and meters were a pair of twelve-inch magnetic pole faces with a two-inch gap between them. Samples had to fit into special 5 mm test tubes that fit into that gap. NMR was not yet the user-friendly, computer-operated, laboratory tool it would become.

During the late 1940s and 1950s, NMR research focused on examining a variety of substances in minute samples. With the installation of the machine at Caltech, chemists, led by John D. Roberts, branched into the study of organic compounds. Soon other researchers began exploring small slices of tissue from once-living creatures, such as rabbit nerves and rat muscles, by examining the water in the tissues. In 1959 a major threshold was crossed when Jay Singer at the University of California at Berkeley was able to measure the rates of blood flow in mice with NMR, proof that the technique could be successfully used to study living creatures without harming them.

It was becoming obvious that NMR could be an excellent medical tool, but it was not clear precisely how. If it could measure blood flow and track water in tissue, there had to be a way to use it in the clinic.

Extracting an Image

MRI grew from the shoulders of NMR through the epiphany of one man and the zeal and determination of another. There was nothing inevitable about the leap from NMR spectroscopy to medical imaging. But once it had been demonstrated that NMR could yield images of previously hidden regions within the body, a remarkable race for priority began.

The first entrant was Raymond Damadian, a dynamic research physician at New York's Downstate Medical School in Brooklyn. Damadian had grown up in nearby Forest Hills, Queens, the son of a French-Armenian mother and an Armenian father who had fled from Turkish persecutions at the turn of the century. He earned a bachelor's degree at the University of Wisconsin, then returned to New York where he studied medicine at the new Albert Einstein

Medical School, and went on to postdoctoral work at Harvard before joining the faculty at Downstate Medical Center.

In the late 1960s Damadian had become intrigued with the still controversial theory of biologist Gilbert Ling, who argued that water in malignant cells differs in organization from water in healthy cells. Damadian decided to analyze the water in different kinds of tumors using NMR. In 1970, he brought six tumor-infected rats to the nearest convenient facility, the laboratory of NMR Specialties in New Kensington, a suburb of Pittsburgh. At the lab he sacrificed the rats and removed pieces of their tumors to examine in an NMR machine set up to produce T_1 and T_2 readings. As Damadian had predicted, cancerous tissues differed from healthy tissue. Delighted, Damadian published his results in 1971: he had evidence that NMR spectra could distinguish healthy from malignant tissue. He addressed his research to pathologists, not radiologists, as a way to detect cancer in excised tissue. He did not mention using NMR for extracting an image.

These results, however, gave Damadian the idea for a new machine, and supported by a laboratory full of talented and devoted followers, he went to work. Damadian's group accepted his theory about the nature of the water in cancer cells (which was not accepted by others in the medical community, who could not replicate his experiment and dismissed the theory). Ignoring scoffers, in March 1972 Damadian applied for a patent for an "Apparatus and Method for Detecting Cancer Tissue," and announced he would build an NMR machine large enough to map an entire human body for the presence of malignancies.

At this time geophysicists were using NMR to measure the field of the largest magnet of all—the Earth—as well as large samples within the Earth's field. There was no indication that an NMR machine could be used to examine safely a large living organism, like a person. Simply as a matter of scale, it seemed impossible. Just to analyze a microscopic sample took a machine that weighed a ton. It seemed premature to imagine that a machine large enough to hold a whole human body could fit inside any existing laboratory or hospital.

There was also no evidence, one way or another, that it was safe for a human being to be subjected to powerful magnetic fields. It is true that Purcell had inserted his head into a magnet with a force of 2 Teslas in 1948 when testing NMR, and that he reported feeling only a buzzing emitted by the metal fillings in his teeth and tasting of metal, but his limited exposure was inconsequential in comparison to exposing a patient for an hour inside such a field. What, if anything, magnetic fields do to organic tissue is unknown. Researchers have operated on the principle that magnetic fields are harmless since life evolved and has flourished in one. Alarms have been raised, but generally dismissed, as over time there have been no ill effects reported from the magnetic fields themselves.

Damadian was not at all concerned about magnetic fields as he proceeded to build his machine. Supported by faith in the validity of his enterprise, he worked with a small budget that was supplemented eventually by a short-term grant from the National Cancer Institutes. When that ended in 1976, Damadian felt competition breathing down his neck. Despite the lack of adequate funding, his team pushed on. Then, in the summer of 1977—in the footsteps of Edison rather than Roentgen—Damadian preempted his scientific competitors. He called a press conference to introduce and demonstrate a whole-body NMR imaging machine which he called the "Indomitable."

Whether or not there really were contenders for this particular prize at this particular time is open to discussion. What is not debated is the fact that Damadian, with his vision of a body-size NMR machine, leaped from using magnets only large enough to examine tissue specimens in test tubes to building his own superconducting magnet with a bore (or opening) large enough to encircle a grown human being. No one else had the imagination, or hubris, to skip the in-between steps undertaken by others—examining first small mammals and then parts of the human body—and jump to the construction of a whole-body machine. That machine, as first conceived, would discern malignant tissue wherever it might be in the body, much like a body scan but without an image. In the years it took Damadian to go from filing his first patent in 1972, and receiving the patent in 1974, to building the Indomitable in 1977 and starting his FONAR company, CT had come onto the market and passed through its major developmental phases into the medical workhorse we now take for granted. At the same time, Damadian's original vision of a gigantic all-in-one shot body scanning machine to detect cancer had changed into a machine similar to the new CT scanner that used computers to reconstruct images of slices of the interior of the body.

Damadian's first machine, however, was not a new kind of tomography. That vision occurred to another scientist whose path would cross Damadian's apparently innocuously in the summer of 1971, but never without acrimony again.

Zeugmatography

The chemist Paul Lauterbur grew up in a small town near Dayton, Ohio, where he enjoyed the typical school life of a clever child, starting a high school science club and "doing all sorts of wild and crazy and dangerous things with chemicals."[5] After graduating from the Case Institute of Technology in Cleveland, he began graduate studies at the Mellon Institute in Pittsburgh while he went to work for the Dow Chemical Company. There, in 1951, he learned about NMR when a sales representative from Varian came to talk about developing new applications for NMR. Varian spurred the growth of NMR research because it incorporated the participation of its NMR researchers at conferences in basic science into its marketing plan, and it sent representatives to instruct and encourage chemists in the use of this new technology. Varian also ran an applications lab where sales representatives could demonstrate what could be done.

The approach certainly worked for Lauterbur. His curiosity whetted, he shifted career course abruptly when he was drafted into the army during the Korean War. Lauterbur was relieved to be assigned to the military's medical laboratories in Maryland. Here he had a second encounter with a Varian representative who was giving a seminar at the military lab. When the fiscal year 1954 ended, the lab found it still had money in the budget, and used it to buy an NMR machine.

By this time Lauterbur was well acquainted with NMR, and he continued to work with it while he completed his graduate studies after his discharge in 1955. In 1963 he joined the faculty of the State University of New York at Stony Brook. A few years later, in 1971, he was tapped by a struggling company, NMR Specialties, which was in trouble. NMR Specialties had been founded by a Varian field service engineer to continue producing a device that Varian had discontinued. Lacking a summer grant, Lauterbur accepted the job of both acting president and chairman of the board of the already insolvent Pennsylvania company. NMR Specialties was the company that Damadian had visited to get NMR readings on his six rats.

Lauterbur recalls first encountering Damadian when he discovered an order from Brooklyn for a superconducting magnet. Examining the sorry state of the business, and realizing that the company could not possibly produce the magnet, Lauterbur refused to fill the order. Damadian sees that cancellation as part of a long history of dirty tricks, deliberate sabotage, and outright theft that, in his view, was typical of the obstacles he confronted in his effort to invent MRI.

Lauterbur dropped by the company's lab to see Damadian's results and recalls thinking as he watched that there had to be a better way of using NMR clinically than excising tumor samples.[6] He flinched at the idea that patients in surgery would have "little chunks" cut out so someone could make NMR measurements while they waited. He dismissed Damadian's idea: judging from the rat experiments, it would mean putting NMR machines into operating rooms to do on-the-spot NMR biopsies.

He did not have Damadian's approach in mind at all later that summer of 1971 as he sat at dinner, pondering the fuzzy picture he had seen of a test-tube "phantom"—the object inserted for trial examination. NMR fields have to be as homogenous as possible, so chemists often spin their samples to expose them to a uniform field. He recalled that when an NMR machine is not finely adjusted, all sorts of weird shapes and lumps and line-splitting appear, artifacts that, somehow, have to be eliminated. It suddenly occurred to him that those lumps and bumps carried information, not only about the magnetic field, but about the sample as well.

Then, Lauterbur recalls, the proverbial light bulb went on. "Was there some way one could tell exactly where an NMR signal came from?" he asked. He answered himself, "*Yes!* by using magnetic field gradients." If a magnetic field varies from one point in the object to another, he reasoned, the resonant frequency which is directly proportional to the strength of the magnetic field will vary the same way. So, for example, if he made a magnetic field increase a little from his left ear to his right ear, the left ear would have one resonance frequency and the right ear would have a different one. With that in mind, he plotted out the resonance frequencies and deduced that he'd see a little ripple on one side for one ear and a little ripple on the other side for the other ear. That would give one dimension of information by reducing all the complexity in his head between his two ears to a single trace. But a single trace is not the same as a full image. He could get a full image by applying magnetic field gradients in different directions. How could he work back in three dimensions to a simple scan? Then the answer came to him.

"I ran out to a drugstore that evening and got a notebook—the best I could find—and wrote down these notes which then I had witnessed, September 2, 1971."[7] This was the beginning of what is now known as one-dimensional imaging. He could translate those single points of data from different places along the magnetic gradient into spatial information. This was a quantum leap beyond the kind of image Damadian was getting at this time, which had no spatial dimension. Lauterbur kept thinking about it until a few days later he figured out a better way. "And that is what turned out to be the kind of method Hounsfield later published for CT. Something called an algebraic reconstruction technique using iterative methods for projective reconstruction—I thought I invented a whole new applied mathematics field."[8]

Of course he hadn't. What he had discovered is a way to create images from NMR. He dubbed this technique *zeugmatography,* from the Greek for "joining together." He was describing the joining together of a gradient magnetic field and the radiofrequencing that corresponds to it in a single image.

That evening Lauterbur predicted in his notebook that his technique would supplement, and at times even replace, X-ray pictures. This was 1971, a year before the public debut of EMI's CT scanner. CT was about to appear as a working machine when MRI was only an idea on paper. The mathematics that Lauterbur thought he had invented was the same mathematics that Cormack had been struggling with for decades. As a chemist, Lauterbur was innocent of the problems that preoccupied both physicians and physicists.

Lauterbur's notebook, duly witnessed, is historically fascinating. But it did nothing for Lauterbur, who had written and dated everything with a patent in mind. Not discovered on university time, it was a summer epiphany. Lauterbur decided he should patent it through the foundering NMR Specialties company. A falling out with its lawyers was a costly setback, and when he finally submitted the patent to the university, the administration did not foresee enough return from his invention to repay NMR Specialties' lawyers. By this time a year had elapsed—the time allowed to file a patent after a discovery is recorded—so Lauterbur decided to give his insight to the world.

He sent off a short paper to *Nature,* the leading British scientific journal, which rejected his letter because it was too low-key, too self-effacing. He felt that they had not really understood its implications and dutifully rewrote it, asking for reconsideration, noting, "My manuscript announces a new principle of image formation, with innumerable potential applications in science, medicine and technology."[9] *Nature* responded this time by requesting a few minor revisions and published the paper in 1973. It included a description of rotating the magnetic gradient around the object and of combining the projections using computer algorithms similar to those used in the CT scan. It also included the first NMR picture of a 4.2 mm diameter test tube containing two water-filled capillary tubes.

This advance was followed two years later in 1975 by the discovery of Richard Ernst, a Swiss who had worked in Palo Alto at Varian Associates for over a decade.[10] Ernst, on his return to Zurich, introduced two-dimensional NMR, a way of quickly receiving digital information, which would play the next major role in turning NMR into an imaging technology.

Meanwhile, in Britain

Lauterbur's article attracted enormous attention within the specialized precincts of medicine and biochemistry. But just as Lauterbur had been unaware of Bracewell's and Cormack's mathematics, so the physicist Peter Mansfield at the University of Nottingham had been unaware of what Lauterbur had been up to. Perhaps it was a function of the increased specialization of science, but each discipline subscribed to its own journals, attended its own meetings, and used its own increasingly private vocabulary. Mansfield, a physicist, could not have been expected to read about chemistry, even in an interdisciplinary journal like *Nature.*

Raised in London during World War II, Mansfield had his early education delayed by wartime emergency evacuations. He studied physics at Queen Mary College in London and spent two postdoctoral years at the University of Illinois in Urbana. Finding himself behind his American peers, he buckled down. "It was a very useful period. It's something I recommend everyone do actually. To go off to a hard pile of land and struggle."[11] On his return to Britain in 1964, Mansfield accepted a position at Nottingham, where he continued studying the physics of NMR imaging.

His objective was remote from Damadian's, which was to map areas of malignant tissue with NMR, and very different from Lauterbur's, which was to focus on imaging liquids. In 1973 Mansfield published his first paper on NMR, "NMR Diffraction in Solids," which describes the principle of imaging of solids to the level of atomic structure. Using a vocabulary that differed from Lauterbur's, he recalled: "We came up with an elaborate mathematical explanation. What we did was we made a lattice. A model lattice of the material with a much coarser gradient. The principles behind that, of course, are exactly that this would have applications in biology."[12]

When he presented the paper at a physics conference in Poland, he "thought [he] was telling the world for the first time about imaging." Then someone in the audience asked if he was aware of Paul Lauterbur's work. He didn't know anything about it. "It was a bit of a bombshell to me," he recalls.[13] Mansfield had come up with the idea of a gradient very much like Lauterbur, only he had described it in terms of the physics of solids rather than the biological framework of largely liquid materials. His audience was aware of the multiple discovery, and unlike Mansfield, was sensitive to the medical implications.

Mansfield was describing imaging in a different dimension. "With the benefit of evolution and time, we introduced ideas in a mathematical framework for imaging so-called k-space. And when you talk to people today about how imaging works, they always talk about k-space trajectories." K-space trajectories, Mansfield says, is a way that physicists talk about imaging in what he calls "reciprocal space" instead of real space.[14]

What is significant is that he had zeroed in on the matter of imaging. After returning from Poland in 1974, Mansfield decided that imaging solids was too difficult, and he, too, turned to liquids—that is, to the human body—as simpler. Two years later his group displayed a good image of a human finger at a conference in Heidelberg. Damadian was also there showing images of mice, and seemed, to Mansfield, to be shocked by the high quality of the Nottingham group's images. In retrospect, Mansfield sees that this shock sent Damadian back to his lab to work even harder. Damadian was in a race with them all, and although Mansfield was not yet aware of it, he, too, was part of the competition. Not that it would have mattered, he recalls. Damadian already had a giant, whole-body magnet with which he intended to image a whole person. With only a small laboratory version, Mansfield was not running in the same event.

Mansfield, unlike Damadian, did not regard Lauterbur as an enemy, or even his major opponent, not because he was above the fray but because he had a raft of energetic competitors at home. He saw the race within national boundaries. There was E. R. Andrews in the neighboring physics laboratory at Nottingham. There was John Mallard in Aberdeen, Scotland, a research physician who hoped to get NMR images equal to those from CT, the standard against which NMR would be measured. (By this time EMI had moved into the third stage of the CT revolution and was selling an excellent machine.) And there was Ian Young at EMI's research laboratory in London who now, by 1982, had produced NMR images of every organ of the body using a different method of enhancing radio frequency signals. While Damadian and Lauterbur had been working doggedly along in New York, the British laboratories had set the pace throughout the 1970s.

Each British group had a special approach. Focusing on imaging large specimens, Andrews built an NMR machine that could accommodate a 10 cm diameter object—ten times larger than the commercial machines then available in Britain. Mansfield worked on speed—getting images in less time—and explored mathematical variations of data collection, that is, getting information from a whole line, or plane, in what he calls echoplanar, rather than from the single individual points Lauterbur had used. A variation of this approach would eventually trigger a second revolution in magnetic resonance scanning. Not yet satisfied that he had explored all the ramifications of NMR imaging, Mansfield's group would eventually explore the production of volumetric images, three-dimensional pictures that are not reconstructions from slices but receive data from three dimensions directly onto the computer screen.

At the same time Mallard, who had previously worked on tracking radioactive isotopes inside diseased patients, focused his NMR research on identifying cancer cells. A physician like Damadian, he, too, was eager to build a clinically useful whole-body machine. In 1976 he convinced the Medical Research Council to pay for the giant magnet he needed and ordered it from Oxford Instruments.

The most explicit arrangement was with EMI, which, while deeply involved in the production and ongoing development of CT, also supported another group of researchers in NMR. Mansfield recalls being asked to give a talk at EMI in London. He went, eager to meet Godfrey Hounsfield, only to discover that Hounsfield had not been told about his visit. EMI kept its research units separate and, unbeknownst to Mansfield, was in the process, as we have seen, of eliminating its entire medical instrument division in order to concentrate on music. But research continued in Britain nonetheless, where the Medical Research Council, encouraged by the privatizing forces in Thatcher's industrial-governing coalition, was willing to work out arrangements with industry.

Across the Atlantic, Again

Government grants were difficult to win in the United States. Damadian, who was not generously funded in Brooklyn, simply forged ahead and built his own superconducting magnet. (This was a gamble since all of his competitors were then using permanent magnets.) Damadian won a small grant from the National Cancer Institutes. So did Lauterbur, who later received additional support from the National Heart and Lung Institutes.

In Brooklyn, Damadian sought money in the private sector by filing at least twenty additional patents and by helping a journalist write a dramatic account of the way he had developed the Indomitable. Money was always a problem, which he solved finally by forming a company, the FONAR Corporation, with financial backing from family and friends. He sold FONAR instruments at radiology meetings but his role as corporate executive as well as doctor-inventor raised the hackles of colleagues whose associations with manufacturers were contractual, and less blatantly commercial.

By the end of the 1970s, physicians and surgeons whose imaging appetites had been whetted by CT scanning had become excited by the promise of magnetic resonance imaging. Ready to use it on patients, they distinguished the imaging technology from NMR, which was a tool for chemical research, and renamed it MRI. It is impossible to pinpoint the actual reason for the name change, or who implemented it. Mansfield believes that there was a major turf battle between radiologists and physicians in nuclear medicine—between those who read images from internal sources of radioactivity as David Kuhl was doing in Philadelphia at this time and those who implanted nuclear isotopes as therapy.[15] The more common explanation is that the change was made to avoid the word *nuclear,* with its connotations of atomic weapons, fallout, and total war.

Whichever the explanation, by 1980 American medical manufacturers eager to jump the line hired some of the best British scientists and engineers to staff their MRI laboratories and start-up companies. The center of activity, despite continued research in Britain, shifted to the United States, especially to the medical school of the University of California in San Francisco. Alex Margulis, chairman of the Department of Radiology at UCSF, had watched leadership in CT scanning in the United States go to the Mayo Clinic, Massachusetts General Hospital, and Columbia Presbyterian Hospital in New York. He was determined that with MRI, UCSF would take the lead.

Taking funds from his department's budget and from medical fees earned on the side, he leased space for this new research "away from Parnassus" (the real as well as metaphorical site of the medical school) in the adjacent municipality of South San Francisco. There he installed the physicist Leon Kaufman, whom he calls the scientific genius of the project.[16]

Describing how the San Francisco laboratory worked, Kaufman recalls that there was very little government interest then in supporting something for which there was no clinical plan. As it had been with CT, save for small grants from the NIH, American scientists, engineers, and physicians depended on private investors for support. The NIH was interested in basic science, not instruments. Kaufman explains, "When you go in for an NIH contract, the first thing they want is what's your hypothesis. Well, my hypothesis is I can make it work. When you're inventing a machine, you don't know *how* it's going to work. . . . Instruments don't have hypotheses."[17]

So in the beginning Margulis got funding from the Pfizer Corporation, the same pharmaceutical company that had marketed Ledley's ACTA whole-body CT scanner and American Science and Engineering's CT scanner with the Stein-Shepp algorithms. But neither scanner had earned any money for the company, so Pfizer quit the imaging business. Margulis then made a new arrangement with Diasonics, one that allowed his department to proceed with clinical research while developing better machines. Eventually Diasonics became part of the Japanese electronics firm Toshiba, where much of the original UCSF team continued to work.

An Englishman who worked with EMI in the 1970s has pointed out that industry and academia were intertwined to an extraordinary degree in the development of imaging machines.[18] While the basic ideas were largely in the public domain by the time industry entered the picture, industry developed them by subsidizing advanced research and hiring away experts in exchange for having a show-window for what it expected would be its new product. Large corporations invaded the field, notably Siemens and General Electric. The same companies that had exploited the X-ray earlier in the century stood ready and very able to refine these new machines and offer them to those doctors and hospitals with whom they had established generations of rapport.

Hovering in the wings, Damadian's FONAR Corporation attacked the giants more than once. Perhaps taking EMI as an example for its decade-long protection of its CT patent, FONAR used the courts continuously. But unlike EMI, FONAR did not successfully bluff its opponents into settlements. FONAR ended up in court with mixed results. It sued Johnson & Johnson over a cancer-detection patent and convinced the jury, only to have the judge set aside the verdict. In 1995 FONAR was awarded over a hundred million dollars in a suit against GE for patent infringement on the MRI, and is awaiting GE's appeal of the decision. Damadian continues to be a controversial figure in the world of medical instrumentation, and FONAR remains the "new boy on the block," with a list of products that includes CT machines and ultrasound.

Once Lauterbur, like Roentgen, had explained—without claiming patent protection (although he had tried)—how to take advantage of the irregularities in the magnetic field to reconstruct an image of the body's interior, it was only a matter of time before someone or some group of scientists would produce clinically useful pictures. According to Kaufman at the South San Francisco laboratory, "Radiologists basically will buy anything we make; they don't ask for it. We give it to them and they 'ohh' and 'ahh'."[19] It was simply a matter of someone willing to invest in building the machine.

In 1980, despite some impressive images from Damadian's machine, NMR machines were still not clinically useful. The push was still on to get higher resolution. The San Francisco group achieved this in 1981 when, according to Margulis, they "went clinical," with a system that could get whole-body images with millimeter resolution in a matter of minutes. But Margulis was not satisfied. In 1982, he ordered the largest and most homogeneous-field superconducting electromagnet ever made from Oxford Instruments, triggering a new generation of MRI machines (and incidentally stimulating superconductivity research in physics, coming full circle to where magnetic resonance research had begun).

By the early 1980s, most MRI hardware had been developed and the three theoretical contributions that explain why magnetic resonance can produce images of the body's interior were in hand: Paul Lauterbur's discovery that an image could be extracted from NMR data using single-line projection data—one-dimensional MRI; Richard Ernst's implementation of the mathematics of Fourier transforms that brought in data from two dimensions; and Peter Mansfield's echoplanar application that a decade later led to functional, or fast, magnetic resonance.

The Shadow of CT

Was MRI really powered by a fierce, no-holds-barred race that erupted into the name-calling confrontation that reputedly occurred between Damadian and Lauterbur? Or was Damadian an anomaly among scientists who usually affected a gentlemanly cordiality? The gloss of good manners has been exposed as just that—Roentgen, for example, chafed at Lenard's constant carping—and there are scores of examples across scientific disciplines.[20] Alex Margulis at UCSF has no doubts. "Of course there was a race," he recalls, and the contestants were all aware of it.[21]

A race, but toward what? What were the rewards that lured the participants on? Unlike the original X-ray, which seemed to appear out of nowhere, and unlike CT technology, which climaxed a seventy-year-long effort with grids and tomographs to use X-rays to see through anatomical obstructions, in the early days of NMR no one anticipated that nuclear magnetic resonance could be used to produce uncanny images of the interior of the body. A former student of Lauterbur's notes: "All good ideas seem inevitable in retrospect, but in fact there is nothing more ludicrous than trying to get spatial information out of NMR. If you look at what the goal was before imaging, every power you had was concentrated on removing spatial information from the data."[22]

MRI may not have been inevitable, but today, in hindsight, physicians, scientists, and engineers all claim to have taken it directly from Lauterbur's drawing board to clinical maturity. It is difficult to determine which group deserves primary credit. Damadian, Mallard, and Margulis are doctors who sought clinical applications from the start. They were primarily interested in treating the sick, but they were not oblivious to the money that an imaging system that did not rely on radiation could earn, either for themselves, or for their laboratories. Nor were they fearful that the high price of such a machine would discourage potential customers: the response to CT scanners had proved that the market was there. In 1982 Kaufman predicted a rapid drop in CT sales. "Ironically," he told the *New York Times*, "the acceptance of million-dollar CAT scanners paved the way for the equally expensive NMR imagers."[23]

Most of those involved in developing MRI were convinced early on that it was better than CT. Some begrudged what appeared to them to have been the accidental arrival of CT on the market first, preempting the budgets of many clinics. Paul Lauterbur confesses to a favorite thought experiment.

> If suppose, for whatever reasons, somebody worked out how to do magnetic resonance imaging and it had suddenly blossomed before anyone figured out that you could do similar things with X-rays, and then someone else came to the NIH and to GE and said, "You know, we can do the same sort of things with X-rays. It's going to give people a tremendous radiation dose and the bone is going to obscure a lot of the soft tissue detail and you can't really see as clearly the differences in soft tissues, and you can only figure out how to get transverse planes in the head instead of all these 3-Ds and all the different slices that show up so beautifully in the MRI, but gee, we'd like to develop it anyway." Would the Federal Government have smiled on that? Would the grants have been forthcoming? Would there be companies willing to sink their money in it? Not likely. It would have been stillborn.[24]

From Kaufman's point of view, however, it is hard to imagine MRI without CT. "By '75 he [the department chair] had already gone through two CT scanners, thrown away a $400,000 one and gotten a $500,000 one." So when his group asked for a $100,000 magnet, it didn't sound so crazy. "CT paved the way for MRI by proving that you could sell a very expensive piece of equipment to this market. Without CT there probably would be no MRI. It's the frame of mind. It's not technology."[25] An economic frame of mind.

Marketing MRI

The frame of mind in every self-respecting emergency room and every radiology department by 1980 demanded at least one CT scanner. Never before had hospitals been willing to spend so much on a single instrument. Budgetary priorities had changed—not everywhere, but in the United States where a consumer-driven system did not ration medical dollars in any systematic way. (In all other medically sophisticated nations, governments oversaw spending.) Manufacturers could count on consumers to help push early models into obsolescence as they demanded the latest machines from their doctors.

MRI sales representatives liked to point out that MRI has few moving parts. Once installed, MRI machines can be upgraded by changes in software. Nevertheless, the early instruments, especially those with superconducting magnets that used liquid helium as a coolant, cost two or three times that of a CT scanner. For that price, MRI had to reveal a great deal about the interior of the body that X-rays couldn't.

In the first years of MRI, many hospitals were reluctant to invest in yet another expensive machine, because they were still paying for their CT scanners. Besides, many MRI machines were clumsy and the images often fuzzy. Compared with CT they were slow, expensive, and the final images, though usable, were simply not as clear.

While it is true that MRI machines last a long time, the initial costs are high, depending on the kind of magnet selected, the resolution of the image, and whether or not a special building has to be constructed or a standing building has to have shielding added to protect people and property from the enormous magnetic field. At first there was a generalized fear that the powerful magnets and radiowave frequencies would warp radio reception, even in cars driving past the MRI machine. There was also the worry that metal watches, buttons, paper clips, and even staples would fly every which way in the strong magnetic field (which is true, but only for the immediate area where the instrument is installed). These hardware considerations leveled out or disappeared as the technology reached some kind of equilibrium. But the economics of distribution, investment, and the way doctors practice medicine determines the real costs, and these are shifting.

CT was a hard standard to equal, let alone exceed. Physicians accustomed to CT insisted that MRI produce equally crisp anatomical images. CT bestowed the gift of a high standard of diagnostic picture, but it came with strings attached. Professional independence, long guarded by physicians, had been breached by government in ways that many doctors were getting used to. It began with the inauguration of Medicare and Medicaid, federal funding that guaranteed care to the old and poor, but opened the door to government control over costs. The Food and Drug Administration, which monitors the safety and efficacy of all medical products, initially approved MRIs only for research. And because Medicare and most private insurers will not reimburse for experimental procedures, the FDA's action kept a lid on sales of MRI machines until 1985, when it decreed them no longer experimental.

Another impediment were the certificate of need (CON) regulations passed by states and local authorities to reduce duplication in expensive medical technologies. When a hospital sought to purchase an MRI machine under the 1974 National Health Planning Act, it had to show that nearby hospitals did not already provide the service. Teaching hospitals often received the benefit of the doubt and access to the newest instruments, but in some parts of the country, especially the East Coast, these regulations severely limited distribution of MRI machines. All over the United States the new regulations had unintended consequences.

Just as radiologists had moved into hospitals in the 1920s, so in the 1980s and 1990s, as hospitals slimmed down and out-patient services increased, some radiologists picked up and moved out to independent imaging centers. These freed them from the constraints of CON laws, and in some states proved profitable because imaging centers could be owned by the referring physicians. Within two years of FDA approval, more than half the machines were in imaging centers.

Wherever they are, MRI are expensive. Machines cost over a million dollars (depending on the strength of the magnet). Even if the "pass-through" time the time it takes to get pictures of a single patient—can be reduced from an average forty-five minutes to something more like the fifteen minutes of CT scans, and even if the machines are in use all day, the cost will most likely remain higher than CT and ordinary X-rays for some time. Insurers question their need for routine examinations and they wonder, as they wonder about CT, if some are not prescribed to fill up the time of the myriad machines that seem to flourish in high-rent areas, especially in California, which boasts more MRI machines than all of Canada (with nearly the same population), without a commensurate difference in the level of health and longevity.[26]

About Magnets

Magnetism is to MRI what radiation is to X-rays, the word in the name that denotes invisible power with mysterious ramifications. The strength of magnets is measured in gauss and Tesla units. The magnetic field of the Earth is half a gauss, and there are 10,000 gauss to a Tesla. The magnet in a telephone earpiece is capable of producing about 30 gauss. The first machines used permanent magnets (except for Damadian's).[27] Since then most instruments use superconducting magnets whose strength ranges from one-half to 4 Tesla, that is, from 10,000 to 80,000 times the magnetic field we are exposed to in the ordinary course of things. The most powerful magnets produce images with the highest spatial resolution. Spatial resolution is a function of gradient steepness and field homogeneity. Powerful magnets improve the sensitivity of an image, but they can obscure that same image by producing chemical shift artifacts—ghosts of things that are not really there. Machines with as much as 10 Tesla are used in laboratories with animals and provide

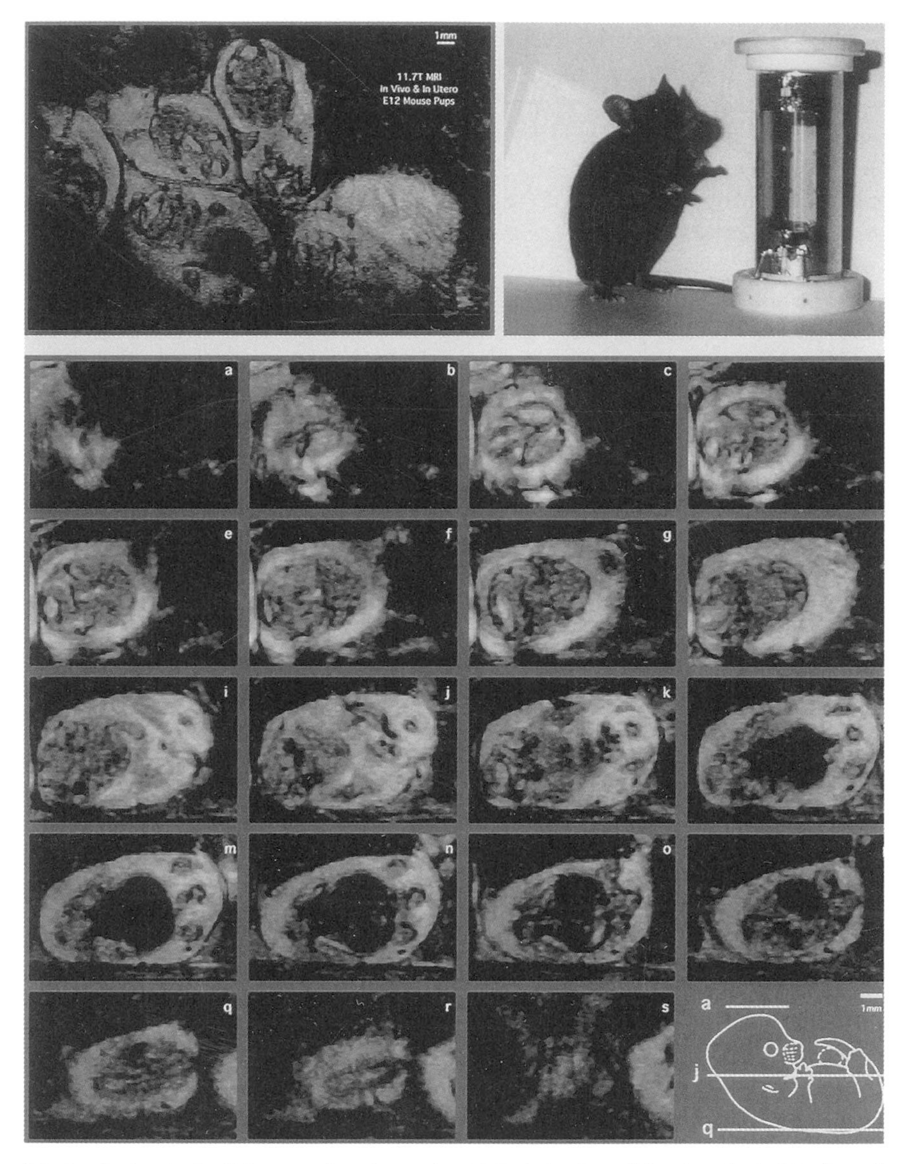

34. Fetal mice in the living womb as imaged at 12 Tesla by Russell Jacobs, Mark O'Dell, and Pratik Ghosh. Courtesy of John Allman, California Institute of Technology.

appreciably better resolution than machines used clinically. This degree of resolution is not necessary to image a knee or elbow, but could conceivably revolutionize the study of disease—if high magnetic field strengths could be shown to be harmless to the patient. So far, exposure to fields up to 4 Tesla seem safe.

Researchers in medicine and in neurobiology may volunteer to be scanned by MRI a hundred times, but they are reluctant to use the instrument on pregnant women because of the unknown effect on fetuses. Likewise, the

FDA has limited the strength of magnets that can be used clinically for adults, and made the strength less for children, without explaining its reasons for these limitations. And these standards differ from country to country, the British allowing stronger magnetic strength for clinical use than the Americans. These limits are drawn from negative results. So far nothing has happened from short-term exposure to any strong magnetic fields.

But like exposure to ionizing radiation, the long-term effects of intense exposure to strong magnetic fields may not be discernable for many years, and even then it may be hard to determine causality. On a more practical level, experience has already demonstrated that high-powered magnets do not have to be located in deserted lots, although they do have to be buffered to protect computer equipment and other instruments that are susceptible to distortion from magnetization. Accidents resulting from a lack of respect for the power of magnets occurred episodically from the late 1980s through the early 1990s.

All of these were attributable to human error, the most common being a result of the blind persistence of people to behave as if what cannot be seen is not there. A common fault has been people simply ignoring the warning signs that ask everyone near an MRI machine to stow all metal objects. From time to time random individuals, including doctors, technicians, and support staff, have been sideswiped by flying objects caught in the magnet's powerful field. The list of incidents is long, but no one has been killed by an object swept into the magnet. Close calls have involved the introduction of an oxygen tank into the MRI room, which became a missile, crushing the patient's face;[28] and the crash of a forklift, with its operator aboard, drawn into the side of the machine—about which incident one witness observed, "You really have to work at it to be that stupid."[29]

During its formative years MRI developers witnessed other problems, including excessive heat that could, and did, raise a patient's temperature, and excessive cold, when the helium that cools superconducting magnets accidentally boiled off, producing a "quench." A quench could (but has never) suffocate everyone in the room.[30]

Horror stories pervade the lore of MRI. Although they are mostly fantasies of might-have-beens, occasional real incidents keep physicians alert, such as two cases in California. The first occurred in San Jose in 1990 when a metalworker entered an MRI machine for a brain scan, and came out blind. The presence of microscopic metallic particles in his eyes caused irreparable damage when exposed to the magnet. (Since then all candidates for scanning are quizzed about their exposure to metal grinding.) The second happened in 1992 when a seventy-four-year-old woman with multiple medical problems arrived in a California facility to have her head scanned.[31] The neuroradiologist had been dubious about the procedure because he doubted the usefulness of the scan and because he knew she had an intracranial aneurysm clip in an artery from an operation fourteen years earlier. When the patient was still four feet away from the gantry, but well inside the 1.5 Tesla magnetic field, she complained of a headache. She was immediately escorted from the room and placed on a

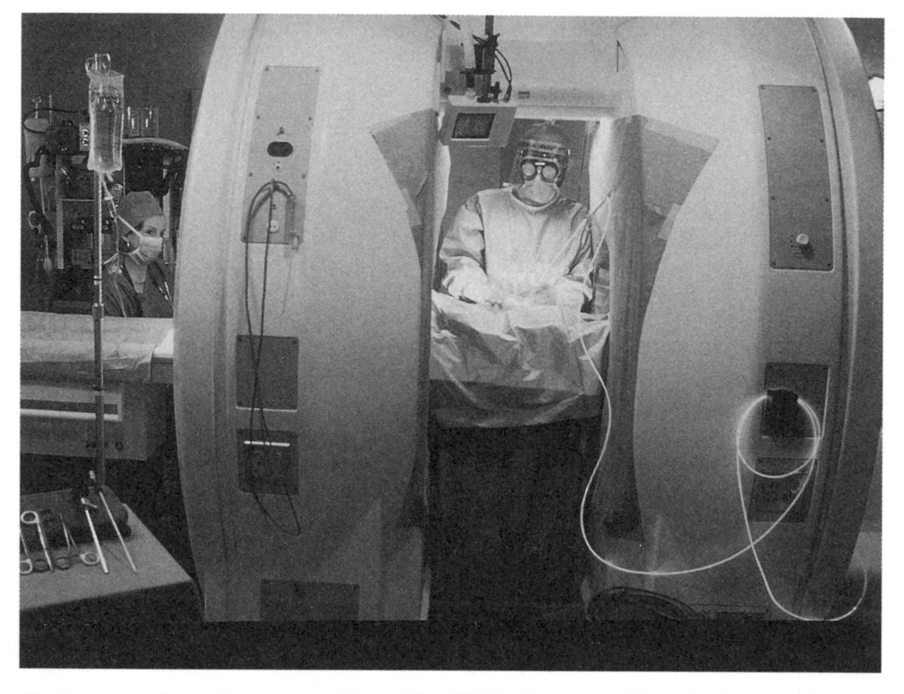

35. Surgery performed in an open MRI machine (1995). Courtesy of GE Medical Systems, Europe.

stretcher. She soon was unable to speak, sank into a coma, and within twenty-four hours had died. The autopsy revealed that the surgeon had misrecalled the kind of clip he had used. The clip contained stainless steel and, in the strong magnetic field, had pulled free of the artery, causing the fatal hemorrhage.

Eventually it should be possible to eliminate all metallic devices (excepting pacemakers) from the physician's armamentarium, and then these accidents will become historical oddities. Surgeons are already beginning to operate with nonmetallic tools inside of new open MRI machines. These machines are constructed so there is space to work within the magnetic field. Whole new sets of tools have had to be developed to avoid all magnetic metals, and the GE system does not use liquid helium.[32] Hardware aside, the major leap has been in computing, which produces almost real-time images on a screen so that the surgical team can actually see their instruments inside the tumor as they work to remove it.[33]

It is comparatively easy to keep iron objects away from MRI machines, but the presence of naturally occurring iron is problematic. Iron, of course, is plentiful in the human body, most notably as ferritin (an iron oxide) deposits in the brain and as part of the hemoglobin molecule in red blood cells. The amount of ferritin increases throughout life, visible first in MRIs of six-month-old infants, and especially visible in patients with Alzheimer's disease (a condition which has been described as the "rusting of the brain").[34] But ferritin is not magnetic and not susceptible to the effects of a powerful magnetic field, nor is the iron in hemoglobin.

However, magnetite, sometimes called lodestone, is. And this is the kind of iron crystals that Joseph Kirschvink, a geobiologist at Caltech, has found in the bloodstream and isolated from the human brain. In 1992 his laboratory isolated brain magnetite for the first time. The amount synthesized by the brain is small—5 nanograms per gram (5 billionth of a gram)—but discernible. It may be vestigial, but it, too, is known to increase with age, whatever that may mean, and may account for some of the "blips" in MRI images of the brain. Kirschvink is still trying to identify the particular brain cells that contain the miniature magnets, and to see where the magnetite is inside those cells. Elsewhere he has found significant quantities of magnetite—500 nanograms per gram—in certain tumors. The role of magnetite in the body and the effect, if any, that powerful magnetic fields may have on human health is still unknown.[35]

For the moment, MRI looks very good, but not perfect. There may be inherent limitations. The procedure is usually slow and most machines are not suitable for emergencies. It is difficult to image patients hooked up to larger machines, such as ventilators that enable patients to breathe. Another group of patients who present a challenge are those with pacemakers which must be inactivated before allowing the patient inside the magnetic field, and still others have metal artifacts inside their bodies. Part of the population is claustrophobic and cannot endure the enclosed machine, although here, too, open MRI machines may alleviate this problem.

Users looking at the two technologies, CT and MRI, might well weigh the dangers of both instruments. The memory of the X-ray martyrs is powerful, and their ghosts hover over every imaging machine. On the one hand is the familiar beast of ionizing radiation. Although the individual collimated X-ray beams in CT scanners do not often endanger the area around the target with diffuse radiation, it is still radiation, and no thoughtful physician would routinely order CT scans without judging the health costs of exposure.[36] The shadow of the first decades of X-ray machines is a reminder that there may be a second shoe here too. The shadow may be larger than the machine, for with the exception of avoidable incidents, MRI has not harmed doctors, technicians, or patients, and many people can and have been scanned frequently, with no evidence of any lasting effects.

The MRI Brain

Just as the court in Rouen in 1896 was able to use the X-ray to convict the brawler of attempting to kill the milkman, MRI scans have provided damning evidence of a condition that once did not have a name, and of a crime that went unmentioned. That crime is baby shaking; it causes acute brain damage, and often death. It was first described by John Caffey, a New York pediatrician who became a radiologist and coined the appropriate, but seldom used, acronym, PIT (Parental Induced Trauma).[37] In a landmark paper in 1946, he presented over twenty years of X-ray evidence of injuries and fatalities that could not be explained away as accidents. Caffey wrote: "Physicians refused to believe that the parents, who were often their trusted friends, could be guilty of such dastardly offenses to their own flesh and blood."[38]

Caffey documented the telltale fractures that came from swinging a child by an arm or leg. Eventually CT scans confirmed these multiple fractures—often in the same place on the same limb, but which in the process of healing reveal a pattern that cannot be dismissed as the result of "accidents." Studies of injured children whose histories suggested that they could have been abused showed that CT scans and skull X-rays alone can only detect occasional rib fractures. Caffey speculated that some infant head trauma is a result of abuse, and he documented "whiplash shaken baby syndrome," in a series of cases where infants died of brain damage and intracranial bleeding with no surface marks.[39] He suggested that these children were victims of severe shaking.

This was mere supposition until MRI scans of living, often comatose, infants suffering from severe seizures, retinal hemorrhages, or subarachnoid or subdural hemorrhages in the brain provided evidence of the kind of brain dislodgement which could only occur after violent shaking. Pediatric neurologists disagree about whether the rapid acceleration-deceleration in whiplash shaking can, by itself, cause mortal damage, without leaving external bruises. But, for babies younger than three months, babies whose heads are still large in proportion to their bodies, and whose necks have underdeveloped ligaments and musculature, the evidence of murder by shaking is conclusive. MRI scans can reveal intercranial injuries that indicate that violent shaking alone is enough to cause permanent injury or death. And MRI scans can also reveal a lack of such injuries, exculpating parents who have been wrongfully accused.

The diagnosis is good medicine, but it is seldom sufficient to interfere legally with parental custody. In most instances of child abuse those responsible for the injuries never acknowledge guilt. In one case, however, a mother who was convicted but given a suspended sentence for involuntary manslaughter lectured from her own experience on the dangers of baby shaking. As much as 10 percent of all mental retardation and cerebral palsy in the United States may result from this kind of abuse. MRI provides excellent diagnosis, but offers little hope to the tiny victims.

MRI brain diagnosis has benefited thousands of other patients, including those suffering from the once mysterious history of attacks of partial paralysis, blurred vision, and blind spots that had been diagnosed tentatively as multiple sclerosis. Until MRI, the confusing symptoms of MS could only be verified by autopsy. X-rays cannot show the destruction of the myelin sheaths around diseased nerve endings, but the white areas of lesions on the myelin show up clearly with MRI. MRI can discern the number and location of lesions and to some degree predict the course of the disease, and the possibility that a case may respond to new treatments.

MRI can also successfully identify a condition called normal pressure hydrocephalus, a dementia most common in older patients that mimics the loss of mental powers of stroke and Alzheimer's victims. This dementia, however, is caused by excessive flow of cerebral spinal fluid that, in effect, deforms the brain, and once the cause is detected, the relatively simple procedure of inserting a brain shunt allows a patient who may have been demented for years to walk away from the hospital as if reborn with renewed mental acuity.[40]

While the average MS patient visits eight doctors before getting an accurate diagnosis,[41] the average person with Cushing's disease could visit twice as many doctors. Cushing's and the related agromeglia (gigantism) are diseases of the pituitary gland, the small bean-shaped organ locked inside the sella turcica (the part of the skull at the base of the brain). The pituitary controls almost every body function by regulating the thyroid gland and sexual hormone production. A pituitary tumor can affect growth, causing gigantism, dwarfism, or

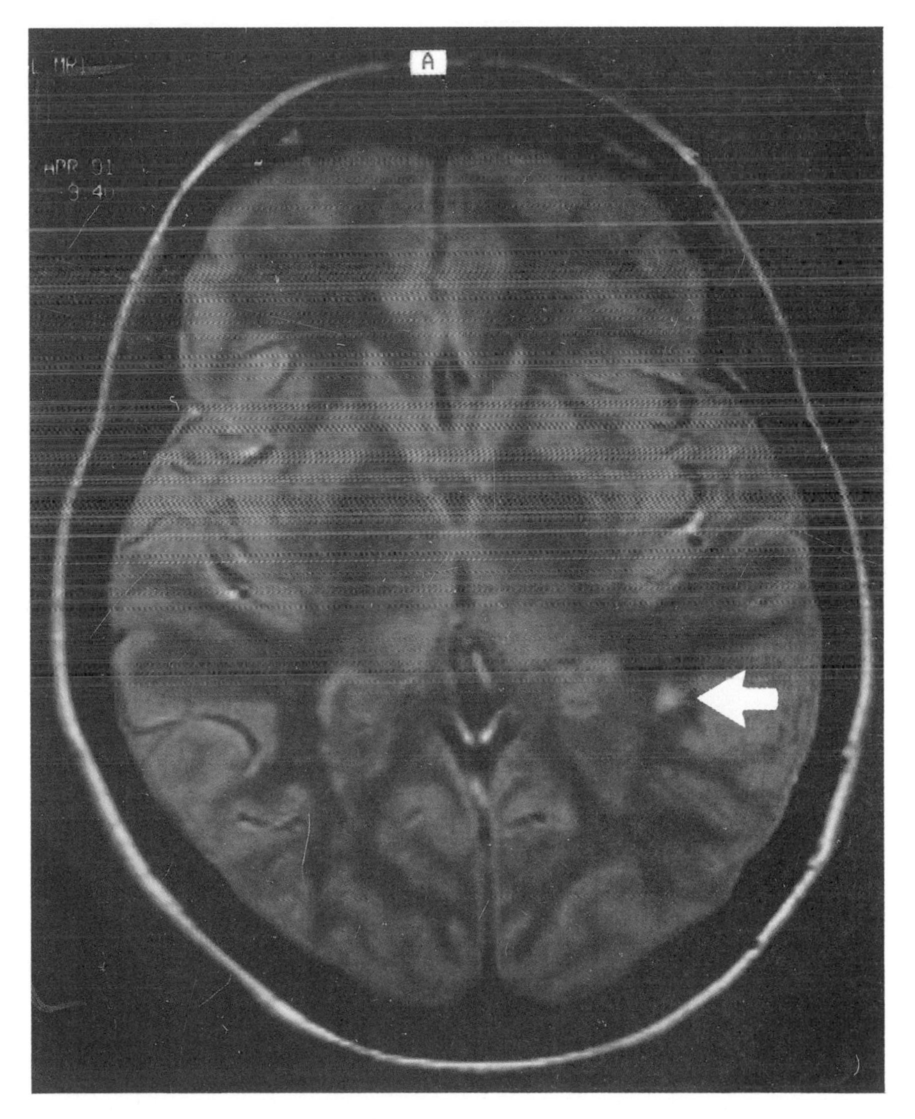

36. MRI of multiple sclerosis. Lesions in the brain are shown with arrow. Courtesy of Dr. William G. Bradley, Memorial MRI Center, Long Beach Memorial Hospital, Long Beach, Calif.

huge weight gains that put life-threatening pressure on the heart. Symptoms vary and many people wander through a maze of referrals before they find the medical detective, usually an internist or endocrinologist, who, suspecting severe pituitary problems, sends the patient for an MRI. Pituitary tumors are visible only by magnetic resonance, but once they have been identified and removed, the patient returns to life as it was before the gland went awry.

Unaided, MRI gives remarkable images. Blood—hemoglobin—is a natural contrast agent. But the use of chelates (compounds that combine with metals of rare earths), especially gadolinium molecules, as contrast agents enhances the scope of MRI in a way that parallels the introduction of iodine-based contrast media for X-rays during the 1920s. Gadolinium salts are paramagnetic (they act like magnets) compounds that by themselves are toxic, but when surrounded by a chelate can remain in the system as long as twenty-four hours with little effect on most people. Gadolimides act like an arrow targeting diseased tissue in the MRI-generated magnetic fields, so they produce a higher resolution.

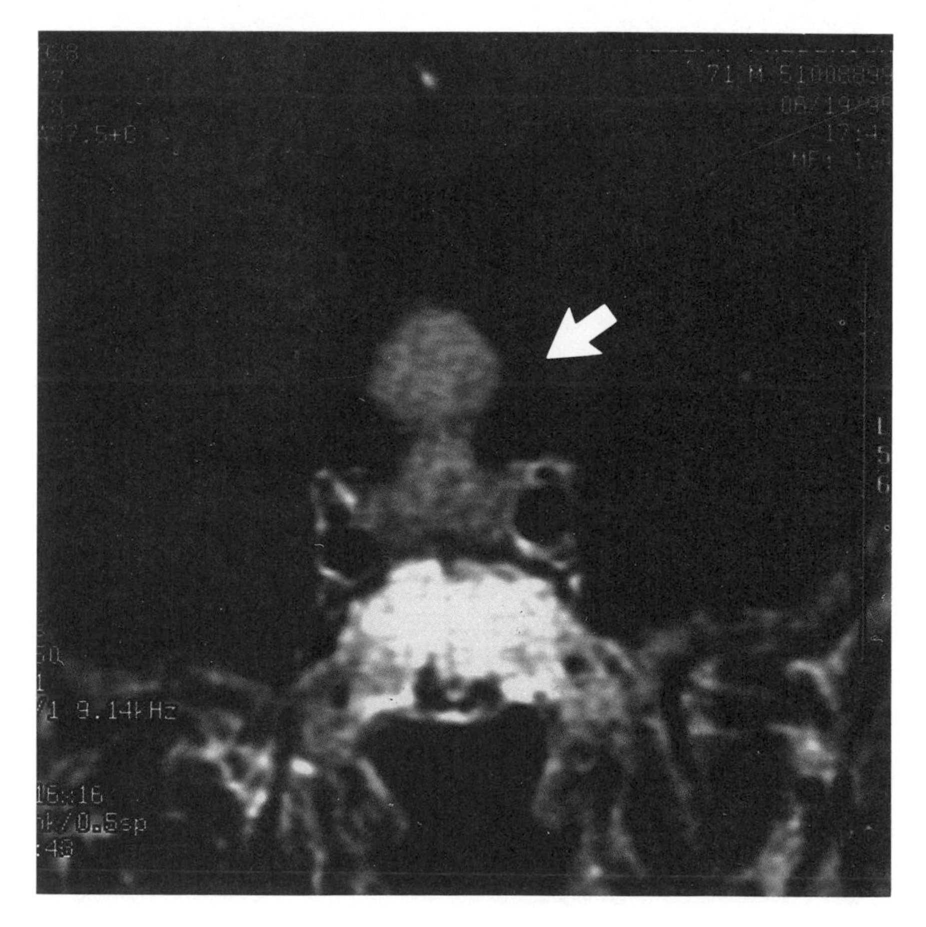

37. MRI of brain with pituitary macroadenoma. Arrow indicates the large tumor (1995). Courtesy of Dr. Martin H. Weiss, Department of Neurosurgery, University of Southern California.

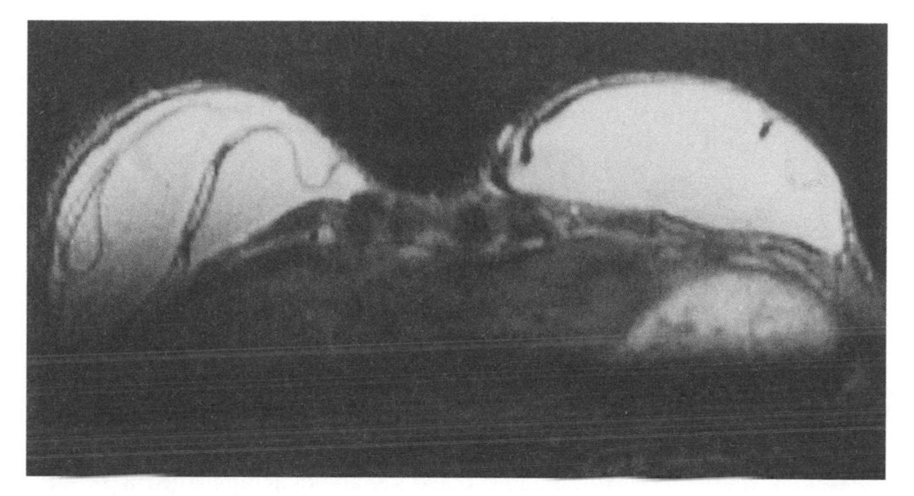

38. Ruptured silicone implant in right breast (left in image). Courtesy of Dr. William G. Bradley, Memorial MRI Center, Long Beach Memorial Hospital, Long Beach, Calif.

Although gadolinium injections increase the cost of the image, they enable MRI specialists to get a more diagnostically useful picture.

MRI deploys images from body territories which had remained dark to other kinds of illumination. The list is awesome: soft tissue cancers spring to light under MRI, as do knee injuries, breast lesions as well as the paths of escaped silicon from breast implants. Wherever there is water in the body, MRI can detect its presence and get a picture. MRI is another level of vision, exposing the workings of the most hidden, vital—and soft—organs, the brain and the heart. MRI has shifted our sense of transparency so that we can see those structures whose form and function had previously been the domain of poets and philosophers.

Fast MRI

Orthodox MRI images are very sophisticated tomographs, cross-sections or planes inside the body, and unless colorized, are black and white like Roentgen's original pictures. Anatomical snapshots of living tissue, they are exactly what surgeons need to plan operations, but they do not show the organ functioning. For that purpose researchers managed to develop a technique akin to the fluoroscopic images that were captured on film in the 1930s: fast magnetic resonance imaging (fMR). Using sophisticated MRI machines with computers able to handle complex algorithms, fMR captures these fast-flowing pictures on a computer screen. At 30 to 100 frames per second (faster than the 24 frames per second of motion pictures), this speed enables MRI to capture biological or metabolic processes in the living brain.

The possibility of such rapid images was suggested by Peter Mansfield's echoplanar method in 1977. Whereas ordinary MRI data is acquired line by line, fMR acquires and processes data from an entire plane through the body at one time. Speed is advantageous because it can avoid distortions caused by the motions of living like breathing, heartbeats, blood flow, intestinal movements; or by movements of patients too ill, or restless (like children) to keep still during an ordinary MRI examination, which lasts about an hour.

Aware of the rewards of rapid imaging, MRI research teams all over the world, including Mansfield's in England and several in the United States, explored approaches to getting "snapshots," or movies, of vital processes. Using upgraded MRI machines with powerful computers, they took off from the knowledge that brain activity stimulates blood flow.

The initial breakthrough in the race for fMR came from Seiji Ogawa, a physicist at the AT&T Bell Laboratory in New Jersey.[42] Using animal models in an MRI machine, he wanted to see what happened to the radiofrequency signals when the brain functions; he knew the change had to be very small, but he suspected it could be detected. Unlike Mansfield, who was looking for a way to image the beating heart, Ogawa was interested in understanding the nature of the MRI signal itself. Beginning with an effort to understand the signal, he ended up, in 1989, publishing a paper about gradient echo MRI in the brains of rats.

He worked with the knowledge that activated brain cells use more oxygen than cells at rest. When someone performs a task, the brain cells involved summon oxygenated blood, which, after giving up the oxygen, becomes deoxygenated. This venous blood, lacking a bound oxygen molecule, is paramagnetic, and when placed in a magnetic field changes the magnetism all around it. The amount of change depends on the supply of deoxygenated blood. This distortion of the magnetic field, in turn, affects the magnetic resonance of nearby water protons. It amplifies their signal as much as 100,000 times. Ogawa called this effect BOLD—Blood Oxygenation Level Dependent—contrast imaging. From looking at the signal, Ogawa had discovered a key to rapid MRI. The proportion of oxygen was reflected in the hydrogen in the water molecules. The fMR images, especially those acquired with magnets stronger than 4 Tesla, offer remarkable images of the brain in action.

In 1991, Ogawa collaborated with neuroscientists at the University of Minnesota who were doing research with human volunteers. Knowing that mental stimulation increased blood flow, the team was able to image increases in signal intensity in five- to ten-second intervals after their subjects had seen flashing lights or made figure-eight movements with their hands. At the same time, an MRI group at Massachusetts General Hospital in Boston was successfully using a gadolinium-based contrast medium with similar computer software to capture fast images. They eventually adopted the BOLD approach instead of the contrast agent because it is totally noninvasive and can be used on subjects for as long as they can hold still in the claustrophobic MRI machine. BOLD was the breakthrough to fast MRI. According to the neurobiologist John Allman at Caltech, "There were a lot of us up at bat, but Ogawa made the home run."[43]

Ogawa's method may yet be replaced by another approach, but he and his colleagues are the first to have found a way, without using contrast agents, to track not only *where* brain activity occurs, but *how* it works using MRI. How much activity is involved, and what exactly is being measured, is still not completely understood. But fMR's conquest of speed, reduction of background noise, and elimination of unwanted artifacts is enabling physiologists to track metabolic processes in the heart, the brain, and in the fetus without any apparent deleterious effects.

Developing in tandem with MRI, which focuses on imaging hydrogen nuclei, is MR spectroscopy (MRS). The nuclei of all elements with uneven numbers of protons will theoretically respond to an appropriate radio frequency. MRS, which is largely experimental, images phosphorous, hydrogen, carbon, and nitrogen molecules. It has been used to study cell death as well as cell rejuvenation. In cases of children resuscitated after near death from drowning, physicians are able to track the changes in the lactate levels, predicting either recovery or further brain deterioration.[44]

When a seventeen-year-old Navajo girl with an eight-year history of progressive muscle weakness was examined with MRS that tracked the phosphorus in her blood, the study revealed a tremendous deficit in phosphorus metabolization. Once identified, her deficiency was treated with vitamins K and C which enabled her to attain almost normal muscle control. Tracking phosphorus enabled physicians to see the malfunctioning of her system at a molecular level, and to prescribe treatment that was not a cure, but a way around the problem that enabled the patient to live in reasonable comfort.[45]

MRI technology is developing on several fronts: spectroscopists and computational experts are working on increasing speed and increasing signal-to-noise ratios to get sharper images; engineers are developing safer and less costly magnets using liquid nitrogen instead of liquid helium to cool high-temperature superconductors; Mansfield and others are developing volumetric images that differ from orthodox MRI imaging by producing real-time images that are not reconstructed from slices, but process data from three dimensions.

A team at Caltech has pushed the limits of Constant Time Imaging, another three-dimensional volumetric approach to imaging solids.[46] They used an 11.7 Tesla NMR machine to reveal the three-dimensional structure of a molar removed from the fifty-year-old skull of a young woman. The image exposes the layers of the tooth down to the dentine, in resolutions of 100 microns (a micron is a millionth of a meter). They have successfully demonstrated that a powerful enough magnet, over a long enough period of time, with the right mathematical algorithm, can extract information from a laboratory specimen that has a mere trace of water and obtain a volumetric, three-dimensional image of a solid object.[47]

MRI, with its multiple imaging possibilities for both structure and function, promises a future of radiation-free opportunities to see the interior of the human body. The enthusiasm of its researchers is contagious, and they well may have a completely risk-free technology whose only limitation is the properties of the protons themselves. The actual images that MRI provides cannot be understood by amateurs, but the educated eye grasps a vision of a world without supports—organs floating on their own in a black sea.

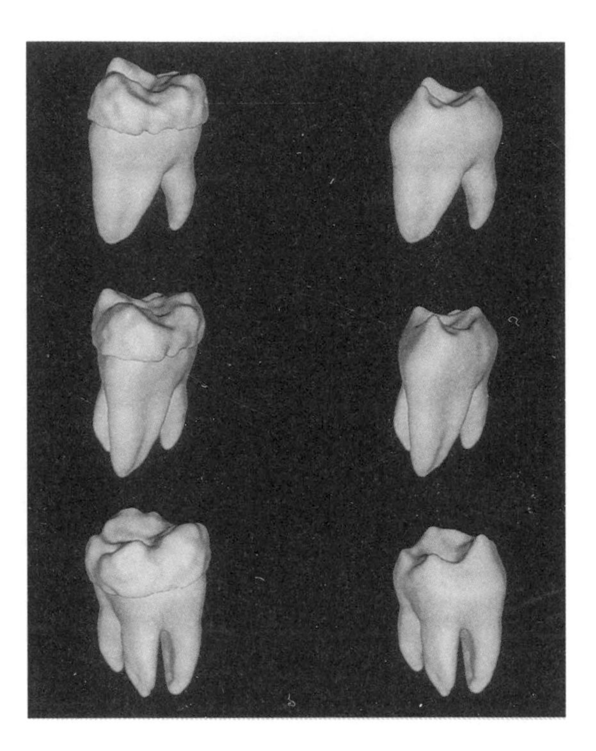

39. MRI of human molar by Pratik Ghosh (1995). The roots and air-dentine-enamel interfaces are easily distinguished. Computational removal of the enamel crown allows direct examination of the morphology of the dentine cap; it is here that the structure of the crown is initially determined as tooth development progresses. Courtesy of Pratik Ghosh.

In a bow to the cabarets in 1903 that featured dancers carrying glow-in-the-dark radium-filled cocktails, MRI has even found its way onto the New York stage. In 1994, the Feld Ballet featured a new production called *MRI.* In this abstract dance, the figures moved up and down in a metal cage because, as Feld explained, "changing the relationship of gravity changes the nature of time."[48] One critic likened the ballet spiritually to Auden's poem about "the body beneath the skin."[49] Another, more scientifically, wrote, "By referring to the medical diagnostic technique magnetic resonance imaging, Mr. Feld reportedly wanted to present the equivalent of objective data, to reveal images hidden below the surface without commenting on them."[50]

By 1994 MRI had become a catch-phrase for all medical scans. Representing the general confusion of the educated public, the critic in *New York Newsday* thought she was clarifying the technology when she commented: "MRI stands for 'magnetic resonance imaging'; you may have seen the initials if you've ever had a CAT scan." MRI had become synonymous with all imaging innovation and with its intimations of mystery, new age spiritualism, and hi-tech machines.[51]

Nine

From the Inside Out

PET (Positron Emission Tomography) in Nuclear Medicine

George Hevesy, a young Hungarian physicist, arrived in Manchester, England, in 1911 to learn the new techniques that the great Ernest Rutherford was using to study electrons. When he was asked to separate the radioactive isotopes of lead from a pile of ordinary lead ore—a procedure we now know is impossible by chemical means—he was stymied. But making the best of a bad situation, he grasped triumph from the jaws of defeat by turning the radioactive isotopes into tracers.

Hevesy had found a room in a boardinghouse and, familiar with such hostels, he suspected the integrity of its cuisine. One Sunday evening to satisfy his curiosity he performed an experiment. Bringing the laboratory to the dinner table, he added a speck of the radioactive metal to the fresh meat pie. The following Wednesday he brought an early radiation detector, an electroscope, to dinner and demonstrated to the collected guests that the leftover meat—marked with radioactive lead—had survived the chopper and the oven and been returned to the table in the form of a soufflé.[1] By "tagging" the pie, Hevesy had "traced" the meat through the kitchen back to the table. Some decades in the future similar tracers would enable scanners to obtain images of the body, from the inside out.

Seventeen years later and half a world away, the neurosurgeon Harvey Cushing at the Peter Bent Brigham Hospital in Boston examined a patient who complained of headaches, failing vision, and most curious of all, a loud blowing sound inside his head whenever he used his eyes. Cushing operated but could not remove the vascular malformation he discovered near the man's visual cortex; when he closed the skull, he left a small bony defect sticking out beneath the scalp. This protrusion enabled Cushing to hear, and even record, the blowing sound (called a *bruit*) which increased in volume every time the man used his eyes to read. In the annals of brain research, this case remained a unique demonstration of the close connection between blood flow and cerebral function until 1983 when radioactive tracers, which Hevesy had pioneered, were used in the form of PET (positron emission tomography) scans to record and map the functioning of sight.

The development of PET is the story of the merging of two separate technologies: the first, which began with Hevesy, is the creation and manipulation of biologically safe and useful radioactive tracers that have to be swallowed, inhaled, or injected into the body; the second, which began twenty-five years later, is the construction of instruments to detect those radioactive sources inside the body and from those signals extract tomographic pictures.

PET differs from the other computerized imaging technologies in the preponderance of physicians, or scientists employed in or collaborating with medical laboratories (who were sensitive to the hazards of radioactive isotopes) among its inventors. They solved the initial ethical dilemma of finding a human subject by following the medical tradition of experimenting on themselves. Hevesy was the first person to swallow radioactive deuterium. Indeed, some of these isotope pioneers were surprised, as the years passed, to discover that the radiation illnesses they had presumed would occur, never, in fact, did.

When Hevesy began his research in earnest after World War I, he was limited to a handful of naturally occurring radioisotopes, like the lead he had used to expose his landlady's recycled leftovers. Physicians in the 1920s simply moved their new Geiger counters manually over the surface of the patient's skin to track where these substances had gone. Like Bell's effort to "sound out" the bullet inside President Garfield, doctors listened to, rather than watched, the signals from their detectors.

In Copenhagen, and later in Freiburg, Germany, Hevesy explored the uses of radioisotopes by growing bean plants in a solution containing radioactive lead. At intervals, as the plants matured, he measured the radioactivity of their roots, stalks, leaves, and beans, in effect following the course of the leaded solution through the growing plant. This simple experiment, for which Hevesy received the Nobel Prize for chemistry in 1943, established three crucial principles: first, that radioisotopes of elements participate in biochemical and physiological processes in the same way as the chemicals they have replaced; second, that organisms absorb material selectively—the bean plants only absorbed the lead that was in the nutrient they needed, not as much nutrient as was available; and third, that there is metabolic turnover, that organisms continually cycle the substances they absorb—the lead isotope, having entered the plant, did not stay there indefinitely but passed through at a predictable rate; moreover, while it remained in the plant, it decayed at a predictable rate.

This discovery had a practical application after the disastrous meltdown at the Chernobyl nuclear power plant outside of Kiev, Ukraine, in 1986. One of the radioactive isotopes released was iodine. Polish health authorities distributed potassium iodide to people living beneath the path of the radioactive cloud, because it concentrates in the thyroid gland. They knew that once the thyroid was filled with as much potassium iodide as it could absorb, there would be no room for any additional iodine from radioactive fallout, that the "good" iodine would remain in the thyroid long enough for the "bad" iodine to lose its radioactive punch.[2]

Hevesy continued to work with naturally occurring radioisotopes, using lead, bismuth, thallium, radium, thorium, and actinium as tracers, but none of these elements plays a role in the normal development of living organisms. Then, in 1934, Irène and Frédéric Joliot-Curie bombarded the nuclei of nonradioactive elements with high-energy atomic particles and produced the first artificial radioisotopes. Then everything changed. Within a short time there were radioactive isotopes of sodium, phosphorous, and iodine.

The next year Hevesy fed these radioisotopes to laboratory rats and established, on autopsy, that the isotopes had, in each case, gone to particular organs and tissue. This demonstration triggered what would become an avalanche of new radiopharmaceuticals—radioactive isotopes that home in on and label specific organs. Physiologists were able at last to trace specific metabolic functions inside the human body.

At the same time, Ernest Lawrence at the University of California's Radiation Laboratory in Berkeley used his ingenious new cyclotron—a circular accelerator—to bombard a host of elements with high-speed neutrons. Inspired by the Joliot-Curies, Lawrence produced a radioactive isotope of sodium which could be introduced harmlessly into the body, and over the next few years he manufactured another seventeen biologically useful radioisotopes.[3]

John Lawrence, Ernest Lawrence's physician brother and an ardent supporter of the use of radioisotopic tracers, recalled the feelings of excitement and apprehension that accompanied this work in the mid-1930s. He could not forget the tragedies of radium workers and remembered making trips to New Jersey to confer with the doctor who had attended "the radium dial painters who later developed aplastic anemia, osteonecroses, and osteogenic sarcomata." These visits convinced him that artificial radioactivity would not produce the same diseases because these isotopes were not permanently deposited in bone or tissue.

All the same, no one knew what the biological effects of working with the cyclotron might be. One study made in 1935 predicted the postnuclear reactions of victims exposed to enormous dosages of radiation such as those at Hiroshima, but these developments were only theoretical. In 1955, John Lawrence wrote, "As a matter of fact, in the 20 years since we first used artificially produced radioisotopes in humans, we have not run into delayed effects or complications as some of the skeptics predicted we would."[4]

In 1939, physicists in America mulled over the implications of a German report that when uranium atoms were bombarded by neutrons, they released energy as their nuclei broke apart. The discovery of nuclear fission stimulated physicists in the United States to consider the possibility of a nuclear explosion and to initiate what became the Manhattan Project to build an atomic bomb. Among the accomplishments of the project was the creation of nuclear reactors which produced, as by-products, short-lived radioisotopes.

World War II was not a radiologist's war, but the development of the atomic bomb was to have important repercussions for medical imaging technologies. After the explosions in August 1945, the United States was in the nuclear weapons business. At the Manhattan Project, Colonel K. D. Nichols foresaw a "virtually unlimited production" of isotopes and suggested they be distributed to "outsiders," by which he meant doctors.[5] The Atomic Energy Commission (AEC) agreed and announced in *Science* magazine on June 14, 1946, that isotopes were now available for research. On August 2, the AEC shipped radioisotopes to hospitals around the country.[6] Medical use of radioactive isotopes became the tip of the iceberg of nuclear research, the part that the public could see and that the AEC wanted to talk about. These isotopes became the cornerstone of the public relations program that became the "atoms for peace" program seven years later during the Eisenhower administration.

Positrons Are Different

Extracting an image from radioactive isotopes was not part of the original plan. That plan focused on distributing isotopes that could be used in therapy, such as iodine, which would go immediately to the thyroid and destroy tumors there. The instrument that would eventually extract a tomographic image from an internal source of radiation began to evolve in 1951.

In 1975, positron emission tomography scanners reached the clinic. The term *positron* refers to the particular particles that the scanner records. Detected for the first time in 1932, positrons are the positive antiparticles of electrons, having the same mass. In the course of radioactive decay, positrons are emitted from the nucleus of some atoms along with protons and neutrons. The positron travels a short distance and collides almost instantly with an electron. They annihilate each other, and in the process produce two photons, or gamma rays, that shoot off at 180-degree angles from each other.

This "coincidence" phenomenon is the key to the way a PET scanner works. A ring of electronic detectors, connected to a computing system, surrounds the body which has absorbed radioisotopes. Whenever two detectors at opposite sides of the ring are hit by photons at the same time, we can infer that a positron must have been emitted from inside the body. Then, using the same mathematics developed for CT, the computer reconstructs a picture of the spatial density of the area where the radioisotopes have come to rest.[7]

Emission refers to the place where the signals originate inside the body. Unlike CT or MR, the PET technique involves putting something into the body—radioactive molecules—and then tracking their position on the inside from the outside. Emission imaging differs from both CT and MR because, in PET, the source that emits radiation is also the site that is being imaged. In contrast, CT and MR are *transmission* techniques.

The T stands for *tomography,* in that PET makes images of planes through the body. But unlike either MR or CT, the aim is not to produce images of anatomical structures of the particular slice of the body being observed. Instead PET tracks metabolic functions. The image itself is a kind of graph, a two-dimensional map on a computer monitor. Each pixel corresponds to the projection of a unit of volume in the body. Each pixel also represents a third dimension, a quantity, presented in the form of brightness, color, or grayscale that reflects the rate of flow of the radiopharmaceutical over a period of time.[8] This allows physicians to watch the flow rate of blood or the position of the tracer in the heart or lungs. Most astonishingly, they can track the way different parts of the brain use energy in the course of a mental process, recalling a particular face, doing a calculation, reading an unfamiliar word—in short, thinking.

Toward a Machine

The first step toward PET was a machine built by the physicist Benedict Cassen at the University of California at Los Angeles in 1951. Cassen, a man of many interests, was a good friend of William Oldendorf, with whom he would chat often about the engineering problems of medical, especially radiological, instruments. Flush with the gift of radioisotopes from the AEC, the UCLA medical physicists focused on the best way to track and record radioactive emissions mechanically. Cassen's idea was to link isotopic readings with the new photomultiplier tube.[9]

The photomultiplier tube (in the image intensifier) had just revolutionized the whole practice of radiology by, among other things, allowing ordinary movie cameras, at last, to capture moving pictures of fluoroscopic images from the new, extremely bright, scintillating screen.[10] Cassen replaced the hand-held Geiger counters with photomultiplier crystals, and harnessed them to a motorized arm attached to a pen. The automated pen recorded the relative number of gamma rays emanating from the isotopes inside the scanned area of the subject's body, moving back and forth over a grid placed on top of the area he was studying, zigzagging down, a line at each sweep, like a television beam. Cassen's "scintiscanner" produced a crude picture of the spatial representation of, for example, a radioactive thyroid gland, as tracks on carbon paper.

The scintiscanner was the state of the art until replaced by the "photoscan," which was invented in 1954 by David Kuhl, who was then a medical student at the University of Pennsylvania. Kuhl would later make the first transmission image of the lungs of a naval astronaut. But the transmission scan was only a detour for Kuhl on his way to perfecting *emission* images.

Throughout the summer of 1954, and over the next few years, Kuhl spent all his spare time tinkering in the hospital basement. Kuhl's photoscan captured the image of a patient's thyroid by sending the output from the photomultiplier tube directly to a moving beam of light and from there to a sheet of photographic paper or film. The photoscan registered different intensities of light, producing images that radiologists could examine in the conventional X-ray viewing boxes that they were accustomed to using.

Kuhl had actually begun to think about medical imaging while still in high school in Berwick, Pennsylvania. As a teenager, he had explored the distribution of uranium compounds in the bodies of mice by autoradiography. This is a process in which the experimental animal is injected with radioactive material, then sacrificed and its freshly killed body laid out in slices on X-ray film.[11] The exposure provides an image of the distribution of radioactivity similar to images now generated by CT. The clarity of those images remained a goal as Kuhl continued to build increasingly sophisticated emission detecting machines.[12]

Applying for a grant to the National Institutes of Health in 1959, Kuhl described his vision as "a whole new concept of scanning body organs in a manner analogous to body section radiography" using radioisotopes.[13] In the next few years he built a series of scanners, all bearing the name Mark, such as Mark I, Mark II, and so on (a tradition carried over from the military, he supposes). He was especially encouraged by the work of two of his former teachers at the University of Pennsylvania: Louis Sokoloff and Seymour Kety.

Sokoloff had practiced his first specialty, psychiatry, while on active duty in the army in the mid-1940s, but he became disillusioned with the talk therapies then in fashion. Convinced that mental illness arose from biochemical disturbances, Sokoloff returned to Penn to work with his former teacher, Kety, a pioneer in measuring cerebral blood flow. Sokoloff continued Kety's investigations when Kety became the first scientific director of the combined research programs at the National Institute of Mental Health and the National Institute of Neurological Diseases and Blindness, and in 1953, joined him at the NIH. During his years in Washington, Sokoloff developed the technique of using radioactive isotopes to track blood flow as well as the concentration of labeled substances in the brain. In 1955 his studies of the effects of retinal stimulation in cats were the first examples of imaging local cerebral functional activities.

In 1957 Sokoloff began experimenting with a radioactive analogue of sugar, a molecule with the awkward name "2-deoxyglucose," that approximates glucose consumption in the brain. He suggested it could be used as a tracer for studying cerebral blood flow because, like glucose, it would go to whatever part of the brain needed energy most. Almost twenty years later, in 1979, Kuhl and two colleagues, Alfred Wold and Joanna Fowler, figured out how to attach radioactive fluorine to deoxyglucose. This new radio-labeled chemical, FDG, quickly became the most frequently used short-lived radiopharmaceutical because it enabled PET to image the brain at work.

By the 1970s, the pharmaceutical branch of what was now called *nuclear medicine* had successfully pioneered the use of oxygen isotopes to track blood flow throughout the body. The instrument makers were hard at work, too, and increasingly better detectors suggested that emission methods would take the lead in medical imaging. The teams, scattered in hospital laboratories throughout the United States and Europe, were unaware that EMI was about to launch CT, and alter the playing field.

Nuclear Imaging and SPECT

The simple mapping of internal organs with radioactive tracers for medical purposes began with Hevesy in the 1930s. The development of injected radioactive tracers was accelerated by the discovery of technetium in the new Berkeley cyclotron before the end of that decade. But radioisotopes were not used routinely until 1961 when, starting with technetium, which became the warhorse of scanning, radioactive isotopes were radiotagged to chemical carriers, creating radiopharmaceuticals. Thus tagged, radiopharmaceuticals are used to scan almost every vital organ. These scans are not glimpses of the insides of the body, and are not really images. Rather, they highlight "hot" or "cold" areas, recording either functional or anatomical changes. They resemble silhouettes rather than three-dimensional pictures of the body's interior.

The invention of actual three-dimensional emission imagers began with the announcement of the first SPECT machines in 1968. SPECT (Single Photon Emission Computed Tomography) was the most versatile, convenient, and relatively inexpensive imaging technology of this new generation of machines and the first triumph of emission imaging. It evolved out of SPET (Single Photon Emission Tomography), Kuhl's first system for mapping photon emissions from internal radioactive substances, which did not use computers. He used cameras, which he kept steady while rotating a patient. The cameras recorded photons as single lines of data which were back-projected onto a film cartridge that rotated in synchrony with the patient. These projection strips were then built up into pictures, as Bracewell had done with data "strips" of sunspots.

By adding a computer (and eventually a rotating camera with an immobile patient), Kuhl turned SPET into SPECT—the C standing for the computer—and got a crude, but useful, three-dimensional image of the distribution of radioisotopes in an organ.[14] In 1972 Niels Lassen, in Copenhagen, began using SPECT to track blood flow in the brain to map function, especially the way movements by the right hand activated areas in the left cerebral cortex. Lassen also introduced the use of color into the computer-reconstructed images.[15] Ever since then the use of color in all computerized imaging has been a matter of controversy. Those who defend it point out that there is no light inside the body so that there is no "real" color or real illumination to be reproduced and the use of color dramatically delineates one kind of tissue from another. Opponents deride its use, asserting that color exaggerates the differences between tissue and is really used for public relations and to attract investors.

Two years later at Berkeley's Donner Laboratory, Thomas Budinger presented the first study of a patient with quantitative SPECT. Budinger, who had earlier in his career studied oceanography and helped map underwater icebergs, found his interest in visualization redirected to a different kind of unmapped territory—the brain. Under his direction, Berkeley's lab would perfect SPECT and, turning to PET, generate the highest-resolution images of any PET scanner.

SPECT, which provides a generalized tomographic image by using rotating cameras (or a single camera) to detect and reconstruct gamma-ray emissions, can use only a limited number of radioisotopes.[16] Relatively inexpensive and easy to operate in a clinical setting, SPECT is the most frequently used emission-scanning technology all over the world.

Yet SPECT has major drawbacks. Its images have only half the spatial resolution of PET, and in some instances individual pixels are so large they give the impression of a Cézanne landscape.[17] This limits its use for delicate organ mapping. Moreover, SPECT exposes the whole body to small doses of radioactivity for periods as long as several days. The length of exposure is a result of using isotopes with a shelf-life long enough to be shipped to hospital pharmacies. These over-the-counter isotopes are a cheaper, but less subtle tool.

The Center of the Road: PET

In the United States, with the blessings of the AEC, scanning experiments with positron detectors were part of the research protocol beginning in the 1950s at the National Laboratories of Brookhaven in New York, the Donner Laboratory in Berkeley, and at medical-school laboratories in St. Louis, Los Angeles, and Philadelphia. During a joint trip to Brookhaven, Gordon Brownell, a physicist at MIT, and William Sweet, a neurosurgeon at Massachusetts General Hospital, became fascinated with the possibilities of positron detection. By 1952, they were operating the first positron scanner to image brain tumors in patients. They would place the patient between two detectors, one on each side of the head, and the machine recorded data when both detectors were hit simultaneously. Alan Cormack tried then to interest the team in his computerized tomographic algorithms, but Brownell was indifferent. Like Kuhl at Penn, that failure to see that there was a connection between transmission scans and emission scans contributed to the delay in making PET until EMI demonstrated the CT scanner in 1972.[18]

British physicians, who also had access to cyclotrons, were likewise interested in emission tomography. London's Hammersmith Hospital, with its tradition of medical instrument innovation, attracted Americans interested in postdoctoral research. It was there that two American visitors who would play leading roles in PET scanning, Michel M. Ter-Pogossian and Henry Wagner, met in 1964. They discussed working together to develop PET, but they couldn't raise enough money. Wagner went on to head the PET program at Johns Hopkins University, where almost twenty years later, under his leadership, the first imaging of a dopamine neuroreceptor, the focus of degeneration in Parkinson's disease, took place.[19] Ter-Pogossian went on to head a program at Washington University in St. Louis, where the first PET scanner would be built eleven years later.

Research in nuclear medicine continued apace in Great Britain, France, and Scandinavia where radioactive isotopes were available from their respective national nuclear power programs. There would be constant feedback between the European and North American laboratories with a surprising lack of secrecy or overt competition, perhaps because clinical applications did not seem promising, and there was relatively little money invested in the research. Chemists manufactured radiopharmaceuticals where medical facilities had access to cyclotrons, which in the United States meant that PET research was centered at UCLA and Berkeley in California, at Massachusetts General Hospital in Boston, and at the Mallinckrodt Institute in St. Louis, all laboratories attached to research-oriented medical schools.

The breakthrough occurred in St. Louis in 1973. Ter-Pogossian had installed the first hospital-based cyclotron there in 1964 and had pushed ahead with research in positron scanning. By 1972 his group had built a cumbersome positron imaging device that looked like a helmet spiked with 26 detector probes. Everyone called it the "lead chicken."[20] The chicken did not capture much of a picture because the researchers had to process the data manually. They did not yet have the algorithms that would make a computer useful.

A year later, following Hounsfield's publication of his description of the CT system, PET investigators like Kuhl realized that the image-retrieving formulas that worked with *transmission* tomography—passing rays through the body—would also serve *emission* tomography—tracking the radioactive source within.[21] Then it was only a matter of time before two assistant professors in Ter-Pogossian's laboratory, Michael Phelps and Edward Hoffman, both chemists, disassembled the clumsy lead chicken to salvage its probes and rearranged them as a hexagonal array. Phelps and Hoffman linked the hexagonal detectors electronically so that a positive signal registered only when two opposite detectors picked up a positron at the same time. The computer stored these signals and then processed them mathematically, employing formulas like those used in CT scanning—first an iterative algorithm and later Fourier transforms—to reconstruct a slice. This process was dubbed PETT (positron emission transaxial tomography) in a paper published by Phelps and Ter-Pogossian in 1975.

Phelps, a former Golden Gloves boxer whose pugilistic skills may explain his combative approach to science, had worked out the considerable computational and engineering problem of PET. But he clashed with the hierarchy in Ter-Pogossian's laboratory, which he described as having a different ethic because it was medical rather than purely scientific, and where he, as a junior member of the staff when he solved the PET instrument problem, had to share credit with the laboratory director. In 1975 he and Hoffman left to join Kuhl at the University of Pennsylvania. The following year, 1977, Phelps, Hoffman, and Kuhl moved to UCLA where they secured a strong beachhead for PET and nuclear medicine.

Throughout these improvements in theory and practice, the symbiotic connection between the development of the PET machine and the development of radioisotopes continued. The usefulness of the machine depended on the ingenuity with which complex molecules were tagged. Detectors became better at extracting data and reconstructing images as radioisotopes underwent a revolution of their own. Once thought of as "throw-away" by-products of nuclear reactors whose very short half-lives made them useless therapeutically, short-lived radioisotopes came to be recognized as ideal tracers. Ter-Pogossian, for example, had encouraged his laboratory to use isotopes like Oxygen N15, which decays in two minutes, and Fluorine N18, which decays in two hours, because he recognized them as excellent ambassadors to diseased organs that could be used with the cumbersome "lead chicken."

Researchers first targeted the iodine-hungry thyroid gland, then moved on to the heart, and then to the brain. The next major advance came from the 1979 production of the radiopharmaceutical FDG, or deoxyglucose, the key to both clinical explorations, especially of Parkinson's and Huntington's diseases, and activational studies of the working brain. The subsequent development of additional radiopharmaceuticals targeting specific neuroreceptors has helped in the study of Alzheimer's disease, depression, anxiety, schizophrenia, pain, and drug addiction.

By the mid-1980s the hardware of PET scanners and radiopharmaceutical manufacturing had reached a stage where the emphasis shifted from invention to fine-tuning and simplifying the machinery to make it less cumbersome and simpler to operate. Well ensconced in government laboratories, PET thrived as a research tool; but the efforts of its advocates to move it into the world of clinically accepted procedures that are reimbursable by Medicare and private health insurance were not very successful, and for that reason PET remains an expensive option.

The Market

PET faced a series of problems that neither CT nor MR confronted when it moved into the world of the clinic. First of all, PET requires more skill to produce and to interpret, and skill is not cheap. Because the radio-tagged molecules used in PET have very short half-lives, the intensity of the radiation they emit rapidly diminishes as the molecules move through the body. All the time that the isotopes are accumulating in the targeted areas, they are losing radioactivity. Figuring out precisely how to measure the fading radiation of short-lived radioisotopes as they head to their targets requires complex kinetic mathematics, which translates into dollars to pay for mathematicians.

PET was also different from CT and MR in its financial base. Where the other technologies developed on the margins of state subsidies and had to wait for the right moment to win private investment, from the start PET was funded, organized, encouraged, and distributed by the U.S. government. The AEC (later the Department of Energy, or DOE) funded the research at the Argonne National Laboratory in Illinois, the Brookhaven National Laboratory in New York, the Oak Ridge National Laboratory in Tennessee, the Donner Laboratory at Berkeley in California, and at Los Alamos in New Mexico. The DOE eventually supported work at universities including UCLA and UC Berkeley, the University of Chicago, Harvard's Massachusetts General Hospital, the University of Michigan, University of Pennsylvania, University of Rochester, and Washington University in Missouri.

In 1979 the National Institutes of Health gave grants to support research in clinical applications, complementing DOE's support for improved instrumentation and the transfer of PET technology to industry. Although sales of PET scanners never ballooned like the sales of CTs, they held steady until 1995 when the market for all medical instruments sagged. The major PET producers are now the same companies whose names have been associated with imaging for almost a century, Siemens and General Electric, who, by the end of 1995, had placed a PET scanner within two hundred miles of most Americans.

It is doubtful that there would have been any PET without considerable government support. However, what the government provided with one hand, it withheld with the other. While the NIH and DOE used PET in research, the Health Care Finance Administration, which administers Medicare and Medicaid, did not cover any PET procedures until 1995. Many private health insurers did pay, however, impressed by PET's ability to distinguish different kinds of heart disease, to determine the viability of heart tissues in preparation of bypass surgery and transplants, and to identify metastatic cancers.

PET and Cancer

The newest generation of PET scanners in the early 1990s introduced whole-body PET into the imaging competition. It was often a matter of comparing apples and oranges, and PET found itself competing with other forms of nuclear scans, such as SPECT, where the resolution is several times larger but the expense several times smaller, or with the other functional imaging technique, fMR. Whole-body PET is used almost exclusively for cancer detection; it can discover metastatic tumors as well as track the functional development of cancers. Moreover, PET can monitor the success or failure of chemotherapies as the various drugs are introduced in the body, rather than waiting weeks for symptoms to appear.

In treating a malignancy such as a brain tumor, PET provides information about the regional chemistry of a tumor and can detect changes before any structural signs are visible. This kind of early diagnosis precludes evaluations

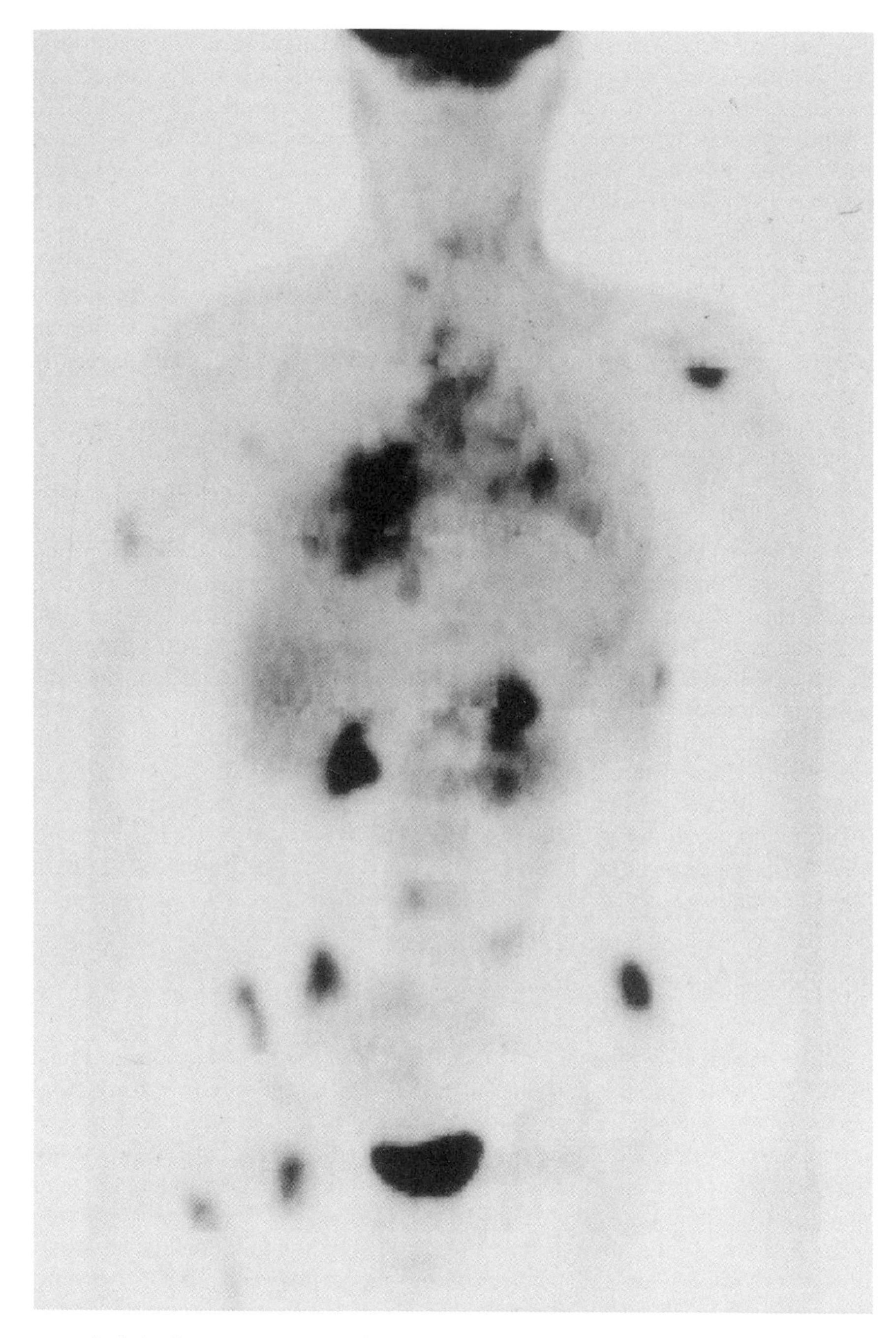

40. Whole body PET/FDG study of patient with widely disseminated anaplastic thyroid carcinoma (1992). Courtesy of Dr. Peter Conti.

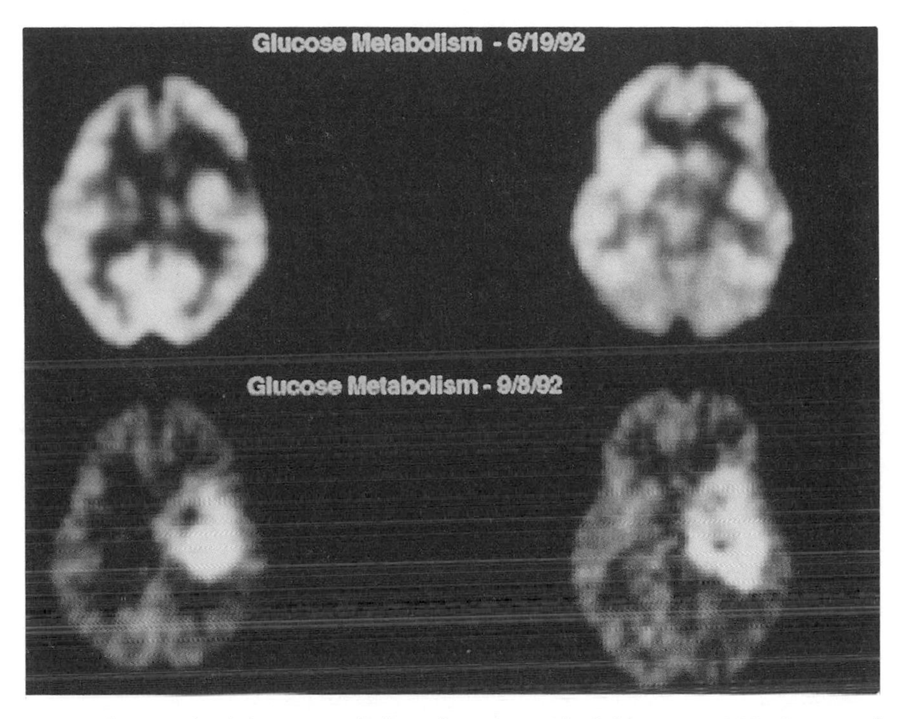

41. Serial PET study of glucose metabolism of a patient with glioblastoma (1992). Courtesy of Dr. Peter Conti.

based on biopsies and clinical responses. Oncologists can assess the effectiveness of surgery, radiation, or chemotherapy in treating tumors early, and modify treatments if necessary.[22]

Research has shown that tumors are seldom homogeneous in the same patient, and a combination of radiotracers injected serially offers an opportunity to profile multiple biochemical processes. These have included markers O^{15} for water, and FDG for glucose. This list may, in the future, be expanded to measure other substances that prove appropriate for evaluating particular tumors.[23]

Exploring disease at the molecular level is one of the great advances in modern medicine. The physicist Karl Darrow once said, "One of the things which distinguishes ours from all earlier generations is that we have seen our atoms."[24] PET specialists Henry Wagner and Peter Conti have this in mind when they point out that our bodies are made of combinations of atoms—molecules—which, with PET, can now be tracked. Cancer, they explain, has traditionally been seen as an invasion by something foreign into the body, to be destroyed or excised. Their view is that everyone is constantly in danger of developing cancer, but that normal control mechanisms keep it from happening. They define cancer as a failure of normal controls, and its treatment the restoration of these mechanisms. The real mission of PET, they believe, is to help physicians see the process of restoration as it takes place.[25]

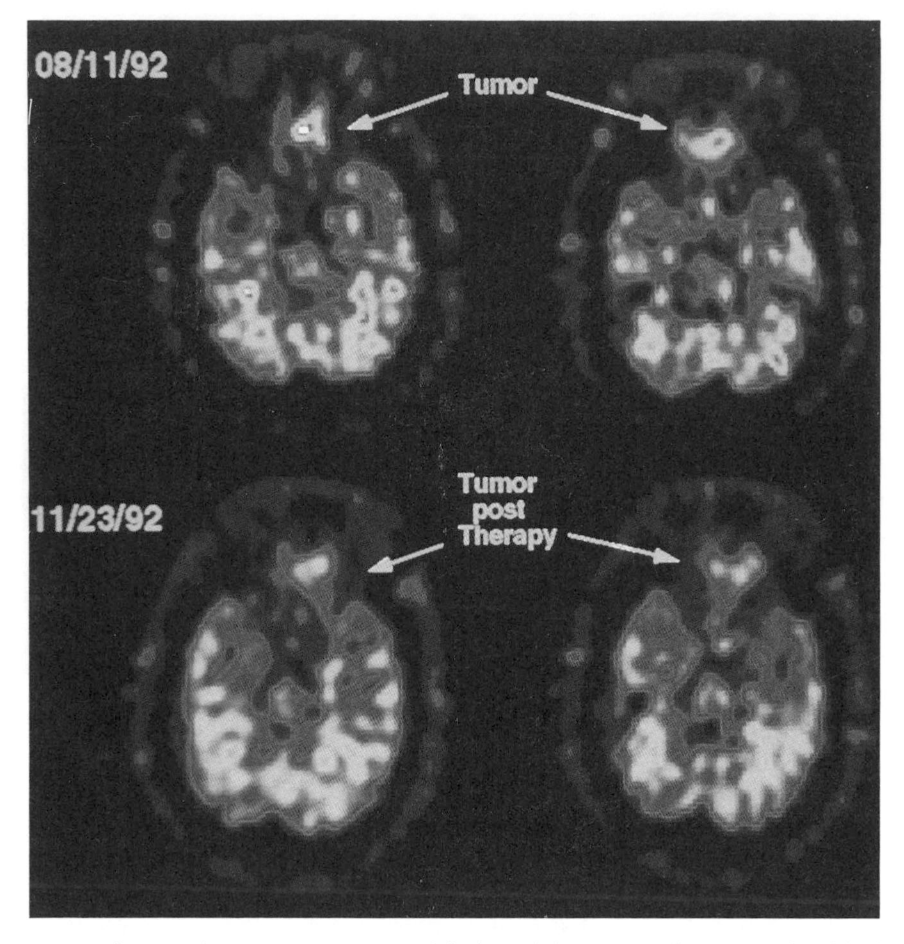

42. Serial PET studies (1992) in patients with high-grade brain tumors being treated with high doses of tamoxifen on an experimental therapeutic protocol. Note reduction in metabolic activity in response to treatment. Contrast-enhancing lesions noted on MRI examination (not shown) were unchanged through therapy. Courtesy of Dr. Peter Conti.

PET in Court

All eyes in the courtroom look to Charles Reese. The jury has convicted him of six counts of premeditated murder. Grasping at the only straw left to save his client's life, his lawyer asks for a PET scan before the jury passes sentence. A computer-generated skull revolves behind a computer monitor, and as the skin peels effortlessly away, the ivory bones dissolve, leaving a naked brain rotating in red and green. A second brain, a "control," appears beside the first. Anyone can see that the two brains are different. A doctor explains why.

Pointing to the first, he says, "These are abnormal patterns without a doubt. . . . What you are seeing is a computer-enhanced image of the chemistry of [Reese's] brain. And what it shows is a picture of madness."

Convinced, the jury sends Reese to a mental hospital instead of the gas chamber. The picture has done what words could not. It has convinced the jury that an abnormal brain scan indicates an abnormal brain in an abnormal person, who is not responsible for his actions.[26] This is the finale of *Rampage,* a 1989 movie that was filmed, in part, at the PET laboratory at the University of California at Irvine, a lab that had made a specialty of forensic PET scans.

Because California law requires a second trial after a guilty verdict when the death penalty is involved, and because the PET facility at this campus is not part of the federal network, its entrepreneurial leaders established amicable relations with high-profile lawyers in the neighborhood. The PET program at the Irvine campus began when the psychiatry department bought a scanner with bank loans, which it repaid, not by leasing its lab as a movie set—that was just a one-time gig—but by fees from providing expert testimony.

By 1993 the vast majority of Irvine's clinical referrals came from lawyers, many of whom sought testimony about the brains and the head injuries of convicted felons for the penalty phase of their trials.[27] Responding to demand, the Irvine physicians began lecturing to lawyers and judges about how PET works until PET became the community standard in Orange County. This dovetailed neatly with the interests of the laboratory's head at the time, Monte Buchsbaum, whose research focused on schizophrenia, and especially the psychiatry of violence. These cases provided him with the data on the brains of forty-four people who, like the fictional Charles Reese, had been convicted of brutal crimes.

The idea of explaining violence by finding evidence of neural malfunctions builds on a 1987 study of four convicted criminals with histories of repetitive, purposeless, violent behavior. Studies of these men with CT, EEG (electroencephalograph, which shows surface electrical activity and comes out of a printer looking like a squiggly line), and PET uncovered curious discrepancies. Two of the men had normal CT scans, but their PET examinations revealed widespread defects in cerebral functioning. There was no instance of a normal PET scan coupled with an abnormal anatomical scan. The authors were tentative in their conclusions, suggesting that PET did seem able to find something awry in the brains of three out of the four men, something that had been overlooked by CT. But whether the findings were indicative, much less predictive, of violence, they could not know. The only claim the authors made is that PET might confirm brain derangement in people who had already behaved violently.[28]

PET has a curious history in American courts in that it stands the Frye rule on its head. The Frye rule calls for the acknowledgment by experts that the technology in question is accurate and measures up to some community standard. PET has measured up to the Frye test many times in its use in Orange County courts, long before it received the blessing of the FDA. Even as it was accepted for use before juries, it was still officially experimental in the medical world. Its history is in some ways analogous to DNA identification, which is challenged in many localities each time it is offered in evidence, but which has long since become a standard tool in medical and biological research.

The experts at Irvine believe that their images are compelling, especially those that contrast strikingly colored pictures of matched brains—the defendant's and a control's. This marketing of PET has prompted John Mazziotta, a professor of neurology and chief of UCLA's division of brain mapping, to write "The Use of Positron Emission Tomography (PET) in Medical-Legal Cases: The Position Against Its Use." Mazziotta argues that PET can currently help clinically to evaluate patients with epilepsy, brain tumors, and some dementias, and while a careful evaluation of a patient with a specific disease should allow a clinician to predict the site of abnormality seen with brain imaging, he says, "The converse is not true. That is, predicting behavior by evaluating a structural or functional image set is far less accurate." He offers the examples of people whose brain scans show Huntington's disease or Alzheimer's disease, but who have no symptoms.[29]

The idea that guilt can be determined by a brain scan he finds "currently farfetched." His reasons are practical. For example, he explains that the "controls" are age-matched normal individuals with no personal or family histories of mental illness, who are made as relaxed and comfortable as possible while being scanned. The defendant, in contrast, is usually transported from prison, anxious and aware that his life depends on the test's outcome. Mazziotta concludes that the use of PET in determining guilt in a court of law is not only unfounded but irresponsible. His reasoning echoes that of physicians in the 1930s who suggested that X-rays in court without the accompaniment of expert interpretation would only confuse and perhaps mislead jurors, the power of images being so great.

Joseph Dumit, an anthropologist exploring PET, offers another explanation for keeping PET out of the courtroom. Alluding to the power of images in contemporary culture, Dumit coined the term "biotechnopower" to describe the attribution of agency to technology by treating it as more objective than the experts who interpret it. The fictional jurors were swayed by PET images in the film *Rampage,* Dumit points out, despite expert testimony to the contrary, because an image is more powerful than words. As for words, Dumit notes the difference between schizophrenia, or any mental disease for that matter, which is a medical definition, and insanity, which is a legal term. PET's ability to reveal changes in the brain that are invisible with CT and MR scans demonstrates to the satisfaction of part of the public, as well as the medical community, that mental illness is a disease. It is not something "in the head," which is inexcusable, but in the *brain,* which is.[30]

Brain Scanning

Less in contention is the ability of PET to reveal several kinds of brain dysfunction. PET can show areas of the brain where glucose is being metabolized, indicating high activity. This happens, for example, if the subject is asked to raise an arm or scratch an elbow. PET can also reveal reduced activity, as for example between seizures in epilepsy. A visitor to the Donner Laboratory in 1992 found Thomas Budinger excited about a patient who at the age of forty-five had suffered a radical drop in I.Q., and for whom anatomical scans had revealed nothing. The PET scan revealed an area of extremely low activity. Although the patient's condition had not been thoroughly diagnosed at the time, he could be assured that the problem was visible and that he was not neurotic—there really was a functional problem—and that he did not have AIDS, or Alzheimer's, or any known brain disease.

PET also shows the location of electrical storms, or seizures, inside the brain. Readers of the January 1987 *National Geographic* magazine's article on brain imaging saw the photograph of three-year-old Ryan Peterson, along with PET scans illustrating decreased metabolism on the left side of his brain. Ryan had suffered his first seizure eight hours after he was born in Washington, D.C., in 1984, and he had continued experiencing jackknifing convulsions throughout the next sixteen months as his parents sought help at pediatric centers along the East Coast.

On a Christmas visit to California in December 1985, Ryan, who in his year and a half of life had never held up his head or played with a toy, experienced an increase in the duration of his seizures—each one lasting as long as forty minutes. In desperation his parents brought him to UCLA's Pediatric Neurology Clinic, where the neurologist Harry Chugani observed that the seizures always started on the right side. CT and MRI scans revealed no structural abnormality in Ryan's brain. Chugani ordered a PET scan which revealed that, contrary to earlier EEG results, the damage was confined to Ryan's left hemisphere. PET tracked the electrical storms (categorized under the catch-all term *epilepsy*), to the cerebral cortex. The cortex is where higher functions like vision, language, and speech take place. Chugani suggested that because drugs had not helped and because Ryan's condition was deteriorating rapidly, the child undergo a radical procedure—a hemispherectomy—which Warwick Peacock, the newly arrived head of pediatric neurosurgery, had successfully performed on children in his native South Africa.

In February 1986 Peacock removed the entire left hemisphere of Ryan's brain—everything except for the deep structures: the basal ganglia, the brain stem, and the thalamus. Postoperative microscopic examination of the excised tissue revealed abnormal cellular development that, prior to surgery, had only been visible in its effects—the disturbance of Ryan's brain function. Within a year Ryan was talking, and walking with a brace on his right leg. Eventually, he attended public school.

Seven years later, four-year-old Brandy arrived at UCLA. Her seizures had started two years earlier and her condition, too, was deteriorating. She had a PET scan and then underwent radical surgery, which, by this time, had been refined by the lessons drawn from about fifty hemispherectomies. Electrocortography was performed on her exposed brain in order to save the motor areas so that she would not experience the weakness of the arm and leg on the side of the body opposite from the diseased brain tissue.[31] But a week after the initial procedure, Brandy's seizures continued, and in a second operation Peacock removed the rest of the diseased hemisphere. Brandy, too, is in

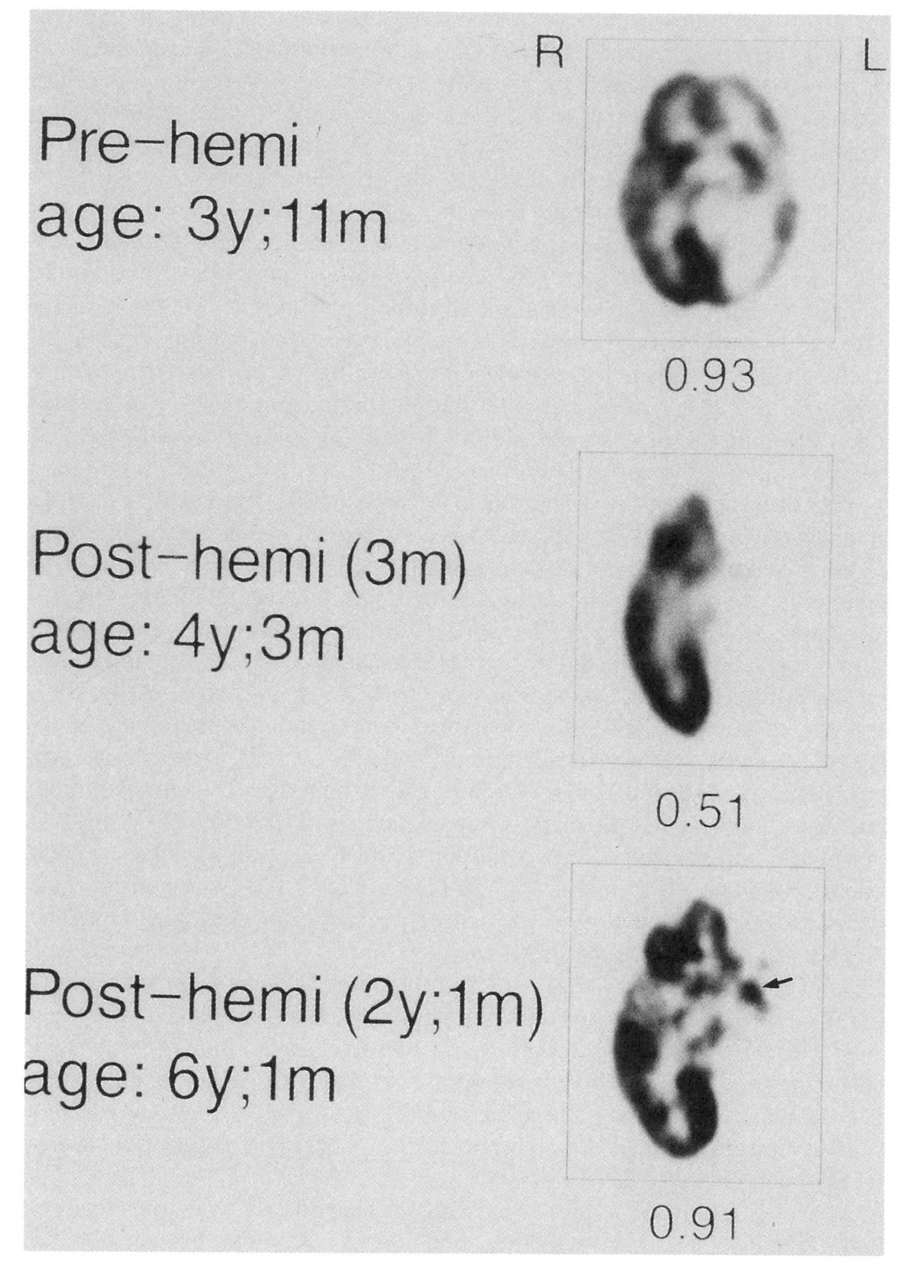

43. Pre- and post-hemispherectomy PET scan of child from age three to age six. Courtesy of Dr. Harry T. Chugani, Wayne State University, Children's Hospital of Michigan.

school now, one leg weaker than the other, but still able to dance with her classmates.

At the end of his first decade at UCLA, Peacock stated that "we would not have operated on so many children if it were not for PET scanning."[32] It enabled the surgical team to pinpoint the trouble spots, areas that look perfectly normal with anatomical scans, but where PET reveals malfunctioning. The children who have had half of their brains removed have shown remarkable improvement. Studies with these children reinforce studies at UCLA with cats, which reveal that the brain in its first years has a huge capacity for making extra connections and can actually compensate for much of the lost cells.

Using PET scans, Chugani, Phelps, and Hoffman at UCLA constructed a visual encyclopedia of the way the normal brain develops throughout life. There was no shortage of adult volunteers for scans, but it would have been unethical to use normal children, so Chugani used studies of twenty-nine patients who had suffered transient neurological events that did not interfere with their normal development. His results confirm the plasticity of the infant brain and fit into a larger PET study of the built-in neuronal redundancy that lasts through the first eight years of life, the years in which children learn an enormous number of skills.

Through PET scans, Chugani (now at the Children's Hospital of Michigan) and his colleagues tracked the use of glucose by the brain and mapped the

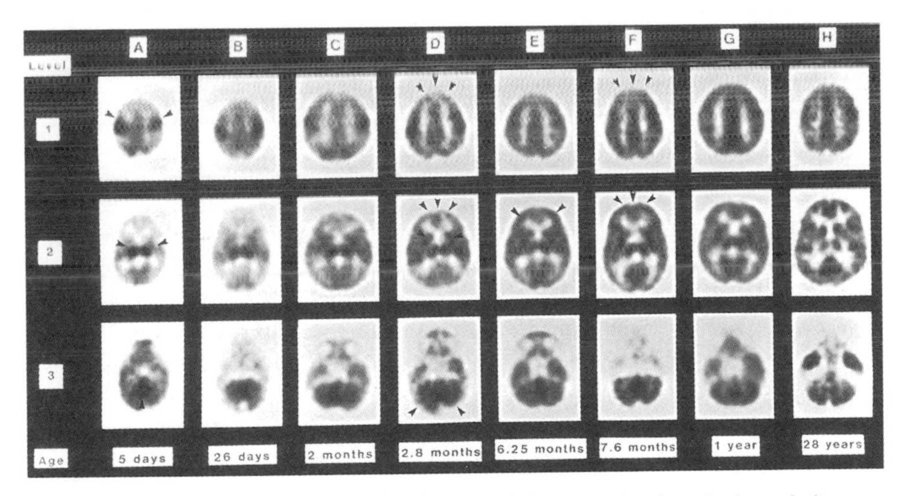

44. PET/FDG-glucose study illustrating developmental changes in local cerebral metabolic rates in the normal human infant as compared to the adult. In the five-day-old, lCMRGlc is highest in sensorimotor cortex, thalamus, cerebellar vermis (arrows), and brainstem (not shown). *(B), (C),* and *(D):* lCMRGlc gradually increases in parietal, temporal, and calcarine cortices; basil ganglia; and cerebral cortex (arrows), particularly during the second and third months. *(E):* In the frontal cortex, lCMRGlc increases first in the lateral prefrontal regions by approximately six months. *(F):* By approximately eight months lCMRGlc also increases in the medial aspects of the frontal cortex (arrows), as well as the dorsolateral occipital cortex. *(G):* By one year, the lCMRGlc pattern resembles that of adults *(H).* Courtesy of Dr. Harry T. Chugani, Wayne State University, Children's Hospital of Michigan.

number of synapses between brain cells in newborns—these are relatively few but multiply rapidly, reaching adult levels by the age of two—and continuing to increase until about the age of ten. The cells begin to decrease at this point until they drop down to adult levels by the age of sixteen. An example of the potential clinical use of this research is the observation that the use of glucose in the visual cortex declines between the eighth and tenth years: this corresponds to the clinical observation that the best time to treat "lazy eye" by patching the "good" eye to let the weaker eye develop is before the patient reaches the critical age of eight.[33]

Chugani suggests that future research using more selective radiopharmaceuticals may reveal inborn errors of metabolism and neurodegenerative disorders, paving the way for treatment. Eventually PET probes may reveal metabolic causes of learning disorders in children, and in adults as well.

PET has already successfully identified disorders that occur principally in adults, such as problems identified by Dr. Parkinson in 1817 in an *Essay on the Shaking Palsy.*[34] Before PET, Parkinson's disease was diagnosed by clinical symptoms and ultimately confirmed by autopsy. Today PET can image the degenerating cells, opening the door to treatments; these include monitoring medication with L Dopa, a synthetic dopamine that increases the amount of dopamine synthesized by the patient's brain. A few patients have benefited from the grafting of fetal cells onto their dopamine receptors, and follow-up studies with PET have revealed vastly improved motor coordination.

More promising now and in cases where cell grafting is not feasible is a procedure called *pallidotomy.* As PET enables neurologists to see in greater detail the areas of reduced function, this stereotactic surgery has shown remarkable results in advanced cases where the efficacy of synthetic dopamine has decreased. In a description of his personal experience as a patient, Edwin W. Salzman, a surgeon and staff member of the *New England Journal of Medicine,* explains how PET and MRI located the area of his basal ganglia that had to be destroyed. That area seems to account for most of the symptoms of the disease, but is so deep in the brain and so close to the optic nerve that only the detailed map provided by PET enabled the surgeon, with the patient's assistance, to oblate the troublesome cells without damaging his vision. Although surgery does not affect the course of the disease, it does alleviate symptoms. Salzman testifies, "On August 9, 1995, I underwent a pallidotomy with electrophysiologic monitoring. By the end of the operation, most of my motor symptoms were gone. On September 1, I awakened at dawn, hopped out of bed, and drove myself to my favorite fishing spot. Independent at last!"[35]

PET has, to some extent, delivered on William Randolph Hearst's 1896 challenge to "see the brain at work." Using specially designed goggles, volunteers help researchers follow the impact of an image on the retina toward its final connection in the visual cortex. At the University of Iowa College of Medicine, Hanna and Antonio Damasio have mapped and explored the brain from the visual cortex through a section behind the ear on the left side known as Wernicke's area. In a 1992 experiment they and their colleagues monitored a volunteer who conjured up mental images of familiar faces with his eyes shut while his head was inside the doughnut hole of the PET scanner. Hanna Damasio had aligned the PET scanner so that it matched an MRI image taken earlier. PET images do not give anatomical detail precise enough to identify each brain structure, but when superimposed slice for slice with their MRI twins, PET serves as a map to the brain's activities.[36] Mapping these activities is feeding our curiosity to see more deeply into the mind. Researchers elsewhere have tracked the effect of repetition on learning, discovering that repetition reduces the time necessary for the brain to do a given task. Others have mapped the many different areas of the brain that contribute to performing a single task. PET is literally spelling out the neural pathways used for carrying out relatively simple brain functions, such as recognizing colors or listening to music.

If You Had to Choose?

The story of PET began at the same time as its companion imaging systems. PET has overlapped with them occasionally, but has never taken off with the same momentum. As CT and MR moved into the center of modern medicine, PET remained on the fringe. From year to year PET has seemed about to disappear altogether, or on the verge of joining the others as a mainstay of clinical as well as experimental work. Expensive and complex, PET depends on more skilled personnel than MRI and CT. To the lay viewer, the almost painterly PET image is qualitatively different from the crisp slices produced by CT and MRI.

PET has stood at the brink of breaking through to everyday use ever since 1989, when the FDA said that it was safe and effective to use trace rubidium to image coronary artery flow. In 1992 the imaging advisory committee approved its use for diagnosing epilepsy and a short list of other conditions, which permitted some Medicare reimbursement.[37] While they waited, some states got around the problem of reimbursement by categorizing PET as a justifiable pharmacological procedure. But every time one hurdle was overcome, PET has had to surmount new ones. While PET continued to serve as a major research instrument at the NIH hospitals, quietly breaking ground in cardiac and cancer studies, the FDA decided to regulate radioisotopes as drugs and put them through the same lengthy, and expensive, efficacy tests that medicines have to pass.

PET practitioners have responded by explaining that, by definition, tracers have no effect as they pass through the body so swiftly. FDG, for instance, has a half-life of two hours. This argument has not persuaded the FDA.

Spokespersons at the Society for Clinical PET suspect that the enormous impact of MRI on the Medicare budget made government agencies in general and the FDA in particular gun-shy about anything as costly as PET. While the government built new obstacles to reimbursement, all major private insurers agreed to pay for PET, including CHAMPUS (Civilian Health and Military Personnel), the government's insurance for military dependents. With Medicare and Medicaid alone in not picking up the bills, for a while it seemed that only the poor and elderly would have no access to clinical PET. Should the radiotracer part of the partnership fall to the regulations of the pharmaceutical industry, all bets are off regarding PET's viability in the clinic.

In that event, it would remain a research tool where its value is, at the moment, unchallenged. However, lobbyists for PET are hoping to short-circuit the review process by asking Congress to remove them from what they regard as the clutches of drug regulators.[38]

Part of the promise of the 1990s—the "decade of the brain"—has been the creation of a detailed, three-dimensional model of the brain using every available form of imaging. The project includes radiographs, CT, MR, and PET images, each adding something special to the ultimate picture. Which is best? In 1985 a spokesperson for the Radiological Society of North America had described "the difference between using MRI and conventional X-ray techniques, including computed tomography CT scans," as "like the vast difference between

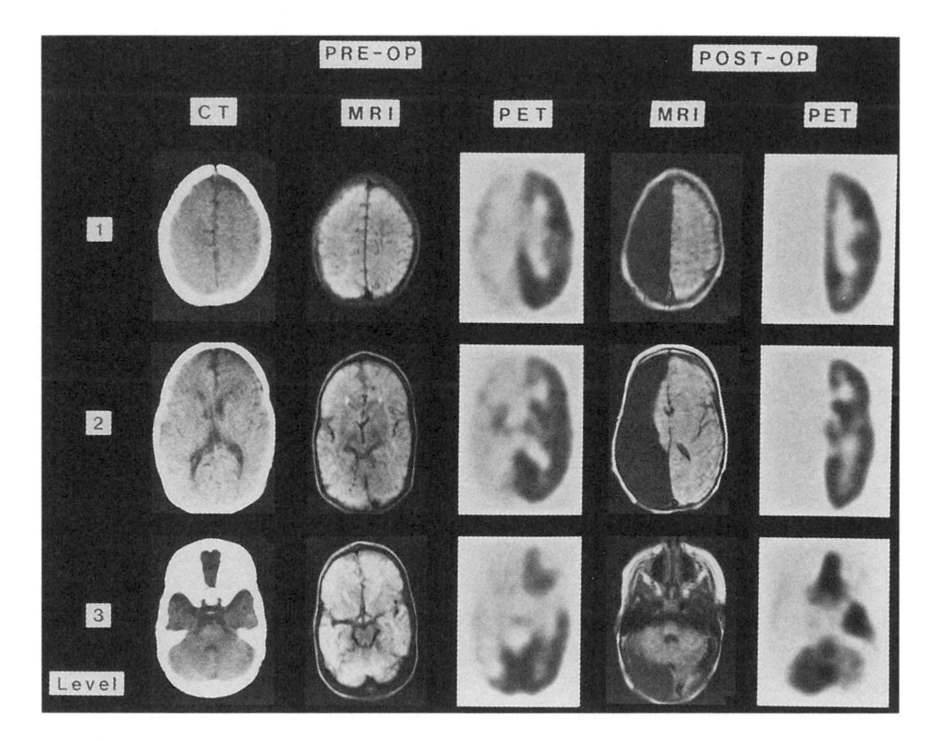

45. This photograph compares CT, MRI, and PET/FDG brain images from an infant with epilepsy beginning at eight hours of age. At age fifteen months, CT and MRI scans were normal, but PET revealed severe diffuse hypometabolism of all supratentorial structures in the left hemisphere. EEG showed diffuse left hemispheric spike-wave discharges. Following left cerebral hemispherectomy (sparing basil ganglia and thalamus), all seizures ceased and the infant began to show rapid diffuse hamartomatous malformation. Prospective MRI scan was normal for the remaining hemisphere, and six months later, PET revealed normal pattern of lCMRGlc in the right hemisphere. Courtesy of Dr. Harry T. Chugani, Wayne State University, Children's Hospital of Michigan.

operating a 747 jet and an automobile. Think of the number of steps in getting the plane off the ground, as compared to getting into your car, turning the ignition, putting the car in gear, and using the accelerator."[39]

The speaker was correct on one level. But a decade later CT has become almost as standard as conventional radiographs. By this time MRI had also achieved images of extraordinary high resolution and been simplified for ordinary clinical use, so that anatomical imaging with MRI can be adjusted to look for particular kinds of tissue depending on the patient's symptoms.

Functional imaging, which had been PET's monopoly, is now possible with fMR. Functional MRI, though still experimental, can track blood flow and the changes in oxygen within the bloodstream faster than PET and with at least ten times finer resolution. Its earliest experiments imitated PET's, using PET as a map and a validation of its own capabilities.[40] What fMR cannot do yet, and may never be able to do, is home in on the molecules that identify specific disease sites. Functional MRI is limited to imaging hydrogen while PET is limited only by the ingenuity of radiopharmacists—and they are still going strong. Their specially designed probes go directly to target molecules in the particular area where trouble is suspected, and they can detect subtle chemical changes that do not change blood flow enough for fMR to measure.

PET had a hard time moving into hospitals outside of the ring of federal largess, where the expense of privately supporting an on-site cyclotron seemed daunting. However, creative financing is solving some of these problems. While the Irvine campus of the University of California supports its PET center through legal referral fees, the PET center at the University of Southern California has found another solution. In cooperation with Syncor International, Inc., a commercial radiopharmacy, USC's PET center serves satellite facilities to which it flies radiopharmaceuticals within two hours' flight time of Los Angeles. This defrays the costs of production while enabling hospitals that can not afford their own cyclotrons to offer PET scans. Meanwhile, cyclotrons have become smaller, and some come with their own radiation shields and new computer programs that simplify the production of radiopharmaceuticals.

PET boosters are passionate about its future. GE and Siemens now manufacture user-friendly PET machines which they are offering to hospitals in North America and Europe. The installation of a new PET facility can cost anywhere from $2 to $7 million, and the cost of operating a center is about $1.8 million a year.[41] The preferred reimbursement may be a set fee: the figure reached by a group of Southern California insurance companies is about twice the cost of MRI. But this may be a matter of comparing apples and oranges. PET can bring down the cost of caring for patients with epilepsy, heart attack, and some kinds of cancer in a way that MRI cannot.

But cost really means relative cost. A PET scanner alone costs about the same as a good MRI machine, but the accompanying cyclotron costs the same amount again, thereby doubling the price. Moreover, PET centers have to pay three skilled crews—one to maintain the scanner, another to run the cyclotron, and another to produce radioisotopes. Costs are reckoned in several ways, of course, and change according to pass-through time (how fast a scan is and how many can be handled a day). At the moment PET scans can be done in five minutes while an MRI scan can easily take an hour. Costs also include upkeep, the price of replaceable parts, computer upgrades, and new software.

A second factor is the competition. PET no longer has the realm of functional imaging to itself. Both fMR and magnetic resonance spectrography, a technique which also tracks specific molecules, are developing rapidly.

A third factor is safety. PET scans use radioactive isotopes, albeit in minute quantities. The amount of ionizing radiation is negligible, but it is present. On the one hand, unwarranted fear of radiation frightens away some patients who might benefit from it. On the other, the radiation is real, if minute, and physicians are careful not to submit patients to multiple PET scans when not essential. Society's fear of anything radioactive has kept nuclear imaging in a kind of technological limbo. PET advocates dismiss possible hazards, pointing out that the low dosages compare favorably with exposure to radiation during flight in an ordinary jet airplane. Its advocates regard PET as "noninvasive" because the quantity of radioactive material and the length of time it remains in the body are negligible. The advocates are probably right, yet their behavior reveals conflicted attitudes. They volunteer themselves as guinea pigs, but will not scan children for research because they consider the unnecessary use of radiation unethical. These precautions notwithstanding, PET has produced remarkable images of metabolic function—and dysfunction—without causing radiation-induced diseases among those who developed the technology or in those who have been scanned.

In the best of all possible worlds, each technology, as well as others that are moving off the drawing boards and into production, would be available both for research and in the clinic. When economic constraints limit choices, the advantages and limitations of each give an idea of which will prevail (see table 1). If the price tag does make the difference, ways have to be found to judge real cost. One expensive image may replace two cheaper ones, or eliminate routine X-rays that are often followed by CT. There are also nonmonetary issues: many people would happily pay for allayed anxiety, comfort, and what has been referred to as quality of life. All of these technologies will last through this decade, but the ultimate survival of any or all of them will depend as much on the economic and social fabric as on the technological breakthroughs of the twenty-first century.

Many hospitals already blend two or three imaging technologies, superimposed or combined to present an amalgam of anatomic and metabolic information, in order to diagnose and decide on treatments, or prepare for surgery.

Most people only care about diagnosing disease when they are ill. But almost everyone is interested in seeing the way their minds and bodies work. Although CTs and MRIs have filtered into popular culture as anatomical images, PET offers a chance to see the heart actively processing oxygen, the brain registering a familiar word, or rage ripping through a criminal's brain as in *Rampage*. The moving image has a special place in our psyches. In 1896 visitors to the

TABLE 1 – Advantages, Drawbacks, and Uses of Imaging Technologies

	X-rays	Fluoroscopy	Ultrasound	CT scan	MRI	Nuclear medicine	SPECT	PET
Imaging source	X-rays	X-rays	Sound waves	X-rays	Magnetic fields	Radioactive isotopes	Radioactive isotopes	Radioactive isotopes
Advantages	• low-cost • minimally invasive (depending on machine and procedure)	• real-time imaging • low-cost	• low-cost • noninvasive • real-time imaging	• speed • scans bones and cartilage	• soft tissue • inside bony structures • noninvasive	• functional organ visualization • helps define space-occupying tumors • uses "nuclear cow" that produces Technicium	• assesses function • real-time imaging • images blood flow/metabolism • uses over-the-counter radio-active isotopes	• assesses metabolic function • real-time imaging • variety of radio-tracers
Drawbacks	• does not image all organs and tissues well • ionizing radiation • does not image behind bones	• more ionizing radiation over time of exposure • image not detailed	• does not image areas around the lungs • image not clear	• high-cost • limited application • limited tissue definition • ionizing radiation	• high-cost • does not image bone • time-consuming (except in experimental modes)	• poor anatomical definition • significant radioactivity	• time-consuming • no spatial definition • limited number of isotopes • exposure to radioactive isotopes up to 24 hours	• high-cost • research-oriented • low spatial definition • complex • needs on-site cyclotron
Frequent and specialized uses	• broken bones • chest/tuberculosis • cancer • mammography • dental	• motion study of organ systems including: gastrointestinal tract, intestinal tract, vascular systems, kidneys, gall bladders, and angiography	• fetus • heart • breast • premature infants • kidneys	• blood clots • fractures • operating/emergency room • brain tumors	• brain diseases/tumors • pituitary tumors • multiple sclerosis/myelin deterioration • soft tissues • knees	• brain • kidney • abdominal region • bones • lungs • specialized parts of the heart	• bone cancer • blood flow in the brain/heart/liver • detects acute myocardial infarction	• epilepsy/seizure disorders • malignancies • cancer • Parkinson's • Alzheimer's • brain-mapping research
Number of scans in U.S. per year*	207,753,747	no data	51,680,190	20,810,208	4,335,646	12,385,383		

*Source: From 1993 Part B Medicare Annual Data (BMAD) procedure file

Electrical Exposition watched their moving fingers exposed as bones in a fluoroscope. Physicians preferred looking at their patients' bodies as moving images through a fluoroscope, despite their own exposure to radiation, rather than examining a static radiograph. They wanted to watch the living lungs, stomach, and heart. Today PET scans track a finer path, imaging not just the movement of food through the digestive tract but seeing how invisible nutrients are metabolized in specific organs. Motion is the message. As superfast CT offers images of the heart between beats, and fMR and PET capture the brain as it processes a visual signal, another technology, ultrasound, has transformed the nature of pregnancy, adding snapshots of the developing fetus to the family archives, and a new patient to the clinic's clientele.

We cannot know which, if not all, of these technologies will survive in the armamentarium of clinical medicine, and which will become historical curiosities. As the first century of "X-ray vision" comes to a close, the races within each technology pale in comparison to the race among them for survival. And there are still new candidates crowding the horizon.[42]

By the mid-1990s, imaging technology had evolved so swiftly that parts of some hospitals had become imaging museums. A neurosurgeon at County General Hospital in Los Angeles, touring the aging facility, points nostalgically to a sheeted gamma-ray detection unit. When it was new, he recalls, everyone was awed that "it could get across the blood-brain barrier and you'd get a hot spot that you could pick up on a scanning machine—that was dealt with in the sixties. It was created by a gamma counter and [the machine] created a picture for you."[43] He walks on. "That was *it* until the radio-nuclei brain scans came about. You had a crude picture of a round structure. Nothing with precision at all." Then he points to the shell of a pneumoencephalograph—a streamlined version of Dandy's 1920 invention, the first instrument to enable X-rays to image the inside of the brain, by injecting air into the base of the spine. "It cost half a million dollars in 1973, and was almost immediately obsolete. That was because of the CT scan. They got one of the first which was made by EMI in England in 1975. It was crude by today's standards but it made what came before instantly obsolete." He rings for the elevator. "Then came MRI. There is no question that MRI has supplanted CT in the vast majority of neurological imaging studies. But not completely." He walks swiftly to another, newer building. The MRI machine is there, along with the cyclotron and PET scanner. "There's still PET. It does brain activation studies in five minutes and images activity that is invisible to the other scans." The PET Center is its own universe of radiologists, technicians, and patients.

Which of these methods of extracting tomographic images from inside the body is best? When should we choose one over the others? The surgeon suggests looking at who is asking and who is answering. As a rule of thumb, the surgeon warns: anyone wedded to a single technology cannot help but have a vested interest in its value. "I always say, 'If the only instrument you have is a hammer, the whole world looks like a nail.' "

Some of the most loquacious defenders of PET choose color over the gray scale when they give presentations for fear that PET will not "sell" on its unadorned image. Truly an amazing depiction of metabolic function, PET is an enigma to the untrained eye. Along with MRS and fMR, also functional images, PET has changed the visual expectations of specialists. The delicate tracery of Pupin's image of the patient's buckshot-riddled hand in 1896, and the 1995 MRI of a malignant brain tumor, each exquisitely detailed, are more alike than either is like a PET scan. In clinical situations, the different kinds of images are understood as complementary, and are often merged graphically.

PET's uncanny ability to record the brain in action has opened a new level of discourse about the meaning of mind.[44] It has also, because of its dependence on trace quantities of radioactive substances, alerted activists against all things nuclear. Advocates of competing technologies in an era of limited investments in medical instrumentation raise the ghosts of the radiation martyrs and the downwind victims of nuclear testing in Nevada and Utah—red herrings when the real issue is money and the promise of cost-effective clinical success.[45]

Ten

Looking through Women

The Development of Ultrasound and Mammography

In 1986 Roger Sanders, chief of ultrasound at Johns Hopkins University Hospital in Baltimore, fielded a telephone call from NBC Television's Washington affiliate asking him to come to their studio and examine a group of mysterious ultrasound images. Sanders, a British-educated radiologist, had emigrated in 1970, and as his specialty became central to the practice of obstetrics and gynecology, he became a leader in the field. The images NBC showed him for comment turned out to include views of empty uteruses, bladders, and fecal material. On some of the sonograms Sanders made out the crude drawing of a baby that did not correspond to any real structure. What he did not see was any sign of pregnancy. Fed up with looking at one picture after another with nothing of interest, he erupted. "There is only shit there, there is no baby!"[1]

Off camera, the producer explained the pictures, and the events that led to the downfall of Cecil Jacobson, the fifty-one-year-old geneticist who, while on the staff at George Washington University's medical school, claimed the distinction of having performed the world's first amniocentesis. Jacobson had since then quit the university to establish the private and lucrative Reproductive Genetics Center in Vienna, Virginia. Now four of his patients were charging fraud. They had sought independent ultrasound confirmation of pregnancies that Jacobson had assured them were healthy, but had learned, as Sanders confirmed, that there were no fetuses.

The fertility doctor had bolstered his "proofs" of pregnancy by injecting his patients with HCG (human chorionic gonadotrophin), a hormone that imitates pregnancy on blood tests. (The NBC producer took the same shots and discovered that his urine also tested "pregnant.") Jacobson had followed chemical confirmation of pregnancies with displays of the sonograms Sanders had examined. Jacobson had no training in ultrasound and the machine he owned was old. This did not stop him from showing his clients their "babies" with beating hearts and nonexistent thumbs in nonexistent mouths.

Jacobson had indulged in "voodoo vision," leading people to see what was not there. Ultrasound lent itself to this kind of deception because ultrasound images are hard for an amateur to decode and easy to misinterpret, especially for someone desperate to see a fetus. Yet Sanders is still amazed that so many people could have been tricked into seeing something that wasn't there. He has forgotten what the shadowy pie-shaped images that characterize ultrasound look like to the uninitiated. Most people need guidance to make out whatever the physician or technician points to on the screen. Early X-rays had also been confusing, even to doctors who were supposed to be familiar with anatomy. The expectations raised by the crisp edges of X-rays make it even harder to understand the fuzzy ultrasound pictures. The untrained eye still needs a guide.

By the mid-1990s sound had joined radiation and magnetism as the operative power behind a formidable new way to extract images of the interior of the body. Ultrasound had as long and distinguished a history as any of the other imaging technologies and as wide a list of applications. But it found a special place in the lives of women because it became widely available just as a wave of feminism (called at the time "women's liberation") began to shake up, and sometimes shatter, the social order in which middle-class women sought counsel from male experts for spiritual and medical decisions. Suddenly women questioned the advice of all the men in their lives and authority in general. Women who were reading works like Betty Friedan's *Feminine Mystique* became particularly distrustful of the way male experts dealt with health issues that only affect women, such as pregnancy and breast cancer. The technologies that revealed the interiors of the uterus and the breast are different in kind, and they provoked very different responses: a whole class of reasonably well educated women felt empowered to take back control over pregnancy, but the implications of breast cancer provoked a different kind of reaction.

While some women in the 1970s looked at sonograms of their developing fetuses, other women met in consciousness-raising groups where they explored their own vaginal spaces with speculums, flashlights, and mirrors. They had dared to *see* what had once been territory familiar only to midwives, a profession that had almost vanished then in the United States, and to usually male gynecologists. Like Jacobson's patients, they believed that *seeing* was the key to power. The deceptive doctor had understood this and made a mockery of it. Seeing might mean power, but seeing was not as simple as they had been led to believe.

Ultrasound images have never been sharp and neat like X-rays and fluoroscopes. The images on inexpensive machines are apt to look like very old home movies, jerking as the hand-held transducer moves across gel-covered skin, grappling for a good view of its moving target. The fetus is indistinct, especially at an early stage of development. These images resemble nothing so much as socks and shirts tumbling inside a front-loading clothes dryer.

Even in the 1970s, ultrasound rapidly became part of the diagnostic checklist for heart and kidney diseases, brain and eye disorders, and vascular problems, often as an adjunct to the work of the cardiologist, nephrologist, or neurologist. But only in obstetrics did it become a cultural as well as a clinical necessity. Women all over the world came to expect to see their fetuses.

Jacobson exploited the anxiety of his patients, convincing them that the crude pictures on the monitor included the bean-sized fetuses they expected to see. His elaborate scam kept infertile women paying until one grew suspicious, sought an outside opinion, and brought down his entire house of cards. In fact, Jacobson, a geneticist, did not know himself what an embryo looked like on a sonogram. Only gynecologists did.

The occupied uterus was one of the first targets of X-ray examination as far back as 1896 when a pair of Philadelphia doctors captured the first image of a pregnant woman with a fetus, albeit a dead one, inside her body. The practice of X-raying live fetuses did not catch on for another decade because the fetus did not show up on X-rays during the first six weeks of gestation.[2] Even then, there wasn't much to see. By 1910, however, detailed radiographs of human fetuses (miscarried or stillborn) from four weeks gestation onward provided enough information for fetologists to label every bone in the diagram of a near-term fetus with the date of its appearance on X-rays.[3]

In 1926 an X-ray exam of a pregnant woman could take as long as an hour. There was so much tissue in the way, and the image before ten weeks gestation was so vague that this "meant that the patient had to lie on her back with her pelvis elevated and with between 1.5 and 2 litres of carbonic gas injected into her peritoneal cavity." This was no light matter, for "occasionally it killed the fetus, and maternal death, even, has resulted from this procedure."[4]

But the procedure improved, and by 1930 many obstetricians suggested routine prenatal pelvic X-ray examinations. The development of the rabbit test in 1931 to verify pregnancy diminished the use of X-rays from the protocol of early confirmation. Obstetricians continued to use them, however, to estimate due dates and check on fetal condition.

For more than half a century, the risks of radiation to mother and fetus were generally ignored. Although doctors at the turn of the century cautioned against X-raying the fetus, X-rays were used nonetheless to check problem pregnancies or to verify the suspicion of multiple births. The impact of radiation on the developing child would not gain universal attention until 1956, when Alice Stewart, an epidemiologist in Oxford, England, correlated deaths from cancer in children younger than fifteen with their mothers' prenatal exposure to X-rays.[5] (By 1960 the results of this study were well known, and radiologists found their obstetrical referrals plummeting.)

But what was bad news for X-rays was good news for the emerging technology of ultrasound. By 1970, when Roger Sanders arrived in Baltimore from England to start a practice, ultrasonic images of the fetus and placenta were beginning to revolutionize pregnancies all over the world. Obstetrics provided

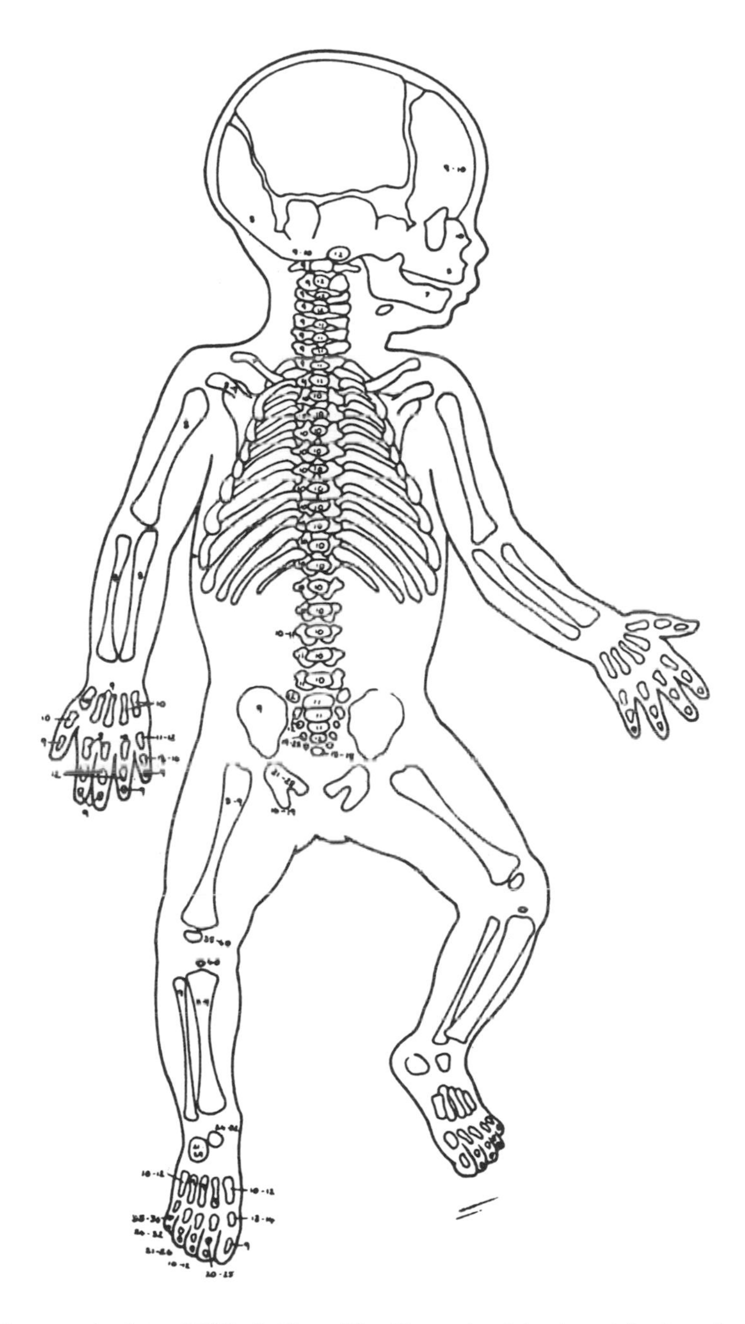

46. Diagram of a fetus (1917). (J. Hess, "The Diagnosis of the Age of the Fetus by Use of Roentgenograms," *American Journal of Diseases of Children* 14 [1917]: 397–423.) Courtesy of the American Medical Association.

the first solid base to a subspecialty that had not found a footing within any other single medical fiefdom. Until then, some ultrasonographers had directed their energies toward identifying cancers wherever they occurred in the body, while others were using the technology to image specific organs including the brain and the heart. Ultrasound struggled in the wings of the technological theater for several decades, working out the kinks as it awaited its chance to take center stage.

The Oldest Technology

Ultrasound has its roots in the physics of sound, not light. Sound waves, unlike light waves, travel through a medium. The speed of sound depends on the physical characteristics of the medium: it moves faster through air than water. Ultrasound captures images by manipulating and analyzing sound waves, very high-frequency sound waves like the kind used in dog whistles, as they bounce off surfaces and echo back to the sender. The speed of sound and the direction of movement of what is being examined, such as flowing blood, can be predicted, depending on the medium and its homogeneity.

The idea of using sound waves to get an impression of the shape of a hidden object goes back to Pierre and Jacques Curie in 1877, long before Pierre met Marie Sklodowska, and long before Roentgen's discovery. When Pierre was eighteen, he and his older brother discovered the piezoelectric effect—a phenomenon that occurs when crystals are mechanically distorted by external pressure so that an electrical potential develops between the crystal surfaces, or, conversely, when electricity strikes the faces of the crystals, which are mechanically distorted. The Curies coined the term *piezoelectricity* from the Greek for "pressure-electricity." The crystals convert electrical to mechanical energy and vice versa. The crystals (which include quartz, tourmaline, calamine, topaz, sugar, and certain ceramics) are called transducers. Almost immediately inventors used the piezoelectric effect to develop phonographic cartridges, microphones, and earphones. Today, more than a century after the Curies' discovery, transducers are used to transmit and collect data from pulses of high-frequency sound waves—millions of hertz compared to the twenty thousand hertz in the audible sound spectrum—that have been directed at a specific region of the body, and reflected back to their source.

The idea of getting some kind of image from sound waves was first broached after the luxury liner *Titanic* hit an iceberg and sank in the Atlantic in 1912. Soon efforts were made to protect other ships by detecting submerged icebergs with sound reflection. Spotting icebergs proved to be child's play compared to detecting the submarines that plagued the Allies during World War I. With that problem in mind, the French physicist Pierre Langevin, a one-time student of Pierre Curie, constructed an ultrasound generator. Langevin wanted to see what would happen when he put the quartz transducer into a field of alternating current. As Curie had long ago predicted, the crystal resonated with the frequency of the electric field. Langevin discovered that ultrasound works easily in a uniform substance like water, where the sound path is predictable and irregularities stand out, but he was too late to be of much help in that war. The problem was taken up anew, and successfully solved, during World War II, and the English-speaking Allies coined the term SONAR, an acronym for *SO*und *N*avigation *A*nd *R*anging.

Meanwhile, in the new Soviet Union, S. Y. Sokolov used ultrasound to detect discontinuities in metals using two transducers, one to generate waves and another to pick up the echoes. Between the wars ultrasound technology all over the world had focused on finding irregularities in uniform materials for industrial purposes. During World War II, however, the technology leaped forward when Floyd Firestone perfected the instrument for use in water. An engineer at the University of Michigan, he invented the "Reflectoscope," a device that combined the generation and detection of sound waves in a single instrument.

None of this had much to do with getting pictures of the interior of the human body. The first attempt using sound for imaging was made by two Austrian brothers, neurologist Karl Dussik and physicist Friedrcich Dussik,

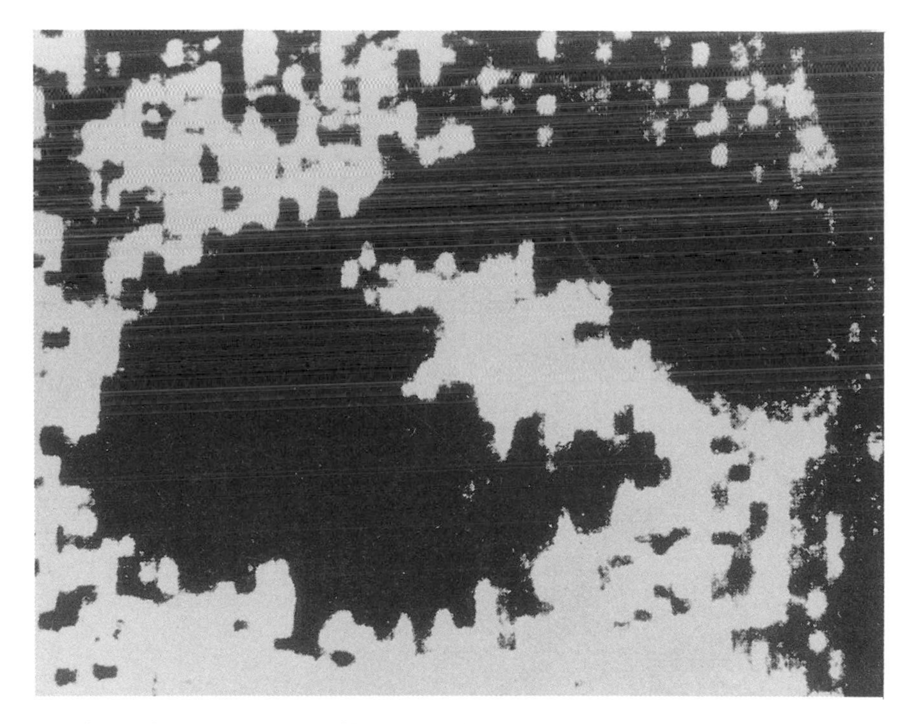

47. A hyperphonogram produced by K. Dussik, F. Dussik, and colleagues. The dark areas, representing areas of the greatest intensity of *transmitted* energy (the Dussiks did not use a pulse-echo technique), were thought by the Dussiks to correspond to the shape of the brain's lateral ventricles, hence, a "ventriculogram." Courtesy of Barry Goldberg, Archives Committee of the AIUM.

who in 1937 transmitted attenuated sound waves through a patient's head. In a manner analogous to getting an X-ray image on film, they put the ultrasound source on one side of the patient and the detector on the other and got a crude transmission image. But just as the skull had foiled Edison's efforts to get X-ray images of the inside of the brain for William Randolph Hearst, the thick bones stopped sound waves from getting a usable image.

Within two years the Dussiks' work was interrupted and accelerated by World War II. While this war is rightfully associated primarily with the development of nuclear weapons, which had a tremendous impact on medicine, it was also a training ground for other scientists, some of whom happened to be doctors, who after the war began to consider applying the principles of SONAR to imaging the body. It would take another twenty years after the war had ended for ultrasonography to become a commercial reality.

In 1945, newly demobilized American, British, German, and Japanese experts in submarine warfare turned ultrasonography into cottage industries in some of the communities and factories where submarine warfare had been a priority. They had access to war surplus materials and knew what to do with them. Some retained military contacts and others had family ties with companies that manufactured devices to detect flaws in metals. They shared the belief that ultrasound could be harnessed for medical diagnosis, but these experts had no connections with each other. And because ultrasound had no connection with radiation, these entrepreneurs served no existing medical constituency.

Free agents, they set about designing what would become the basic modes of ultrasound machines, with differing styles according to their particular medical training—the organs they were exploring, and the conditions they were looking for. Karl Dussik, for instance, had continued working as a neurologist throughout the war. Shortly after the Allies declared victory, Dussik received visits at his clinic in Bad Ischel, Germany, from members of the Allied occupation forces. He understood immediately that he no longer had ultrasound to himself. But before he faded from the scene, he hosted Richard Bolt, a physicist who directed the Acoustics Laboratory at MIT and who in 1948 had learned about Dussik's work from a report out of the Headquarters European Command, USA. Bolt had just enlisted the neurosurgeon Thomas Ballantine from the Massachusetts General Hospital to work with his MIT team. Soon they met Theodor Heuter, a German citizen working for the Siemens Company at a trade show in New York, and asked him to join them first on their visit to Bad Ischel, and then permanently at MIT. What they had learned from Dussik excited all of them, and by the late 1940s they had organized the first of what would become four ultrasound research groups in the United States.

The MIT group was completed with the arrival of George Ludwig, a surgeon who had gone from an internship to the Naval Military Research Institute in Bethesda, Maryland. Ludwig had spent the war working with echo-ranging and underwater detection. He had investigated the fundamental problems of ultrasonic waves and established the standard measurements of the velocity of ultrasound in animal tissues. Still wearing both naval and medical caps, Ludwig developed an ultrasonic probe to locate and remove "enemy" gallstones using flaw detection A-mode ultrasound. *A-mode* stands for amplitude mode, a way of displaying the returning echoes as a line of bright dots on an oscilloscope screen, where each dot corresponds to a point in the body. This linear mode is called one-dimensional imaging.[6]

By 1950, the MIT laboratory had built an ultrasonic brain scanner and tested it on two human subjects—one a healthy member of the research team and the other a patient with a brain tumor. Ludwig's first scanner, like the first CT machine twenty years later, included a ring of water surrounding the subject's head in order to ease the transition of measuring sound waves as they moved from one medium to the other. But the water ring could not eliminate the distortions caused by variations in the skull's thicknesses. So despite the successful research on gallstones that had validated the technique, the MIT group abandoned the research.

The other three groups did not give up so easily. A second American team coalesced around William Fry, a physicist who founded the University of Illinois's Bioacoustics Laboratory in 1946. Fry had spent the war designing piezoelectric transducers at the Naval Research Laboratory's Underwater Sound Division in Washington, D.C. Funded by the navy, Fry, with his brother Francis, led a team developing therapeutic uses of ultrasound. One of the team members was Elizabeth Kelly, who helped in the development of equipment to pinpoint lesions within the central nervous systems of animals. A refinement of this technology was used to explore the human brain. Interested in developing ultrasound as a treatment, Fry designed a sophisticated way of focusing high-frequency sound waves (a departure from the low-frequency sound waves used in physiotherapy).

The Fry brothers founded the not-for-profit Interscience Research Institute in Champaign, Illinois, in 1957, devoted to a two-pronged goal: refining ultrasound instruments to treat human brain disorders, and developing computer-based instruments to visualize soft tissue.[7] Elizabeth Kelly married William Fry but remained Dr. Kelly when she became head of the Institute in the 1960s. With William Fry's sudden death in 1968, Kelly became Kelly-Fry and soon was a leader in adapting ultrasound to the detection of breast cancer.

A third American team formed around Douglas Howry at the University of Colorado Medical Center. After graduating from Colorado's medical school in 1947 and interning in radiology there the following year, Howry began looking for a way to get an image of the abnormalities in soft tissues that X-rays could not see. Ultrasound seemed a good possibility, and in 1949 Howry built his first rudimentary machine from navy surplus SONAR equipment and used bomber parts. In the venerable medical tradition of self-experimentation, he focused the machine on his own thigh and got an image of its tissue.

Satisfied that he was on the right track, Howry built a second, more sophisticated machine which he called a "somascope." This evolved into what is now called B-mode (brightness mode) imaging, a way to produce two-dimensional images by recording sound echoes from tissue interfaces onto 35 mm film. Once filmed, he plotted the positions of the ultrasonic echoes, measuring the distance from the surface of the body to each organ inside the body. These measurements enabled him to construct a compound picture from the cross-sectional images.[8] Howry then arranged a unique system of detectors placed at different angles to convert echo signals from spiked lines (an amplitude response) to line segments or dots (intensity modulations).[9] And he was only just beginning. Howry was interested in mapping soft tissues missed by X-ray machines, and he did not confine his focus to any one organ or part of the body as the easily discouraged brain imagers had done at MIT.

By 1951, Howry was working with Joseph Holmes at the medical laboratory of the VA Hospital in Denver to improve the accuracy of his images. He concentrated on eliminating sonic shadowing and came up with a system that got a good image, but required the patient to sit in a tub of water with lead weights strapped around the waist (to prevent the naturally buoyant human body from floating). The first time around he used a laundry tub for his "patient." Then he discovered it was more efficient to use a cattle watering trough with transducers running along the sides. These were excellent attempts to get images with ultrasound, but he was forced to acknowledge that there were drawbacks inherent in a system that immersed real, presumably sick, patients in water. Howry's group continued to focus exclusively on making accurate cross-sectional anatomical images, the kind of image that became the major interest of diagnostic ultrasound. By the early 1960s, Howry had switched to using contact scanners, or transducers, like those developed by a fourth team in Minnesota.

The Minnesota research was led by John Wild, an Englishman who had emigrated in 1946 with a medical degree from Cambridge and service in the Royal Army Medical Corps. He came as a fellow to the Department of Surgery at the University of Minnesota where, from the start, he apparently fell into personality conflicts with almost everyone he worked with. Both at the medical school and at the nearby Wold-Chamberlin Air Station where he stored his cobbled-together machines, Wild faced a knot of problems compounded of cultural differences (one colleague objected to what he called Wild's arrogant, eccentric, upper-crust attitude) and conflicting personal and medical styles.[10] The British surgical tradition, which Wild had experienced at its extreme on the battlefield, valued manual dexterity and prized clinical applications above theory.

But apart from different national medical cultures, there were conflicts in the way medical specialties trained their own. As radiologists, Ludwig and Howry had had to master physics. As a surgeon, Wild had had to master physiology. Because he happened to be familiar with ultrasonic therapy, Wild knew from experience that continuous high-intensity ultrasound can damage tissue. Eager to get some kind of ultrasonic image of patients but wary of doing them harm, he avoided the danger of unintentionally damaging tissue by the ingenious tactic of sending sound waves in short pulses. Working with A-mode (one-dimensional) scans that projected a linear pattern on an oscilloscope screen

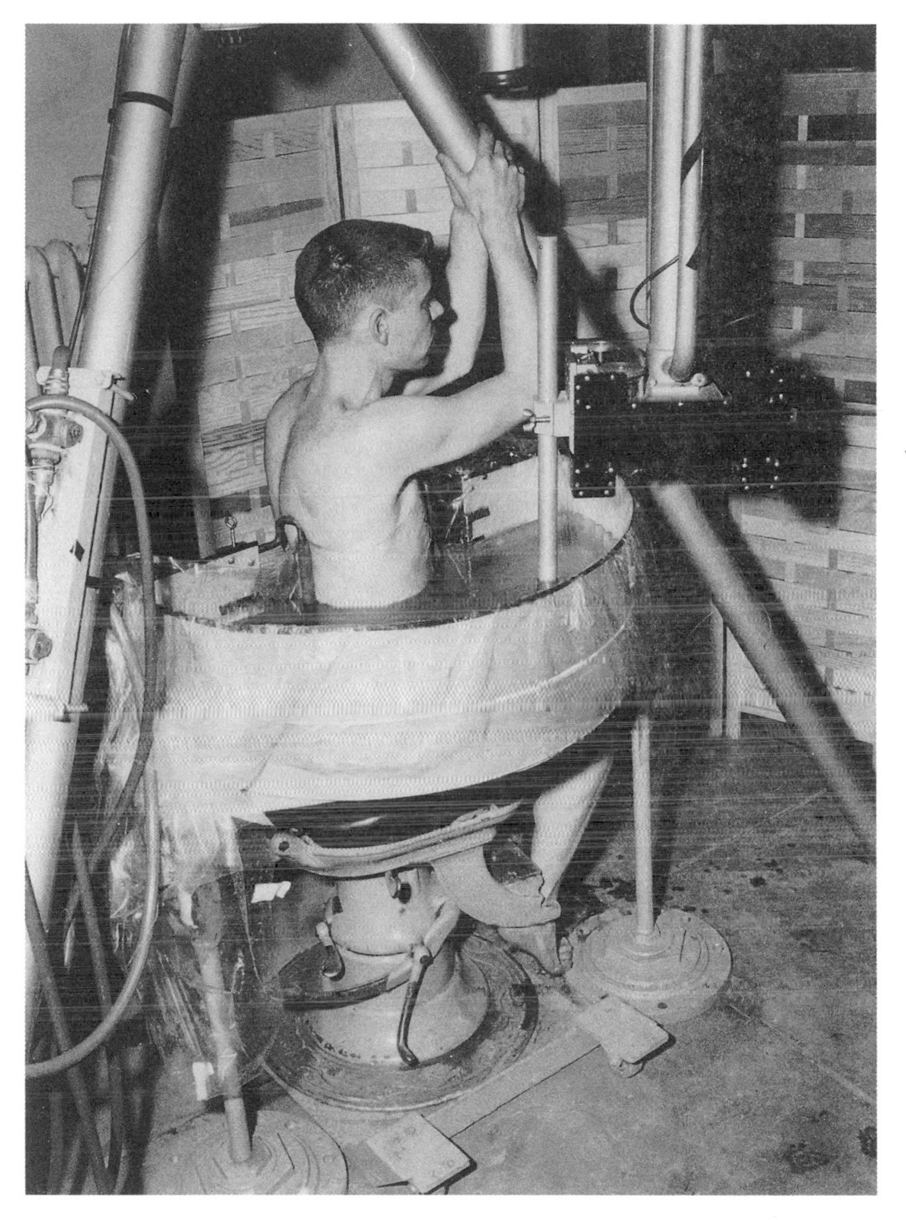

48. A "patient" (actually C. R. Cushman, an electronic engineer working on the project) demonstrating early ultrasound. He is in position in the B-29 scanner, prepared for having his neck scanned. Lead weights on his stomach ensured a consistent immersion level. Courtesy of Barry Goldberg, Archives Committee of the AIUM.

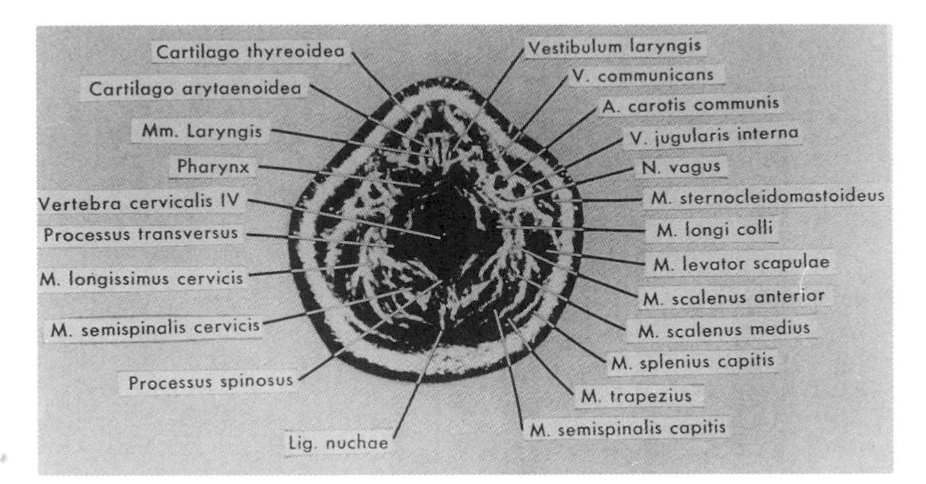

49. Cross-section of the neck with ultrasound, made in the "gun-turret" scanner in 1956. Ten minutes were required to construct the image onto photographic film. The ability to image anatomical structure within the neck in such detail was a technical breakthrough for the Howry team. Courtesy of Barry Goldberg, Archives Committee of the AIUM.

like those at MIT, Wild recorded the echoes in short pulses as they were reflected from the different surfaces within the patient and back toward the generation source. Dubbed the "pulse-echo" technique, it enabled a single transducer to act as both transmitter and receiver, a melding of function that became basic to the emerging technology of ultrasound.

Using his new transducer to measure the thickness of a dog's bowel walls, Wild noticed that signals changed where two different kinds of tissues met. His A-mode imaging provided enough information on the depth and size of the reflecting surface to enable him to determine the dog's condition. He could demonstrate visually, through sound waves, that tumor-invaded tissues are distinguishable from normal tissues.

This chance discovery sent Wild in pursuit of developing ultrasound as a cancer detector. He quickly applied what he had learned from dog bowels to human breast malignancies. Although the problems involved in extracting an image from soft tissue were theoretically enormously complicated, Wild was getting good images. He noted that "a system having a nightmare of complexity to the physicist may be considered simple by the biologist in his blissful ignorance."[11] Donning the cloak of a simple biologist, Wild felt he was ready to test his equipment on patients.

What seemed obviously right to him disturbed his hospital colleagues. They were not ready for him to use human subjects. First the air station and then his department at the university forced him to move his research until his laboratory ended up in his basement. There, between 1953 and 1957, Wild and his team built the first B-mode echoscope—a hand-held device that enabled doctors to image cancers in patients scheduled for surgery.[12] What they saw is the now-familiar pie-shaped image as "the machine swept through the same arc repeatedly, emitting a pulse every few microseconds and recording the

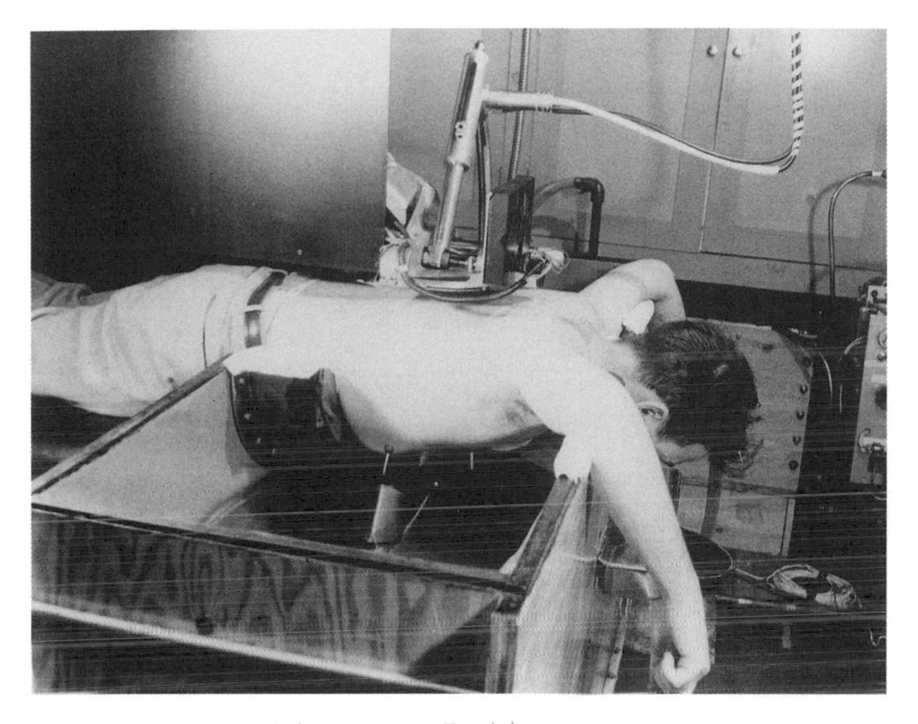

50. Demonstration of Wild's breast scanner. The abdomen is supported; beneath the subject, a transducer and mount (equipped with a guard that would shut the system down if it came into contact with the patient) moved rapidly in a semicircular back-and-forth motion. The hydraulic motor driving the transducer mechanism is at the patient's back. Courtesy of Barry Goldberg, Archives Committee of the AIUM.

returned echo, renewing the image on the screen."[13] To the naked eye the rapidly displayed series of scans looked like a moving picture.

Whatever their goal, each team made important innovations during the 1950s. Wild incorporated a water column sealed with rubber into the transducer, dispensing with the need for immersion baths. And where backscatter—"noise"—caused what Howry had felt were aberrations in the image, Wild captured as much of this "noise" as possible, figuring that the nature of scattering was an index of tissue character.[14] This cleared the way for convenient and relatively discernable images.[15]

Wild's and Howry's approaches were not interchangeable. The images produced by their machines differed significantly. Both researchers imaged tissues beneath the skin, but where Howry sought the best anatomical images he could get of structures that had theretofore evaded traditional X-rays, Wild sought to identify cancers in patients, which added a sense of urgency to his mission. He was impatient with protocols that called for extended use of animal models. Convinced that ultrasound was safe, he ran into trouble each time he went ahead on his own schedule.

Wild continued to make progress, even though more than once he became enmeshed in controversy over grants from the National Cancer Institutes and

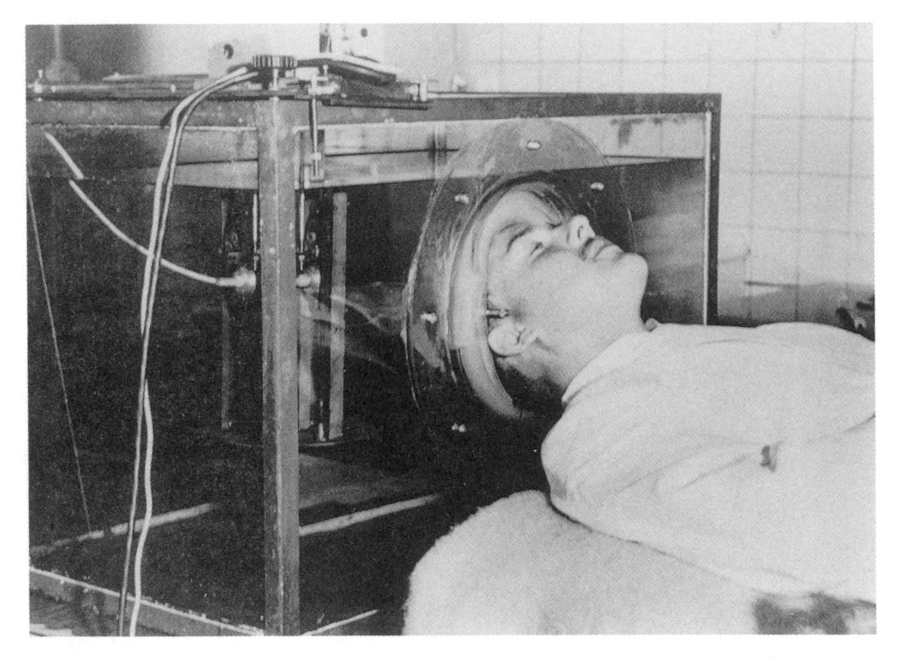

51. B-mode water-bath scanner (c. 1963), with a subject in position for scanning. Note the water bag similar to the early CT water bag machines. Courtesy of Barry Goldberg, Archives Committee of the AIUM.

how they should be administered. Yet many of his contemporaries recognized his genius and periodically came to his aid. In 1951 he worked for a while with the Minnesota Foundation, and he had on-again off-again connections with hospitals in Minneapolis. He was saved from losing institutional connections by the timely intervention of Charles Mayo, at the nearby Mayo Clinic, in 1951, and through the intervention of Senator Hubert Humphrey in 1962.

In 1957, the National Cancer Institutes, which was supporting both Wild's and Howry's research, decided that it was too expensive and duplicative to fund projects that looked very much the same. They insisted that the teams consolidate their efforts and asked Wild to adopt Howry's techniques in detection equipment. Wild would not accept this interference with his work; he saw his approach as incompatible with Howry's. In an early version of the conflict between Lauterbur and Damadian, Howry (like Lauterbur) was focusing on using his approach to make an anatomical map, while Wild, like Damadian, was concerned with identifying malignant tissue.

In spite of Wild's refusal to accept NCI's terms, in 1962 the National Institute of General Medical Sciences, another group within the NIH, granted Wild the then-unprecedented sum of $500,000 to develop a new stage of research—in vivo experiments for malignant tumors in the brain and breast. Once again the project stumbled against Wild's insistence on what some medical colleagues considered premature use with patients. Wild sued the fund that administered his grant and, in the acrimonious aftermath of the legal proceedings, the NIH sequestered his equipment and removed it to Washington, where it moldered into obsolescence behind lock and key. After a long exchange of recriminations and lawsuits (which he finally won), Wild struck out on his own in 1964. Inventive and enterprising, he developed more ultrasound equipment, including miniature transducers for insertion into the vagina and rectum, as well as a system for mass ultrasound screening for breast cancer.[16]

The research by Wild, Howry, and the Frys evoked very little interest from the private sector. Siemens and other medical instrument companies checked in from time to time, but there was no market clamoring for the technology. Perhaps because there seemed little chance of making money from the research, the relations among ultrasound researchers were relatively warm. They exchanged information frequently and published in the same journals. All of them were interested in practical, clinically applicable machines. Unlike the developers of the other scanning technologies, ultrasound pioneers did not approach it as the key to any specific area of basic research. They looked to ultrasound as a practical, clinic-friendly tool.

Seeing with Sound

The brain was the focus of the Dussiks, the first ultrasound clinicians. Still largely a mystery in 1953, the brain was also the interest of Lars Leksell at the University of Lund in Sweden, where he was called to examine a mysteriously comatose sixteen-month-old child. Leksell realized that the skulls of infants, unlike adults, are thin enough for ultrasound waves to penetrate. Desperate to help his small patient, he tried flaw-detection equipment, successfully diagnosed a hematoma, and saved the child's life.

That was the first step. Three years later he discovered an acoustical window into the adult brain. Just above and in front of the ear, the skull is thin enough that a pulse of ultrasound introduced at right angles to the head produces an echo from a place inside the brain called the midline. This is a wall of the third ventricle, located in the middle of the head. When this area is distorted, the echo will not bounce straight back, thus giving evidence of a tumor, blood clot, or some other abnormal structure. The phenomenon Leksell had established is known as the midline echo.

Leksell's approach was picked up by Marinus de Vlieger in Holland, who used a similar industrial flaw-detection device on a patient whose skull had been surgically opened, leaving an unprotected brain. By the early 1960s, midline echo-encephalography was a favored and relatively inexpensive way to explore the intracranial area. Suddenly accessible to sonographic imagery, the brain tempted more explorers to map the still dark continent. They had begun to make progress in the 1970s when the entrance of CT cast them adrift. Ultrasound images of the brain could not compete with CT. But there were other sites where it could, such as the heart.

In 1953 Inge Edler, a physician, and Helmuth Hertz, a physicist, both also at the University of Lund, launched the specialty of echocardiography. They

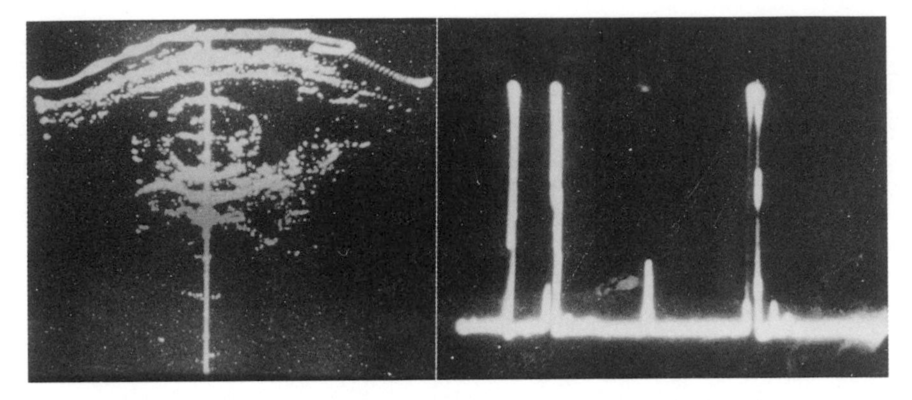

52. A 1964 ultrasound scan of the fetal head, showing the midline echo in the A-mode presentation at right, and cross-section of the fetal head in the B-mode presentation at left. This scan was probably produced by Donald's Diasonograph. Courtesy of Barry Goldberg, Archives Committee of the AIUM.

applied ultrasound to the human heart in vivo, successfully demonstrating that they could get real-time images of identifiable cardiac structures using an approach they called M-mode ultrasound—short for Motion mode. Their system displayed a signal—a B-mode presentation of motion on an oscilloscope screen that they filmed as the echo shifted position. The resulting image, in wave form, reflected the interior structure of the heart through several cardiac cycles. M-mode was a breakthrough in providing structural, anatomical information. It showed a lot of what clinicians wanted to see, even though it did not show a three-dimensional image or the direction or velocity of the flowing blood.

The matter of imaging the direction of blood flow was solved in Japan. Here, as in the West, physicists, engineers, and physicians with wartime experience in ultrasonics cooperated to perfect medical imaging. By the end of the 1950s, several Japanese groups had initiated a new approach to ultrasound imaging of heart and blood flow studies, and despite the postwar occupation, Japanese medicine grew on its own, semi-isolated from Europe and the United States. Like their Western counterparts, Japanese doctors and engineers with military and industrial experience collaborated in several cities at the same time. And like their American and European colleagues they began with A-mode equipment, experimenting with the detection of brain tumors, breast cancers, and gall bladder problems before they moved on to B-mode scanning and the perfection of transducers.

The Japanese were ahead of the West in one critical area in 1955, the application of the Doppler effect to show the speed of the blood as it moves through the heart. This was pioneered by Shigeo Satomura and Yasuharu Nimura at Osaka University. The Doppler effect depends upon the fact that the frequency of a sound wave reflected from a moving object differs from the frequency of the original wave in proportion to the speed of the object. A common example of the phenomenon is the change in frequency of the whistle from a passing train.

The Osaka team used an apparatus that sent ultrasound into a blood vessel. When the blood moved away from the probe, the waves that reflected back were lower in frequency than the waves originally emitted; those moving toward the probe were higher.[17] Because the speed of the blood would be lower if an artery were clogged, the measure of speed would indicate the condition of the heart's arteries and valves.

The idea was brilliant, but premature. Doppler ultrasound, which eventually made ultrasound an essential diagnostic tool, had to await the development of powerful computers to handle all the information generated. But computers were not applied to most ultrasound until the late 1970s.

In the meantime, American researchers began working on Doppler as well. Dean Franklin's bioengineering group at the University of Washington in Seattle began a research effort in the late 1950s that resulted in successful clinical trials in 1964. Doppler ultrasound attracted interest from the Smith-Kline Corporation, which negotiated technology transfer agreements with the University of Washington. At last ultrasound was entering the marketplace.

Eventually Doppler echocardiography developed as an indispensable tool for examining congenital, valvular, and coronary heart disease. Then, in the mid-1980s, color flow mapping was superimposed on the familiar black and white ultrasound image. Coded in color, Doppler measurements noted shifts in frequency reflecting changes in temperature, a sign of infection, as well as changes in the direction of flow.

Meanwhile, as far back as the early 1950s, Ian Donald, a Scottish doctor who had worked with sonar during wartime military service, began experimenting in Glasgow with the possibilities of using ultrasound in obstetrics.[18] The Glasgow group initially used an A mode, flaw-detection device like the one Howry was using in Colorado. Unlike Wild, however, Donald was not interested in cancers. Donald used ultrasound to measure the size of the fetus in the interest of maternal health. Donald kept improving ultrasound machines targeted at fetal imaging through the early 1960s. By 1970 his work was legitimated by the inclusion of a section on ultrasound in *Antenatal and Postnatal Care,* an obstetrical textbook.

At the same time in the United States, a team at the University of Colorado Medical Center also launched the application of ultrasound to obstetrics and gynecology.[19] Making use of a newly invented scanner by a nearby Denver research group, they were able to discern the echo pattern of the placenta using both A-mode and B-mode techniques and make fetal measurements to determine the presence of twins, placenta praevia, and abnormal fetal growth.

Into the Market

Addressing the seventy-ninth annual meeting of the American College of Obstetricians and Gynecologists in 1968, Ian Donald reminisced on his role in launching a new diagnostic science.[20] By then ultrasound was used in major academic medical centers, but it was not widespread and was only sought when there was a suspicion of serious problems. Donald noted that in the nineteenth century obstetrics had led the world into abdominal surgery, "that hitherto forbidden territory"; with ultrasound, gynecology was once again in the lead.[21] In contrast to the excitement raised by Roentgen's original X-ray, Donald said that sonar "crept in behind the maternal skirts of modern engineering . . . behaving, at least until recently, very much like poor cousins."[22] But now that ultrasound was widely accepted, he credited "the Denver team" as "rivals and friends," for having developed sophisticated techniques. When ultrasound came into its own in the 1960s, imaging technology had not yet become a battle of titans and ultrasound was still part of obstetrics or other specialties and not part of radiology.

Radiologists had other items on their plates. Beside the beginnings of nuclear scanning at the end of the 1940s, ultrasound had to compete with the introduction of intensifying screens that allowed radiographs to be increasingly detailed in subtle shades of gray, black, and white, and the subsequent successful introduction of X-ray cinematography. Through the 1950s, B-mode, the best ultrasound could offer, produced only two-dimensional images and was limited to flat black and white. For another decade ultrasound remained the physician's last imaging choice because of its poor spatial resolution and slow scanning times.

Then, in the mid-1970s, as computers assisted X-rays in CT, the computer worked its magic for ultrasound: the computer brought gray-scale and real-time imaging to ultrasound, and its universe changed. Ultrasound now registered weaker echoes coming from diffuse spaces between internal organs and recorded these weaker echoes in subtle shades of gray. Computerized digital scan-converters enabled ultrasound to reveal subtle differences between tissues.

Topping off this rash of improvements was the introduction of real-time imaging, the advance that brought ultrasound machines into the doctor's office. Acting like a movie camera, the new ultrasound projected individual two-dimensional frames at a rate faster than fourteen frames per second (the flicker-fusion rate that makes cinema work because it is faster than the human eye can register).[23] This was a difficult mechanical problem because B-scan ultrasound used a transducer that moved over the surface of the body in a complex series of angular motions. In early B-scan imaging, the transducer took between twenty seconds and a minute to form a static image. After 1975, however, improvements made it possible to obtain images in a tenth of a second, allowing sonography to produce "real-time" motion. By the mid-1980s these machines had become state of the art.[24] Computerization increased the cost of ultrasound, but even with its higher price an ultrasound scan was, and is, about the same price as an X-ray image, about a quarter of the price of a CT scan and an eighth the price of an MR image.

Radiologists who might have benefited from ultrasound gave no sign at the start that they were ready to buy the machines. Ultrasound technologists were caught in the same commercial quicksand as William Oldendorf and

Alan Cormack, who had offered CT to companies like General Electric and been turned down. The inventors may have been "ahead of their time," but that begs the question of when the time is ripe. This seems to be when manufacturers feel sure of their market, because innovation has slowed down enough so that whatever they make will have a respectable shelf life.

Organized medicine withheld making a commitment to ultrasonography throughout its developing years because radiologists had not expressed interest, and there was no single constituency. Before NMR became MRI, chemists liked to say the letters stood for No More Radiologists. They were wrong then, because radiologists quickly expanded their skills to master the arcane principles of magnetic resonance as a sister technology to CT scanning. PET seemed to be heading into the camp of nuclear medicine, but the advent of "imaging centers" allowed radiologists (some now called themselves "imaging specialists") to dominate the specialty. Ultrasound, however, is the one, perhaps, that got away from the control of organized radiology. Ultrasound machines take a much smaller investment than any of the other technologies, and gynecologists argue that patients prefer the comfort and personal contact of a doctor's office to making another visit to a separate imaging center. The American Institute of Ultrasound in Medicine includes not only radiologists, but also ophthalmologists, obstetricians, and cardiologists, and membership is optional. Nonphysicians may be certified by the American Registry of Diagnostic Medical Sonographers, but any doctor can hire just about anyone to operate a machine. It is up to the patient to inquire how much both physician and technician know about what they are doing.

Ultrasound met a cautious market. Given the many parent inventors, there was no uniformity in machinery, and manufacturers were reluctant to begin production when electronic technologies were changing so fast. Manufacturers, including Sperry, Siemens, and Kelvin Hughes, makers of ultrasonic flaw detection equipment, feared entering large-scale medical production because they saw technology advancing so quickly that "an instrument based on available technology would be very rapidly rendered obsolete while the new solid-state technology did not quite seem ripe for exploitation."[25] Picker, in the abdominal-obstetrical field, and Smith-Kline for cardiac applications, were exceptions. In the early 1970s they began developing ultrasound machines earmarked for diagnosis and advertised as essential. Even with the introduction of CT, ultrasound had a market. New companies like ATL, Acuson, and Diasonics in the 1980s introduced computerized ultrasound and combined different kinds of Doppler with gray-scale images. Their bold invasion of the ultrasound market, which they still dominate, distinguishes ultrasound from its companion imaging technologies, which are dominated by the old X-ray manufacturers.

These improvements notwithstanding—computers, color Doppler, and real-time imaging—ultrasonography might not have had a chance in the clinic were it not for two historical events. The first was Stewart's dramatic publication in 1956 of the impact of fetal exposure to X-rays with the deaths of children younger than ten from leukemia or malignancies.[26] The second event was the new voice of women in the political arena who wanted to influence the practice of childbirth and abortion.

Baby's First Picture

Not so long ago an obstetrician's major concern was the mother's life. A British medical historian quotes a Scottish doctor recalling the delivery of a baby when he was a resident in the 1930s. "I hear you did a breech in the middle of the night. How is the mother?" his chief asked the next day. "I said, 'she's fine.' *Two hours later* he came by and added 'Oh, by the way, how did the baby do in that case?'"[27]

Today we give at least equal attention to the baby. When still a fetus, and at a risk which may compromise the mother's health or, at the least, her autonomy, the visual presence of a fetus raises the sticky issue of conflicting interests. At this point the symbiotic connection between mother and developing fetus can become an adversarial relationship. Ultrasonic images have contributed as perhaps no other imaging technology to polarizing attitudes about the personhood of fetuses, embryos, even unfertilized eggs.

For 70 percent of American parents today, the baby album may begin with a sonogram. Ultrasound produces far more detailed, and earlier, images of the developing fetus than X-rays ever did. Where X-rays showed fetal bones, ultrasound, in its finest resolution, displays the fetal heart and all the fetal organs. Pregnancy has changed, and few people would argue for a return to a past of "blind" deliveries.

Ultrasound is not the only change in pregnancy management. The scales have tipped toward interest in the fetus for a number of reasons: since the development of antibiotics women seldom succumb to infections; moreover, careful monitoring of maternal health—where women have access to good food and prenatal care—has, for the most part, removed pregnancy from the class of "disease"—an unnatural condition requiring treatment. Pregnancy, always a process of enormous fascination to women, has been altered by ultrasound. The images offer women an opportunity to monitor fetal development and offer their husbands, who are now encouraged to participate in the delivery, a chance to track the stages leading toward it.

Women unable to bear children have come to feel almost as deprived of the defining experience of pregnancy as they do from not having children to rear. Such women filled the waiting room in an infertility clinic in Santa Monica, California. They were hopeful as they sat filled with hormones that increased the number of eggs they released each month, which they came to watch ripening in their ovaries on an ultrasound monitor. "Harvested," and fertilized in a small petri dish, the eggs will be inserted as embryos in empty uteruses where a small fraction will begin to grow. Their pictures, too, ultrasound images of a cluster of dark dots, make it into the new family album. When the eggs do not become fertilized, grown men have broken down in tears; they mourn the lost eggs like the loss of a child.

Before ultrasound there was no way to see eggs, a developing embryo, or a fetus at an early stage of development. Gynecologists and obstetricians were apt to regard the developing fetus as a kind of uterine tumor.[28] The Oxford report on the long-term danger of prenatal X-rays, however, focused attention on the fetus. It became horribly clear to the public that fetuses could be harmed in utero. The Thalidomide tragedy in 1961, in which more than eight thousand infants were born without fully developed arms and legs to women who had taken the nonprescription antinausea drug in Germany and Britain, underlined the fragility of the fetus in early pregnancy. With ultrasound, parents could know in advance if there were problems and take whatever steps were possible if certain kinds of damage were caught in time. X-rays had already been useful in troubled pregnancies to show fetal position and indicate approximate time of delivery. When ultrasound appeared on the market in doctor-friendly form after 1970, obstetricians turned to it as a safe alternative technology.

Throughout the 1970s, ultrasound improved, and hospitals, clinics, and private physicians acquired ultrasound machines. The relatively low cost of the equipment, about the same as an X-ray machine, undoubtedly contributed to its distribution all over the world.

Ultrasound was only part of the revolution in the new medical specialty of fetology. By 1967 amniocentesis could and did reveal the sex of the developing infant as part of its genetic profile. In the early days this meant the detection of the extra chromosome that indicates Down's syndrome. Today there is a growing list of genetically caused deficits that can be detected, including cystic fibrosis, Tay-Sachs disease, sickle cell anemia, and Huntington's disease.

Ultrasound and amniocentesis arrived in obstetrics coincidentally with women's demands for autonomy, including the right to choose abortion, which followed in the wake of *Roe v. Wade* in 1972, and a strong anti-abortion movement grew to meet the challenge. The rhetoric of both groups used the ultrasound images of fetuses to advance their cause. Where once mothers felt they were carrying dependent, parasitic organisms, that metaphor shifted. In a *Life* magazine article in 1965 the fetus is described as an astronaut attached by a life-line—the umbilical cord—to its spaceship/mother.[29] It shows the fetus as an independent entity attached to its mother by only a thin cord. The drama was established of the independent fetus yearning to continue growing, and the possibility that its mother—still the spaceship with the controls—might decide to cast it adrift, that is, terminate its growth. Women who had reveled in the ability to control their own lives were gradually overwhelmed by new visual documentation—some skillfully rearranged—that the fetus was an independent being, with rights that rivaled their own.

Ultrasound in the 1970s was confined to high-risk pregnancies, but by the 1980s it had become routine in pregnancies covered by most kinds of insurance. In the 1990s, ultrasound has become a necessary confirmation of pregnancy and the "show and tell" object of parental pride. The entrance of ultrasound into obstetrical practice happened swiftly and silently. The few studies of the effects of ultrasound on rodent fetuses, which showed birth defects, were ignored in favor of other studies that showed ultrasound to be harmless.

There were no large-scale tests of the possible side effects of sound waves bouncing off the developing fetus, largely because ultrasound was institutionalized into obstetrical practice so rapidly. There has been no evidence of any damage to children from ultrasound, but it is curious that, with the history of the delayed effects of ionizing radiation so much a part of societal fears, so few doubts were raised about the safety of the new imaging miracle.

What exactly does the pregnant woman see when she has a sonogram? That depends on the kind of image, and on the woman. For high-risk pregnancies, vaginal transducers manipulated by highly trained sonographers can produce uncannily detailed images of eight-week-old fetuses. Routine examinations in an obstetrician's office, however, may show a fan-shaped blur with a dark, undifferentiated bean which the mother is told is her growing fetus.

In reality, however, most ultrasound images are hazy enough so that doctors like Jacobson can get away with suggesting fetal limbs in the mist. Of course, experts can see the fetal heart, the fetal brain, and make out structural defects invisible to the layperson. Likewise radiologists can identify heart and lung problems on CT and MR images that no patient can understand without careful coaching. Experts will occasionally see problems that are correctable by fetal surgery—a process that encompasses surgically exposing the fetus while it remains inside the uterus so that a shunt can be installed in the bladder or brain.

Whether they can see details of their fetus or not, most people feel they

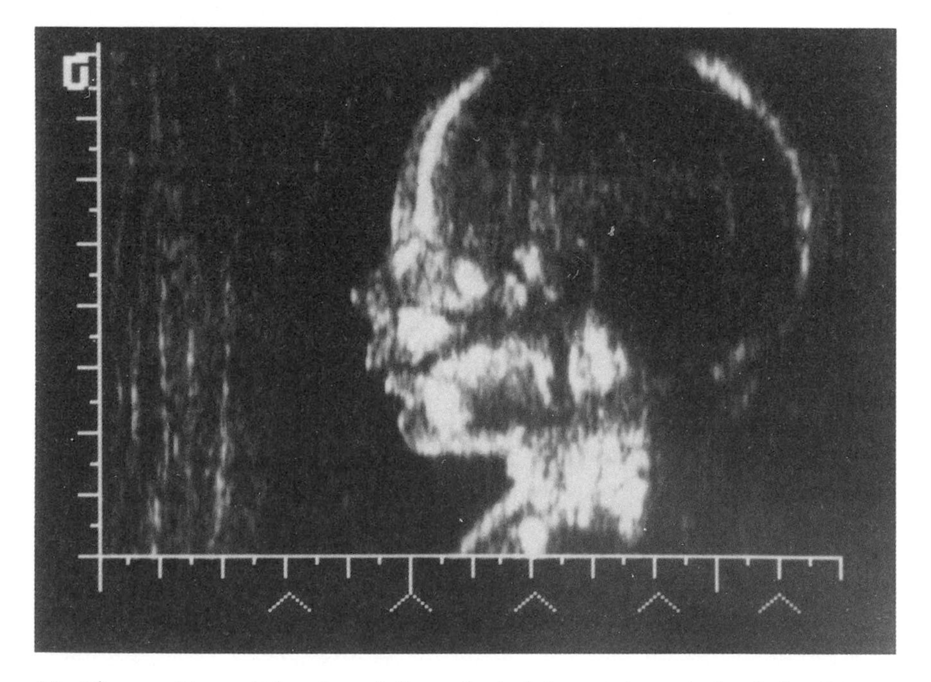

53. Ultrasound image, taken through the mother's abdomen, shows the head of a nineteen-week-old fetus. Centimeter scale above indicates the head to be 5 cm, or 2 in., across (1995). Courtesy of Acuson Corporation.

are entitled to have the picture. Ultrasound is an institution in American life, part of a new pregnancy scenario, and it no longer matters if prospective parents really see anything or not. Most believe they do, and may well "bond" better with their offspring for having glimpsed a tiny hand or foot rather than having to make do, as their parents did, with random kicks sometime after the fifth month. "Expecting" notices in the form of ultrasonograms have become part of our Hallmark culture. Although a study financed in 1993 by the National Institute of Child Health and Human Development suggested that in most instances ultrasound seldom led to any change in the mother's or the infant's health, the survey fell initially on deaf ears.[30] Belt-tightening in medical care, however, has been felt by ultrasonographers; some insurance plans no longer cover routine images and American women are now under-imaged in comparison with women abroad.

What is medically advisable is debatable, but a professor of radiology and obstetrics at Harvard Medical School says, "The ideal situation would be if every pregnant woman got a detailed scan between eighteen and twenty weeks by a very well-trained person."[31] In Europe it is standard for all pregnant women to have at least one ultrasound; in Germany three are the norm, and in England two.

The demand for extra sonograms in the United States has been filled by private vendors who have set up studios, like the early X-ray studios of 1896—often next door to maternity clinics, beckoning women leaving with the prospect of a videotape of their "baby." Many of these "videographers" have no training at all. More worrisome to the medical profession, though, are those professional amateurs, especially obstetricians and general practitioners, who buy an ultrasound machine and use it to generate "free money" by making images that they are unable to interpret properly. There are too many instances of women who almost died from tubal hemorrhage because their ectopic pregnancies were missed, and of babies born handicapped because no one realized there was more than one fetus.[32]

Ultrasound is without doubt valuable as a screening process. Although 70 percent of mothers who have scans don't benefit from them, neither do most of the people who have chest X-rays for TB. The penny-wise advocates of eliminating ultrasound are met by practitioners of defensive medicine. There is no doubt that part of the pressure to maintain scanning comes from the threat of "wrongful" life suits, actions by parents who would have chosen abortion if they had been advised of their child's disability. Other plaintiffs could argue that they were wrongfully denied the option of fetal surgery.

But perhaps nothing has been as controversial in this century of imaging as the suggestion raised in the wake of the 1992 Supreme Court decision in *Planned Parenthood v. Casey.*[33] Casey (representing the state of Pennsylvania) argued successfully that the State has an interest in the protection of the potential life of the fetus while at the same time it cannot unduly burden a woman's right to abort. To this end, the Court discussed the issue of "informed consent." Pennsylvania decreed that before women could elect to terminate a pregnancy, they had to be informed fully, by a doctor, about the procedure.

In the case of a minor, the parents had to be informed as well. The Supreme Court did not think these regulations posed an "undue burden" on the woman even though they add to the expense of the procedure.

If expense is not to be taken into account, and if the true test is information, why not, some legal scholars have suggested, mandate that every abortion seeker see a sonogram of her fetus? That, they assert, would be true knowledge. After all, many doctors use a sonogram in any case to make sure that the fetus is below the maximum age for legal abortion, so such a rule would not add to the cost. All they would have to do is insist the woman have a look along with them.

The assumption here is, of course, that no woman could see a sonogram and go ahead with an abortion, even if the pregnancy had resulted from rape or incest.[34] However, it seems equally likely that if the sonogram showed a defective fetus, many women who had not considered abortion would proceed to have one. The questions only trigger more questions. Is demanding that a woman watch a sonogram the same as forcing a woman to have a procedure she does not choose? Does this interfere with the privacy of the patient/doctor relationship? Does it lead women down the putative slippery slope, that incline that once trod upon leads inevitably to the end, which in this instance might be mandated fetal surgery—or the restriction of medications such as chemotherapies that are harmful to the fetus but whose non-use would result in maternal death? Should such a law be enacted, it would be unique in the history of imaging technologies. At the least, it would alter the intangible feeling of seeing an interior image of your own body from a health-saving procedure to a threat.

Mammography

Breasts—defined as the hemispherical protrusions on the chests of adult women—are not functionally necessary. Among mammals (creatures so named because they boast mammary glands that produce milk to feed their young) human females alone sport full breasts when not nursing. Evolutionists argue over the "adaptive" purpose of the female breast (which may have evolved as a mirror of the buttocks, which is a sexually selective trait among some primates). In Western history breasts have been venerated and exploited, but, whether draped or exaggerated, breasts define women.

Because of this cultural peculiarity, the translucent breast is a special case in the history of imaging the body. During the first half century after Roentgen, breasts seemed to vanish before X-rays, allowing TB screeners to see right through to the lungs. Soft breast tissue was no match for early radiation for diagnosis. The X-rays were only for radiotherapy, as is apparent in Georges Chicotot's 1909 self-portrait where the X-ray tube is suspended above the naked breast of the supine beauty on the examining table.

When X-rays were introduced to the world, the treatment of breast cancer in the United States had been recently simplified to a single procedure: radical surgery following palpation by a doctor's sensitive hands. The powerful voice of William Halstead allowed no debate. Halstead had in the 1890s

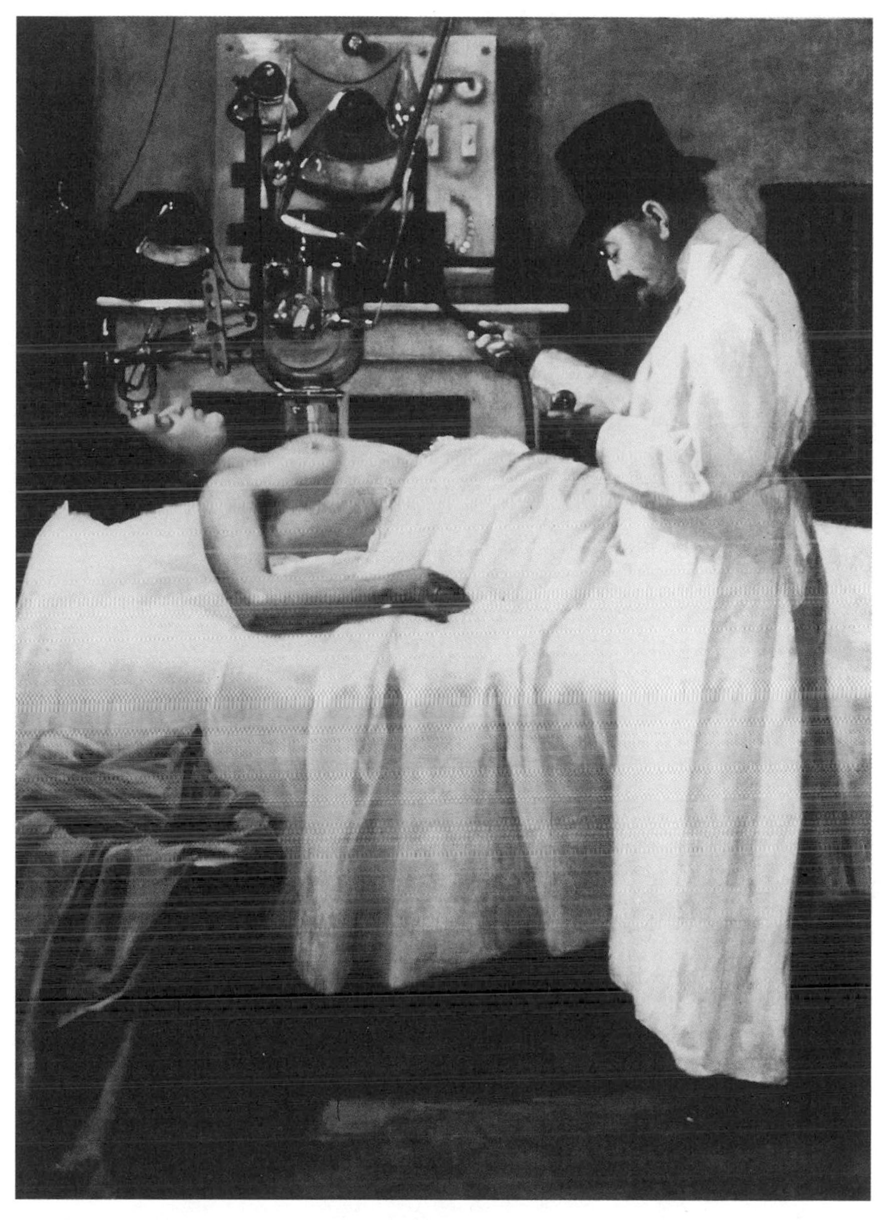

54. *Georges Chicotot* (1909). Self-portrait of Dr. Georges Chicotot, chief radiologist at the Hôpital Herold, doing a radio-therapeutic treatment for breast cancer. In his left hand, there is a timer, and in his right hand, there is a blowtorch to regulate the hardness of the tube. Courtesy of Sipa Press, Paris.

developed the radical mastectomy, a procedure that involved amputating the entire diseased breast and the neighboring pectoral muscles, lymphatic-bearing tissue, and tissue stretching into the chest walls. With that, he declared breast cancer cured. In a medical culture with strong idols and no follow-up studies, the disease remained "cured" until Halstead's death in 1922.

However, in 1913 in Berlin, where Halstead's influence did not reach, Albert Salomon studied breast cancer with X-rays. He examined radiographs of three thousand mastectomy specimens and noticed "small black bits" at the centers of the carcinomas, now identified as "microcalcifications." He was a lone voice in imaging breast cancer for many years, but in the 1930s this line of research was continued in Philadelphia at the Jefferson Medical College.[35] There Jacob Gershon-Cohen decided that the only way to understand the diseased breast was to study the normal breast "under all conditions of growth and physiologic activity" in order to have a norm against which to judge the abnormal, or cancerous, breast.[36] In an article published in 1938, he argued that it was necessary to study the breast throughout the life cycle, but no one responded for over a decade. World War II may have interrupted interest in "civilian, " especially female, diseases, or the suggestion may simply have struck epidemiologists as too difficult to arrange.

Throughout the 1930s and 1940s, however, surgeons in different parts of the world did concentrate on improving the kind of breast imaging needed for surgery. Stafford Warren, soon to become dean of the UCLA School of Medicine, developed a stereoscopic system with a grid for identifying malignant tumors as well as changes in tissue now known as "fibrocystic change."

It was not until 1949 that breast cancer imaging made its major leap forward. It happened in Uruguay, where Raul Leborgne demonstrated the importance of high-contrast breast images: he could see microcalcifications in about 30 percent of the cancer cases he examined. Leborgne was the first to

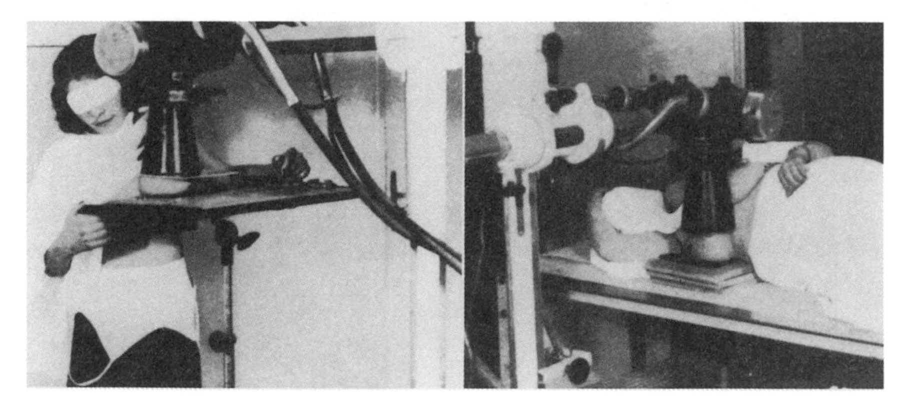

55. Mammography of R. Leborgne (1951). Position of the patient for obtaining a craniocaudal film *(right)* and a lateral view *(left)*. Note the cone and the compression pad interposed between it and the breast below. The film, enclosed in a black paper envelope, is in contact with the breast. (R. Leborgne, "Diagnosis of Tumors of the Breast by Simple Roentgenography," *American Journal of Roentgenology* 65 [1951]: 1–11.) Courtesy of the American Roentgen Ray Society.

emphasize the value of breast compression for identifying both benign and malignant calcification. This proved to be an enormous step toward developing an approach to early diagnosis. Following up on Leborgne's work in 1951, Charles Gros in Strasbourg, France, developed the first radiological unit explicitly designed to examine breasts. Although women now take for granted that there have always been imaging devices designed for looking at the breast (or, in medical jargon, "dedicated" to the breast), in fact, these machines have only been on the market since 1967 when the Compagnie Générale de Radiographie introduced Gros's Senograph at the annual November meeting of the Radiological Society of North America in Chicago. The society's convention had become known internationally for its size, hype, and merchandising power. By the early 1970s, Siemens, Philips, and Picker were also selling special mammography units, and in 1978 Philips brought out the Diagnost-U, a mammography machine that included a system which was a variation on the old Bucky-Potter grid, and by reducing radiation scatter and improving the image, set a higher standard for the next decade.

Breast cancer offered two special advantages to researchers: unlike the stomach, liver, or pancreas, breasts are uniquely accessible to scrutiny. Although a breast cancer might be hidden and not detectable through palpation, breasts are easily isolated for imaging examination and, of course, there are two of them, offering an on-site control. In the 1950s ultrasound pioneer John Wild in the United States tried his imaging efforts on two women volunteers with diagnosed breast cancers, while in Uruguay Leborgne worked on guidelines for locating suspicious areas with X-rays and removing the possible cancer.

Yet imaging the breast—mammography—was still a rare procedure in 1960 when Robert Egan at the M. D. Anderson Hospital in Houston revolutionized the diagnosis of breast cancer by adapting high-resolution industrial film to a mammographic technique. After screening two thousand patients, he reported in 1962, he had discovered fifty-three cases of "occult carcinoma" that had been totally unsuspected.

The new technology was put to the test by the Health Insurance Plan of New York (HIP). Between 1963 and 1966, it organized the first randomized, controlled trial of screening with physical examinations to see if early diagnosis from mammograms could reduce mortality from breast cancer. A five-year follow-up revealed that the women who had undergone mammographies were a third less likely to die from breast cancer than women who had not been screened. The mortality rate remained lower for the next eighteen years.[37] The HIP study was followed by a five-year national study of 250,000 women sponsored by the NCI and the American Cancer Society.

By 1968, radiologists felt comfortable claiming that X-rays had the power to reveal cancer at an early, and often curable, stage.[38] The American College of Radiology responded to the mammogram screenings by conducting a conference on mammography in 1965 and taking over annual conferences from the Public Health Service in 1968.[39] Yet breast screening continued to meet reluctance from primary-care physicians. In the 1970s there was a well-publicized scare surrounding thorotrast, a radioactive contrast medium that had been popular in the 1930s, which turned out to remain in the body, settling into vital organs like the liver, where it caused cancer. It fueled the debate about the pros and cons of X-rays in general and radiation exposure in connection with breast screening. Some experts asserted that the radiation dosage was likely to cause as many cancers as occurred naturally. Was it wise to expose healthy women over and over again to ionizing radiation? Might not the screening mechanism itself be a carcinogenic agent?

The decade of the 1970s saw many other reevaluations of the effects of radiation. Evidence indicated a thirty-five-year lag between heavy exposure to radiation for TB or thyroid treatments, and the appearance of breast cancer. The activist surgeon who headed UCLA's breast cancer center recalls seeing patients in her own practice who had been treated for TB with radiation three decades earlier, and she reports anecdotal support from a study of high occurrences of breast cancer among women in Rochester, New York, who had been given radiation treatment for postpartum mastitis—inflamed breasts—and now had high rates of breast cancer. From what she could ascertain, the risk was dose-related, and only risky to the part of the body that was irradiated.[40]

By the end of the 1930s, the recommended tolerance dose had been cut from 0.2 r (rem) per day to half that amount. The explanation for the change was that the new high-voltage machines had reduced the surface dosage—that is, the radiation that affects the skin—by targeting a specific area deeper inside the body. World War II propelled health physics into center stage and by 1960 the AEC was budgeting $49 million for research in biology and medicine, more than 60 percent of which went to problems of radiation protection.[41] In 1965 the newly organized National Council on Radiation Protection and Measurements, headed by Lauriston Taylor, the physicist who had represented the United States at the first post–World War I international meetings, modernized the system.[42]

In 1940, the international community still had spoken in terms of "maximum permissible dosage," but since then the agencies in charge of the oversight and regulation of radiation have changed, and so have the terms for dosages and our contexts for thinking about radiation.

The world is bathed in radioactivity. Cosmic rays bombard us from space, and natural radioactivity abounds. People who live at high elevations—in Denver, for instance—are exposed to twice as much radiation as people living at sea level. Yet the incidence of cancer is the same in both populations. Currently, most authorities agree that very high doses of radiation are more dangerous than low doses. Moreover, the quantity of radiation that most people are exposed to in diagnostic machines presents less danger than the chance of missing a lesion or carcinoma that an X-ray could reveal at an early enough stage to save lives.

In urging her patients to get mammograms, activist surgeon Susan Love emphasizes that the kind of exposure that led to cancers is on the order of 8,000 rads, while the level of exposure in the occasional diagnostic X-ray for TB or a mammogram is on the order of a quarter of a rad. The negative publicity connecting radiation with cancer kept many women at risk away from the mammographer. Love counters these fears by pointing out that a mammogram in 1993 exposed "a woman to about the same amount of radiation as she would have gotten walking bare-breasted along the beach for ten minutes at noon—or until stopped by an officer of the law."[43]

For all the research on the effects of radiation on living tissue, we still know very little about the risks and benefits of any exposure to ionizing radiation. What we have are statistics in large populations monitored over long periods of time. The answers are very imprecise. Radiologists use the doubling factor. Making an analogy with heat, we know that a temperature of 10 degrees is cold, but safe to people wearing clothes. The same is true for twice the temperature. Even at 40 and 80 degrees we can be comfortable. At 160 degrees we are dead. The same is probably true about exposure to radiation, only we are not sure where to stop doubling.[44] All that can be said with certainty is that the least exposure is the best.

One response to the effort to shorten exposure came in 1966 when John Wolfe at the Detroit Receiving Hospital reported on the advantages of coupling Xerox technology with mammography. The idea stimulated the Xerox Corporation to make a unit specifically for breast imaging. Its commercial unit for xeroradiography was in production in 1971 and for almost twenty years

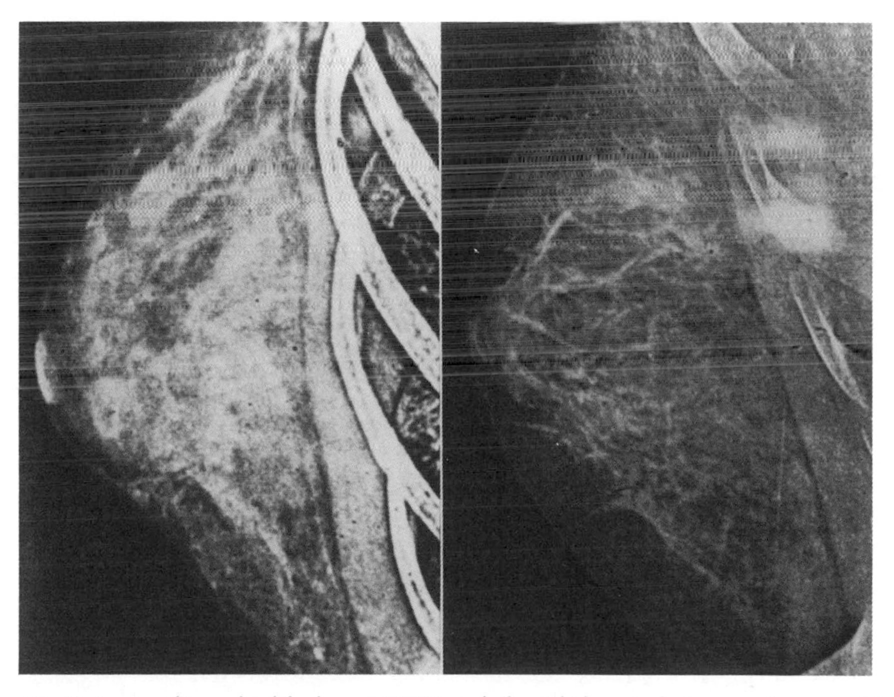

56. First xeroradiograph of the breast (1960). *Left,* the right breast of a twenty-nine-year-old childless woman sharp detail. *Right,* the right breast of an eighteen-year-old mother who was forty-five days postpartum. Individual glands and ducts can be made out without difficulty; the detail is much sharper than with conventional roentgenography in this type of breast. (G. R. Gould, "Xeroradiography of the Breast," *American Journal of Roentgenology* 84 [1960]: 220–223.) Courtesy of the American Roentgen Ray Society.

afterwards women in North America saw their transparent breasts in blue and white. Xeroradiology replaces the film of traditional X-ray imaging with a selenium-coated aluminum plate that was prepared for exposure by being electrically charged. The advantage to the patient was that a short burst of radiation left a latent image that developed on the receptor into a very high quality image, similar to images theretofore obtained only when exposing the patient to a longer period of X-ray exposure. The high contrast of the xeroradiographic image dominated mammography until the old-guard X-ray manufacturers responded to the challenge from Xerox by producing X-ray units built especially for mammography which got even finer images with ever less radiation. (Xerox retreated from this market in 1989, having spurred its competitors toward building that better mousetrap.)

The incidence of breast cancer has increased as the population ages. Yet cancer remained a quasi-unmentionable word (it still is in some parts of the world), and breast cancer even more unmentionable as it affected a part of the body that was so eroticized, until September 1974. That was when Betty Ford, the first lady of the United States, underwent the removal of her right breast, chest muscles, and lymph nodes at the Bethesda Naval Medical Center Hospital. The public was told that, with two of her thirty lymph nodes involved, she had a 62 percent chance of surviving five years. Mrs. Ford followed her surgery with public appearances urging all women to consider frequent self-examination. One month later Happy Rockefeller, wife of the newly nominated vice-presidential candidate, found three small lumps in her left breast because, "like so many women in this country, what happened in the case of Betty Ford made everyone a little more conscious and therefore more careful to check."[45] She underwent the removal of her breast at Memorial Sloan-Kettering hospital in New York, and her doctor predicted a 90 percent chance of recovery. Breast cancer was, in the expression not yet coined, out of the closet. Soon, screening mammograms would be recommended on television. Breast cancer and mammography could at last be discussed in public, and the fear of radiation exposure had entered the arena of public debate.

In 1986 the American Cancer Society and the American College of Radiology met the demand for breast cancer screening by developing an accreditation program and setting standards for physicians and technicians. Some of these centers adopted the American Cancer Society initiative, accepting walk-in patients without physician referrals, and at a lower charge. Soon Maryland and Michigan ruled that health plans had to pay for screening mammograms, and in 1989 a coalition of eleven health organizations, including the American College of Radiology, the American Cancer Society, and the AMA, issued a joint statement urging screening for all women beginning at the age of forty.[46] Breast cancer detection became the equivalent of the tuberculosis-screening crusades of the last quarter of the twentieth century—mobile imaging vans and all. Breast cancer looked like a disease whose eradication seemed possible through early detection that only a look through the body could achieve.[47]

Since the late 1980s, there has been a veritable renaissance in X-ray mammography equipment.[48] The most important improvements were screen-film combinations that reduced radiation dosage by 50 percent. The introduction of automatic exposure controls, better film, film emulsifiers, and processing, and the introduction of digital recording of mammography images have made mammography one of the safest forms of imaging.[49] Another key improvement was magnification mammography in 1977, which permits the technician to magnify the image to twice the size to see detail in suspicious areas.[50]

Improvements, but not foolproof. Mammograms are read by radiologists who miss a full 15 percent of malignancies. Part of the problem is physician education: it was only in 1990 that the American Board of Radiology required a separate section on mammography as part of its oral examination. In part, the problem, not limited to mammography, is the eye fatigue that comes from reading X-rays but is exacerbated by the extraordinary difficulty of spotting subtle irregularities. Despite the great improvement in radiographs, the skill in reading them remains subjective. One effort to sharpen the perception of radiologists was a spin-off of Project Nina, funded by the Department of Defense in 1976 to help pilots detect camouflage. Nina is the daughter of cartoonist Al Hirschfeld, who had delighted young Nina (and millions of *New York Times* readers) in the years following World War II by disguising her name in wisps of hair and folds of clothing in his weekly half-page drawings. Project Nina monitored eye fixation, verifying the well-known phenomenon that you can stare at something and yet not see it. A team of radiologists monitored the length of eye-fixation pauses needed to spot Ninas, and found that teaching radiologists these puzzle-solving skills enabled them to identify the location of lung tumors, a kind of tumor typically camouflaged by overlying structures. When the researchers played back and highlighted the locations of these pauses, they found many missed tumors. By building a computer-assisted visual search system, they were able to reduce error in both lung- and breast-screening X-rays.[51]

In the 1990s X-rays dominate breast imaging, but ultrasound is increasingly used as a companion follow-up approach when a suspicious area is identified. Ultrasound can distinguish between innocent liquid-filled cysts and solid tissue that requires a biopsy. Waiting to be invited to join the breast-imaging pageant are MRI and PET scanners. MRI was used to track silicon leakage in the great breast implant-leakage furor of 1992 and is also being used to screen for early malignancies. PET, too, offers a way of noticing very early tissue changes, long before there is any anatomical evidence, with radioactive isotopes.

By the early 1990s breast cancer, while not epidemic, had become the disease most likely to afflict one in eight women in the United States with the good fortune to survive to the age of eighty-five, of whom half will survive. These figures—gleaned from statistics kept by the state of Connecticut since 1940, and expanded since then to include the entire nation—show annual increases in the number of breast cancer cases reported while the mortality rate has held steady.[52]

Women looked at these figures, recalled the reluctance with which the Pap test was accepted for cancer of the cervix, and wondered about trusting a medical system where, for most of the twentieth century, those men who directed research often seemed to overlook, or trivialize, the needs of women.[53] The women's movement changed the demographics of who practiced medicine as well as who went to the doctor. Women physicians began criticizing the way breast cancer was treated, and women patients found their voices and resisted being left out of the decision-making loop about their own treatments.

Anxiety turned to action in the shadow of the AIDS epidemic. AIDS activists, who were largely, at first, represented by highly articulate homosexual men, served as a model of how to attract research funds as well as hospital and hospice attention. Using AIDS activists as a model, a largely female group calling themselves the National Breast Cancer Coalition (NBCC) persuaded Congress in 1992 to double the money it had theretofore allocated to breast cancer research.[54] The bulk of the $210 million went to the Department of Defense, which had long supported medical research related to the health and battle injuries of its personnel. The NBCC understood the budget-cutting mentality of Congress and agreed that the Defense budget was as good a place as any to place the bulk of the new funding, assuming that it could be used there without interference. Other women disagreed with this arrangement on grounds that the Department of Defense would spend the money on developing better instrumentation to see cancer, rather than on research into its causes. While there is general agreement that imaging accelerates early detection, there is a good deal of disagreement over whether early detection makes any difference in terms of deaths from the disease.

Breast cancer is a political minefield. The studies vary tremendously in every parameter: who participates, what their ages, diets, and histories are, what kinds of mammograms they have been exposed to, and how often. The results are contradictory as to the benefits of mammograms at regular intervals, and for which part of the population. The data on differences in radiation exposure are inconsistent; all the studies are dependent upon image quality of the machines and the skill of the radiologists who read the images. But granting all these problems, a study in May 1995 echoed the views of the AMA and the American Cancer Society that, given the best imaging machines and well-trained doctors, all women over forty benefited from screening mammograms, and that early detection does save lives. The National Cancer Institute departed from its long-standing position and now urges that women should start having routine mammograms only after reaching age fifty.[55]

The experience of a breast exam has changed from simply standing before an X-ray tube to experiencing extreme breast compression in a device described as "appropriate for extracting information from reluctant informants." The compression necessary to get a good image is uncomfortable for women of all dimensions, and while ultrasonic examinations are more comfortable, the resolution is not fine enough to discover microcalcifications. MRI, another possibility, is slow and much more costly, so it is likely that X-ray mammograms will be the image of choice for the foreseeable future.

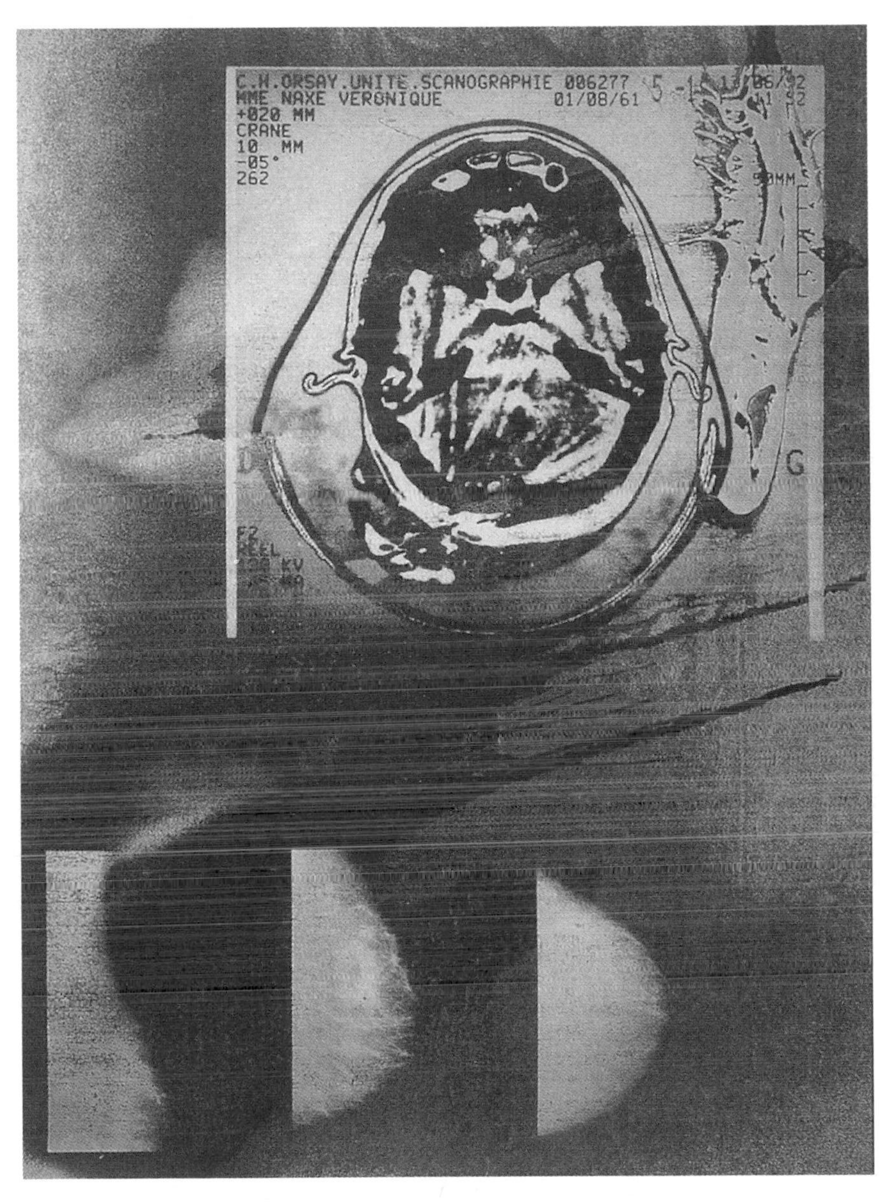

57. Steve Miller, *Portrait of Veronique Maxe* (1993). The artist incorporates a mammogram, which, like sonograms, had entered the culture as icons of the inner woman. Acrylic and silkscreen on canvas, 57" x 86" (144.5 cm x 218 cm). Courtesy of Steve Miller.

The discomfort is not deliberate, although there are those who suspect it might be. All issues connected to women's bodies, especially to peering into them, have become political. Revelations about medical textbooks that defined women's bodies, in general, as ill-formed because they are not male, and about reports of pain and discomfort dismissed as psychosomatic or hysterical have aroused suspicion among many women that the medical profession is conspiring against them. Newly vocal women's health groups bridled at the realization that half the body politic had traditionally been omitted from large-scale health studies because women's bodies change on a monthly basis. They demanded that pregnancy and breast cancer be looked at, and through, with technologies that pay attention to women's biology and way of life.

The politics of pregnancy differs from the politics of breast cancer. A minority of women object to the medicalization of pregnancy altogether; others are conflicted about what they call the "personhood" of the fetus. The ability to see—however imprecisely—its growing presence within the uterus has altered its role not only in medicine (where it has become a patient) but in the public psyche. A fetus may not be a citizen, but those who eagerly anticipate a new family member name it, talk to it, try to educate it, and accept it as soon as they know it is there. This was true, of course, long before the discovery of X-rays, but the experience of seeing the fetus with ultrasound within weeks after conception has altered the fantasies of expectant parents and accelerated the tendency to vest the proto-person with a complete personality.

The popularity of both ultrasound and mammography changed the working vocabularies of twentieth-century women. Women everywhere speak about their breasts, ovaries, uteruses, and endometrial tissues in the language that used to be the purview of specialists. Along with their doctors they have looked at sonograms, X-rays, and mammograms; they are familiar with internal organs that used to have no name, or were unmentionable. Men, too, have benefited from the liberation of being able to see what had been mysterious. Men now accompany women to obstetricians and have also come to look at themselves as deliberately as they look at their fetuses. With familiarity has come a sense of individuality, and sometimes pride. Looking at their body parts, sometimes transparent, sometimes diseased, sometimes simply rich in anomalous lumps and blotches, men and women have been inspired to include these images in a multitude of media, from film to pixels to paint.

Eleven

The Transparent Body in Late Twentieth-Century Culture

X-rays, and later computerized images, did not trigger any revolutions, but they did provide remarkable tools for revolutionaries. We are a more visual culture today than we were a century ago, used to finding information as much from looking at and through objects as from the written word. X-rays and the newer technologies have had an enormous impact on the way individual artists work, on the artist's role in society, and on the popular imagination through cinema and more recently through video. As a culture, we no longer accept surfaces as barriers, but see them instead as smoky scrims through which we know we have access, not just doctors but all of us—patients, poets, and passers-by.

At the end of World War II, the X-ray alone defined the insides of the human body.[1] Thirty years later, the X-ray had lost its monopoly and popular culture had appropriated CT, MRI, PET, and ultrasound images into movies and television (*Hannah and Her Sisters, Rampage, Murphy Brown*), ballet (the Feld company's *MRI*), and the increasingly politically engaged world of the fine arts. Artists no longer avoided technological artifacts but eagerly put their hands on X-ray film and on computer keyboards.

These computer-reconstructed images enlarged the window into the body that the X-ray had opened. At the same time, they increased the sense of fragmentation that comes from seeing parts of our inner selves as transitory patterns on video monitors. Whether anatomic or functional, these new images concentrate on a single organ, continuing the breakup of the body into disconnected parts that began with the original five-by-seven-inch glass X-ray plates and was reinforced intellectually by the movement of physicians away from general practice and into specialties defined, usually, by a part of the body such as the eyes, ears, heart, brain, or kidney.

The new technologies, with the exception of CT, did not image bones. In fact, they scarcely recorded them, muting the long association of glimpses into the living body with premonitions of death, an association that began with Frau Roentgen's fearful reaction to the sight of her skeletal hand in 1895, and continued with Hans Castorp's morbid response to seeing his own living bones in Thomas Mann's 1924 novel.[2] That association was cultural. MRI, PET, and ultrasound images, however, do not image the familiar skeleton and often record functioning that seems to celebrate life.

But right after World War II, the nagging sense that Roentgen's illuminating rays could also be death rays, a suspicion that had begun with William Rollins's 1904 "Notes on the X-light," and had been willfully denied by most of the medical community during the first half century of X-ray technology, was validated by the misery of radiation diseases in Hiroshima and Nagasaki. Yet for all the anguish at the suffering in Japan, it took almost a decade for people to associate the horrors of bomb-wrought diseases with the benevolence of X-ray images. Throughout the 1940s and 1950s American children continued to wriggle their toes beneath shoe-store fluoroscopes. Even after 1956, when the supposedly damaging effects of X-rays on children whose mothers had been X-rayed had been widely broadcast, serious artists did not respond with images of doom. Visions of postnuclear catastrophes were left to pulp fiction and B movies.

At the Movies

Starting with the first fluoroscope, action visible within the body became a narrative. Early cinematographers tried fruitlessly to capture those sequences from the fluorescent screen, and when that failed, learned to simulate moving X-ray images. By the time full-length science-fantasy films were made in the 1940s, they repeated the primordial fears of exposure that had been spelled out in cartoons and music hall jokes since the turn of the century.

X-ray simulations played on the idea that what is opaque can be seen through so that surfaces—like skin—cease to exist. The science-fiction device extends this visual dissolution to all surfaces so that the opaque vanishes entirely. Like "missing matter" in space, the body is still there exerting the gravitational pull of all mass, only it leaves no impression on the eye.

The juxtaposition of solid objects with visually empty space made H. G. Wells's 1897 novel, *The Invisible Man,* popular in print and even more popular in a series of films, the first in 1933, with a sequel in 1940, and a parody, using the same gimmick, in 1992. Like the "visible body" kits that flooded toy stores in the 1960s with colorful plastic body organs inside a transparent doll, the invisible man is recognizable by what is visible inside him. As Wells reasoned in the original story, that would be nothingness surrounded by bandages and clothing. When the hero is naked, his most comfortable indoor mode, the only thing that is visible is the food he is digesting—and that gradually disappears as it is metabolized. Only in the process of dying does his whole body become opaque again as the chemical responsible for his invisibility is deactivated by death. In the 1992 version, *Memoirs of an Invisible Man,* the audience sees different parts of the hero's "invisible" body, as if looking at a scan with a radioactive tracer. The hero smokes and the viewer sees lungs fill and empty as if the smoke were a contrast agent. The digestive system exists alone as well, and there are no bones at all.

Movie makers were so comfortable with X-ray images that they continued to use them exclusively well after doctors and engineers were experimenting with emission images and ultrasound. By 1966, the X-rayed interior of the living body was familiar enough to become the setting for *Fantastic Voyage,* a full-length adventure film built on the premise that the United States has developed a technology capable of shrinking people and things to the size of microbes—but only for about an hour. To save the life of a scientist suffering from a blood clot, a submarine and its crew are shrunk and injected into the scientist's carotid artery. Using a drawing of the sick man's arterial system as a "road map," the submarine's mission is to travel through his arteries into his brain where, with a miniaturized laser weapon, they will blast the clot out of existence. Yet for all the high-tech razzmatazz, the movie is surprisingly old-fashioned in its depiction of technology and oblivious to developments in nuclear medicine that had already made it possible to track a blood clot by seeing inside the body.

Neither are there computers in the film as well, although computers had already entered the workplace in 1966, nor, even more surprising, are there television monitors. The full-size commander in the laboratory communicates with the miniaturized occupants of the miniaturized spaceship in Morse code! The only trace of high-tech machinery that the audience sees is an EEG's spiky lines. Taking itself very seriously, *Fantastic Voyage* is as much documentary as futuristic adventure tale, and an example of a systemic lack of technological imagination in the film industry. Despite its Academy Award for special effects, there was nothing special in *Fantastic Voyage.* It owed its success to its slick adaptation of old scientific imaging, and, for that matter, an old literary device, a twist on Gulliver's or Alice's response to a world whose heroes are minute in comparison to their surroundings.

When *Inner Space,* a spoof on *Fantastic Voyage,* appeared twenty years later (the "Gulliver" character is awake this time and has accidentally been injected with a miniaturized astronaut), the communications are updated but not the imaging technology. This time the Lilliputian communicates directly with the larger world, as well as with the Gulliver character who carries him, by radio, like a tapeworm talking to its host. Yet while Americans had been looking at X-ray images for ninety years, as well as at the newer digitized images, this film, like the one it spoofs, ignores contemporary imaging technology—with its potential for fun as well as imagery—relying on traditional X-rays or on traditional *Gulliver* sets.

When CT finally arrived as the major plot device in a feature film in the 1987 production of *From Beyond,* it was only partially appreciated for its imaging capability. In this adaptation of a story by H. P. Lovecraft, scientists trigger the growth of the pineal gland using a CT scanner. The scanner produces beautiful three-dimensional images of the brain, but it also generates the radioactivity that releases demons who destroy just about everyone in the cast.

From Beyond echoes the century-old tension between *bad* radiation, which generates mutations and threatens human life, and *good* radiation in the form of diagnostic X-rays which expose evil and are, therefore, an instrument of truth. The evils of radiation, as expressed in post-doomsday movies, were a stock element in films made after 1950. Few held much hope for the human future.[3] Radiation had become synonymous with Pandora's punishment, a "gift" from amoral scientists interested only in satisfying their curiosity about matters better left alone. In *Them,* a 1954 movie set in White Sands, New Mexico, giant, man-eating ants appear at the site of the first A-bomb test; the scientist from the Department of Agriculture who is called in for help describes them as a "scientist's dream come true." Radiation-triggered mutations—human, animal, and extraterrestrial monsters—fill American and Japanese science-fiction movies from the 1950s onward.

The *good* X-rays, X-rays used to see through falsehood into truth, are less common in film. Usually they reveal the "other," pseudo-humans as in *The Man Who Fell to Earth,* which exposes an alien passing as a human being. An X-ray reveals that the imposter has no bones. Likewise, the truth about human evolution is exposed in the damage done to one of twenty-three volunteers in *Altered States.* Filmed in 1980, the plot uses an X-ray image of the hero's altered larynx to prove that time spent in an isolation tank, experiencing sensory deprivation and hallucinations, has caused him to regress evolutionarily into a proto-human, apelike hominid, which explains why he can no longer speak.

Our puritan culture had trouble separating the kind of X-ray vision that reveals impostors, who heroes like Superman can see through, from X-rays as themselves a prurient temptation. As recently as 1978 Superman sees all the women at a party topless—but not bottomless. Superman's ability to peer through solid objects has been filmed many times, but his vision remains true to conservative social mores. Although he could see through clothing, he does not use X-ray vision to undress Lois Lane until the mid-1970s. And he has never, yet, been known to look through to the nakedness of men. Superman's X-ray vision is tepid compared to the X-ray machines fifteen years later in *Total Recall.* The 1990 film takes the commonplace experience of carry-on baggage being X-rayed at airports one horrifying step further: all passengers on the subway must pass through giant X-ray machines—and briefly appear as skeletons on giant monitors. In this dystopic future, what chance have the forces of good against such an enormous invasion of privacy?

In mainstream film, medical imaging, like other technologies, is used to add authenticity to place and, occasionally, to plot. But what scientists found exciting—new, three-dimensional imaging of brain and body—did not awe or inspire Hollywood. This is not to say that the public or medical professionals lost interest in new ways of seeing into the body. On the contrary, as computerized images became increasingly refined and entered clinical use, the experience of seeing the interior of one body part or another—one's own body especially—became increasingly valued.

As mass entertainment, movies and television have never been in the business of breaking intellectual barriers. They serve, rather, to reflect the ordinary and the trendy. When Woody Allen has a CT scan in *Hannah and Her Sisters,* the producers feel certain everybody is familiar with CT scanning. When the lawyers in *Rampage* use PET images to prove mental incompetence, the movie-going public has already allocated authority to the new technology. By 1992, when the pregnant lead character in the television sitcom *Murphy Brown* has an ultrasound image taken of her fetus, it can be assumed that seeing a fetus on ultrasound is a virtually universal experience.

Private and Public Property

Movies and television helped familiarize the public with X-ray machines and X-raying as an unveiling process. By the late twentieth century, *X ray* had joined the English language as a noun with two definitions (its original meaning of the beams of particles as well as a synonym for the radiograph itself, now "an X ray"), as a verb (she X-rayed my finger), and as a metaphor for the revelation of hidden things. In a letter to the *New York Times* in 1993, a spokesperson for the American Civil Liberties Union decried the accumulation of computerized information as an invasion of privacy, "an X-ray of our personal lives . . . the most intimate details of our lives . . . our private vulnerabilities, our moral tastes."[4]

The civil libertarian may not have been aware of how recently the right to privacy was defined as a civil liberty. The idea that privacy, particularly private access to the body, is an entitlement is still new to Western thought. At the time X-rays were discovered, slavery and serfdom—a condition in which a master literally owned another person's body—had only recently been abolished. Women and children were, and in many cultures remain, chattel, possessions of the man of the house. The luxury of privacy is inexorably connected to the luxury of owning property. Only when you own your own body, is it yours to do with as you will.

The question of who owns X-ray images is connected with proprietary rights over who controls images of the body—inside as well as outside. The rights of people to control external images has been decided in many courts and almost always in favor of the person whose image has been expropriated. Yet the ownership of medical images has been in dispute for as long as X-rays have existed: the patients who paid for the images, whose body parts are the subjects, have insisted that they own their own images, and the medical world has insisted that they belong to the physician under whose care they were made. Early in the debate doctors cautioned each other to take, and keep, X-rays in the spirit of defensive medicine. When duplicating pictures was difficult and expensive, this argument was understandable. This is no longer convincing, and doctors who insist on keeping images out of the patients' hands now give the impression of greed, or worse, of having something to hide.[5]

While many patients resent the idea that they cannot always see their X-rays, much less take them home, they are outraged at the idea that their images, even unidentified, may end up in a public place. They consider radiographs and scans intimate. To the models of these ostensibly asexual images, their skeletal ribs are as revealing as the nude posture photographs of Ivy League students that were taken routinely during the 1940s and 1950s, supposedly to seek out curvature of the spine or undetected infantile paralysis. The pictures, which their subjects presumed had been destroyed, suddenly surfaced in 1994 in the files of physical anthropologists who had been using them without ever getting permission from the subjects. The men and women whose names were recorded on their photographs justifiably protested their publication and demanded that they be turned immediately, if belatedly, into ashes.

In 1993 a radiologist in San Francisco proudly displayed back-lit radiographs in the foyer of his Craftsman-style home. The decor, published in *Metropolitan Home* magazine, drew extraordinary criticism from art students who sensed an invasion of privacy.[6] Even though photographers routinely display candid images of people in the street, the idea of displaying pictures of patients' bones struck these students as invasive, a breach of faith, far worse than displaying candid nudes would have been. A University of Chicago Hospital study of the reactions of eighty patients to their own body images revealed that, while 90 percent said they would allow their radiographs to be shown in lectures for teaching purposes, 10 percent refused. Referring to a picture of her colon, one patient said, "God didn't put it where everybody could see it," and another affirmed, "What's inside is supposed to stay inside."[7]

In a society where privacy is freely relinquished to the pleasure of public notoriety, where strangers discuss intimate details of their lives in the media, and even members of the British royal family air their sexual histories in public, the details of our interior anatomy may be the last preserve of something private and unique. These images of our interiors are especially personal and forceful because they so often foretell our mortality. In Don DeLillo's 1985 novel, *White Noise,* a professor in the department of American pop culture at a small, rural college has been suddenly overwhelmed by noxious gas from a ruptured railroad tanker. The hero, who knows he has absorbed enough of the poison to compromise his health, muses: "I think I felt as I would if a doctor had held an X-ray to the light showing a star-shaped hole at the center of one of my vital organs. Death has entered. It is inside you. You are said to be dying, and yet are separate from the dying, can ponder it at your leisure, literally see on the X-ray photograph or computer screen the horrible alien logic of it all. It is when death is rendered graphically, is televised so to speak, that you sense an eerie separation between your condition and yourself."[8]

The Meaning of the Message

The sight of cancer-ridden bone on a CT scan is unnerving to the radiologist who fully understands the prognosis. A neuroradiologist confessed, "Suppose a patient's brain scan reveals an unexpected degree of atrophy: we may never speak to that patient in quite the same way again. The light behind the patient's eyes may be forever dimmed in our own."[9]

If experience-hardened physicians question their own responses, it is obvious that patients, too, while less able to understand the image, are deeply affected by the sight of their own interiors. A reaction may simply reflect the patient's ego. One trophy-laden swimmer examined his shoulder on an MRI monitor and, ignoring the fact that pain had kept him out of the water for over a year, marveled at the beauty of the sight. "If it had been in a butcher shop, I would have bought it and proudly served it," he recalls, proud of his richly marbled flesh.

Patients in the Chicago study had mixed reactions to the sight of their own interiors. While one subject felt that "until you see your X-ray, you don't know how ugly you really are," most respondents agreed with the man who, after seeing his own chest X-ray reported, "I feel more knowledgeable about myself. I drew a mental picture of what's in there," or with the woman who knew "a kind of wonder to see hidden things."[10]

Rare and revealing is the insight of psychologist Kay Redfield Jamison, herself a manic-depressive, as she sat in a lecture hall.

> The slides were riveting, and as always, I was captivated by the unbelievable detail of the structure of the brain that was revealed by the newest versions of MRI techniques. There is a beauty and an intuitive appeal to the brain-scanning methods, especially the high-resolution MRI pictures and the gorgeous multicolored scans from PET scan studies. With PET, for example, a depressed brain will show up in cold, brain-inactive deep blues, dark purples, and hunger greens; the same brain when hypomanic, however, is lit up like a Christmas tree, with vivid patches of bright reds and yellows and oranges. Never has the color and structure of science so completely captured the cold inward deadness of depression or the vibrant, active engagement of mania.[11]

A century after the discovery of X-rays, a glimpse of one's own living interior continues to trigger psychological insight. An artist who uses the images in her work explained in late 1993: "I had a bone scan last year and was completely amazed at the self-knowledge I gained from watching my skeleton emerge on the screen. Suddenly, I realized why clothes fit me the way they do and why my shape (short-waisted, long legs) is the way it appears. I am a 39-year-old woman who was finally able to put a skeleton inside a form & understand why it looks the way it does." Then, apparently picking up her pen again, she added: "P.S. I found the technology alienating and exciting simultaneously."[12]

Many people share her mixed feelings. Looking at X-ray or computer-reconstructed images of our own bodies is like a Rorschach test: our responses mirror our general sense of ourselves at a particular time. When the medical problem that called for the image is under control, the reaction reflects the degree of optimism. But a long illness with many scans is more complicated. The repeated experience of being visually "flayed," of seeing the painful reality of a desperate condition, is increasingly common as medical diagnosis races, by necessity, ahead of treatment.

That is how Tamara, a poet, describes her frequent scans. Tamara had been healthy until, without warning, she fell into what seemed like a wonderland of imaging in March 1986. She had left the laboratory where she worked in order to exercise at a local health club. While pedaling an exercise bike, she "felt a little strange"; she woke up in an ambulance with a doctor asking if she knew her name and the name of her health insurance carrier.

The admitting doctor in the emergency room that day happened to be a cardiologist, so he gave her a sonogram, a chance to see her heart on "live TV, like a sea urchin or something, kind of opening and closing, a sick animal with its collapsed microvalve." She said she pitied it—as if it was not part of her, the part actually sustaining her, but an independent creature. But the weak microvalve had not caused her blackout. The emergency room next administered an EEG (an electroencephalograph) that showed something amiss in her brain. Then she had a CT scan, to see if there was a blood clot or a tumor. There was. This got her wheeled across the road to a mobile unit where she had the first of a series of MRIs. She had an oleglioma—a tumor of the glio tissue in her brain. More CT and MRI scans followed, and a visit to the National Institutes of Health in Bethesda, Maryland, in 1990 for a PET scan. All of her scans led to the same diagnosis: a brain tumor that is growing slowly but is not malignant, at least, not yet. The prognosis is vague: the tumor would continue to grow, but how fast is unknowable. The recommended therapy depends on who's being asked. Tamara can be radiated, medicated, operated on, or some combination—or she can follow the advice of her neurologist and do nothing, save take anticonvulsant medication, and go back to business as usual. A fine idea, but it's altogether impossible to ignore a time bomb in your head.

Where a hundred years ago the ostensible reason for most X-rays was surgery, today's rush to see, then wait, rests on new neurobiological maps that are improving almost daily, revealing how each part of the brain works. Wary of the damage even the most skillfully wrought scalpel can do, Tamara's physicians play for time. For her part, Tamara, a responsible medical consumer, has become intimately familiar with the way the interior of her body looks.

"I actually saw my skull for the first time in 1979 when I went to a chiropractor to get a bunch of X-rays. You feel sort of protective. I mean that's how I felt. I thought, 'Oh my poor little skull.' It looked so fragile. On the other hand, there's this dual connotation of skulls and death. One of the things I did when I started seeing these scans of myself was that I became obsessed with the little skull figures that the Mexicans make." But she stopped collecting them seven years ago when the diagnosis was made and she began having semiannual MR exams. "Now with MR you don't actually see your skull that clearly. You don't see the eye sockets." You see another reality, a naked brain without its protective shell.

Tamara is a poet, and like other late twentieth-century artists, she finds these medical images an ideal metaphor for the human condition. A hundred years of peering through the body has accustomed all of us, whether artists or not, to accepting flat black-gray-and-white X-rays as accurate renditions of our internal bones, and over thirty years of ultrasound has trained our eyes to see tiny arms and legs in a fuzzy black and white arc. Our educated eyes peer at an MR image of our brain and dismiss the missing eye sockets as dispensable.

More often than not the image is projected on a video monitor. We are getting used to false-colored three-dimensional images of our brains just as we once got used to enhanced images of the moons of Jupiter, and we walk through holograms of hearts and brains that may be reconstructed from data of our own vital organs, or from idealized models pulled from the ether. In virtual reality we almost touch body parts and move them around. Whether they "pop up" in books or glide, mouse-driven, across glass screens, images of the interiors of the human body are readily accessible to those who want to see them.

The Body in Pieces

Many artists in the years after World War II marched to the powerful drumbeat of abstraction, and like Mondrian and Jackson Pollock, eliminated references to all subject matter in geometrical designs or frenzied swirls and drips of paint. The human body, which for over a millennium had been the focus of Western art, was ignored in the race for representation-free graphic expression. But this rejection was not universal. Of those who continued to paint the human figure, the English artist Francis Bacon did so with a bow to the X-ray. In a series of interviews in 1966, Bacon explained, "I always had in my possession a book that influenced me enormously entitled *Positioning in Radiology* that contained photographs of the position of the body when X-rays were taken as well as the radiographs themselves."[13]

First published in 1939 by the photographer-radiographer Kathleen Clara Clark, the textbook served Bacon both as a manual for the best poses and as a source of compelling images.[14] The poses in Clark's text echo the points of view of neoclassical paintings, because those are the best positions for artists and radiographers alike to get a complete picture of the body. On occasion Bacon literally replicated Clark's artfully arranged models. In other instances he lifted her X-ray images, peeling off the flesh of his subjects, using X-ray-like techniques and the radiographs as his points of departure. Bacon linked the clinic, the zoo, and the gymnasium—three places where animal nakedness dominates the scene—through images that grotesquely caricature the bland figures in the textbook. These models validated his pathological approach to the human body, and his fascination with abnormal pathologies.

In other instances, such as his *Head Surrounded by Sides of Beef* (1954),

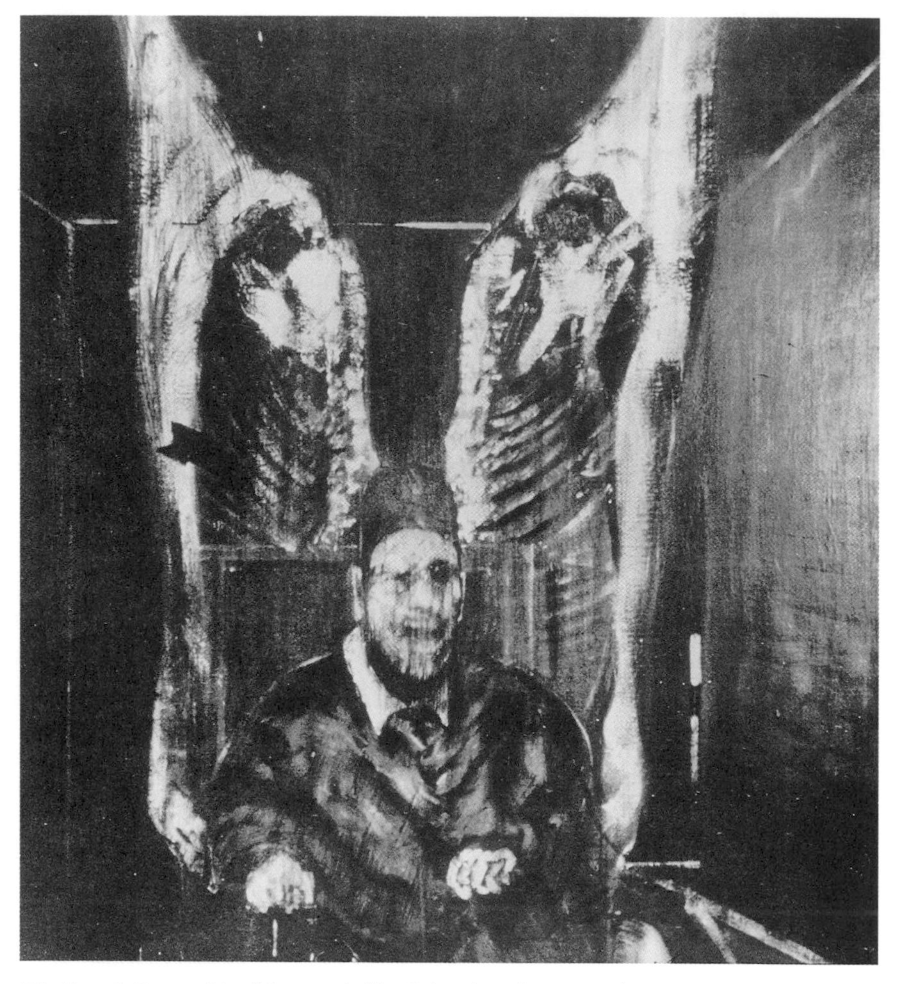

58. Francis Bacon, *Head Surrounded by Sides of Beef* (1954). Oil on canvas, 129.9 cm x 122 cm. Copyright © The Estate of Francis Bacon. Courtesy of the Art Institute of Chicago, Harriott A. Fox Fund, 1956.1201.

Bacon combined different views of his subject on the canvas, just as the Clark text demonstrated how to take X-ray shots of the same subject from different perspectives. Bacon's figurative art is rooted in the well-muscled, heroic tradition of Michelangelo, the proto-cinematic photographs of Muybridge, Picasso's cubist figurative work, and Clark's models. The X-ray, for Bacon, turned a living body into a carcass.

Images in Clark's manual show the patient in a position that Bacon used to model his Christ on the Cross, the rays passing through the patient in planes analogous to the spears passing through Jesus. His *Crucifixion* (1965) conflates the lance wound of Christ on the Cross with a patient receiving therapeutic X-rays. Bacon, a skeptic, found the iconography of the Church a rich source of irony. And just as Christ offered salvation—the final cure—to humanity, so did Bacon (according to his confidant the artist Sir Lawrence Gowing) suggest that X-rays (not Christ) had the power to cure disease.[15]

Bacon approached the Church, in which he had grown up, very personally and found the form of the triptych—the three-panel pictures inherited from Christian altar pieces—especially suited to his vision of the body, especially for his depiction of the body in filmic fragments. Just as radiographs had reduced the body to a patchwork of components, Bacon reinterpreted the panels of the triptych, traditionally used to show different scenes of a narrative, to show the body as a broken narrative of compartmentalized figure elements. Bacon's use of Clark's X-ray models took the X-ray as far as it could be taken as an anatomical guide for painters.

In contrast, a decade later, the American artist Robert Rauschenberg used X ray images as a way of depicting a culture of superficial imagery. In 1967 Rauschenberg embarked on the execution of the largest hand-made lithograph ever made, and he selected his own full-body X-rays as the centerpiece. Rauschenberg asked a radiologist to X-ray him from head to toe—and he pieced together the resulting five separate images to make a six-foot tall lithograph.[16] Like Bacon, Rauschenberg connected fragments to form a complete image, but unlike Bacon, he made no attempt to explain the seams where the fragmented radiographs met. The result was *Booster.*

The original *Booster* expressed the connection between inner man and the external persona: boosterism is the American tradition of self-puffery. The title took on a new dimension two years later when Rauschenberg depicted an actual booster rocket in his lithograph, *Sky Garden.* This print was inspired by Rauschenberg's observations of the blast-off of the Apollo astronauts at Cape Canaveral in 1969. He is clearly playing on words: booster as a fan or supporter of himself, and booster as propellent into space (where the word *garden* suggests manicured, humanized, organic life will spread), and booster as a stage in a rocket that comes apart into sections, like the sections of his lithograph.

Rauschenberg, while interested in producing a self-portrait of inner man in *Booster,* was also piecing together fragments of his own life in time as extracted from the media. By including photographs and charts in *Booster,* he extended his autobiography into the realm of historical document, and by superimposing his X-rayed figure onto an astrological chart for 1967 (Rauschenberg took astrology seriously enough to employ a personal astrologer), surrounded by magazine clippings of athletes and machines, he tried to extend it into some kind of spiritual dimension.

Rauschenberg followed *Booster* with a sixteen-foot-tall triptych, *Autobiography.*[17] This enormous print includes a reduced version of the *Booster* radiographs as well as a panel with a family photo taken in his hometown of Port Arthur, Texas. The triptych, like Bacon's, echoes Christian iconography for a secular purpose. Rauschenberg celebrates himself, using places and events to mark the parables of his own life—including a photograph of the artist wearing an open parachute and skating on a rooftop water tank in Manhattan. By using mass-produced images in the story of his life, Rauschenberg has

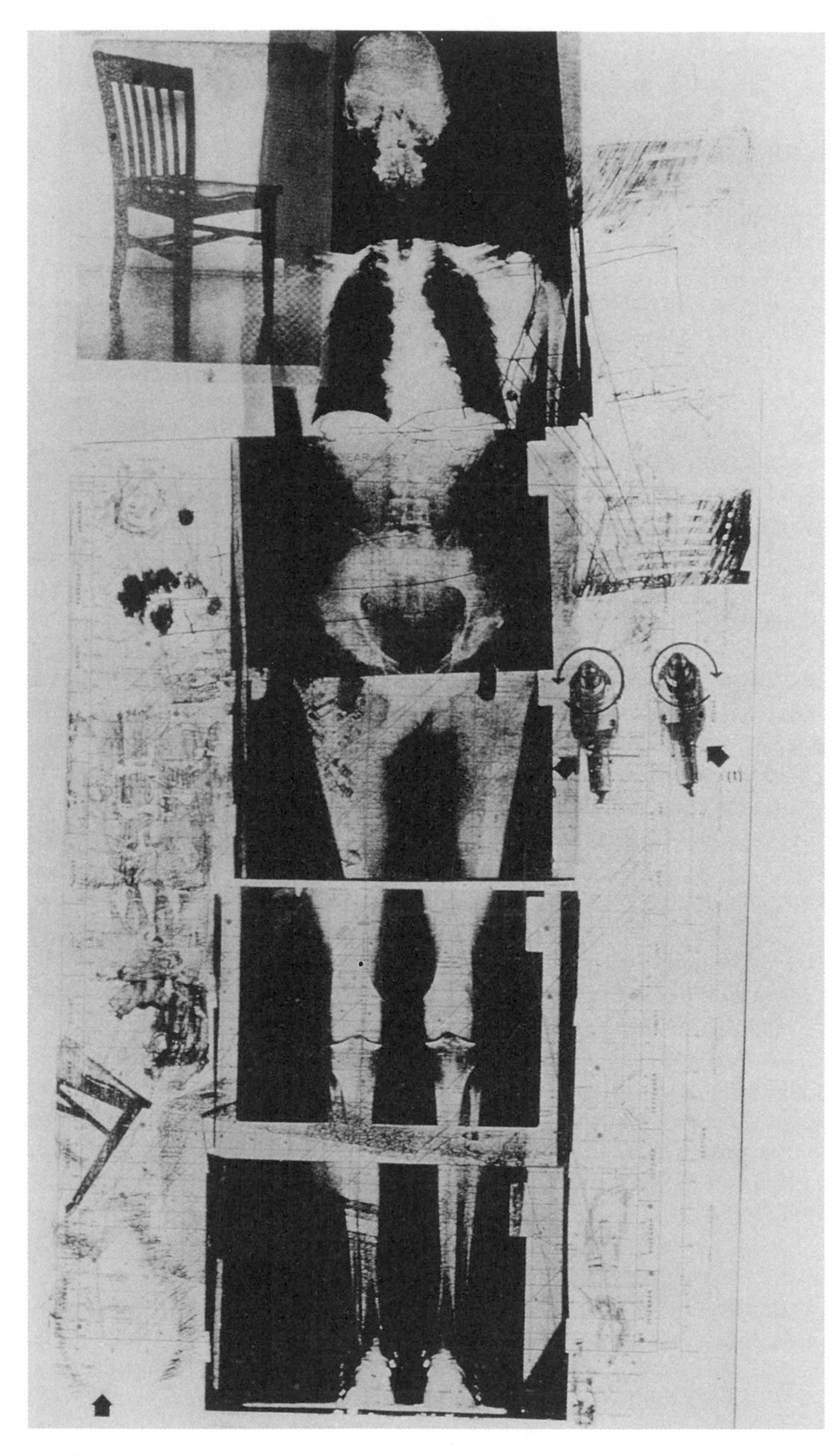

59. Robert Rauschenberg, *Booster* (1967). Lithograph and screen-printing, 72" x 36". Copyright © Robert Rauschenberg/Licensed by VAGA, New York.

personalized modernism, producing a public biography as his version of autobiography. *Sky Garden,* composed around the image of a booster rocket, recycles a fragment of his X-ray from *Booster.* The two lithographs reflect the influence of X-ray technology both explicitly—he uses his own X-rays—and implicitly, as he establishes the theme of layers of images suggesting layers of reality, a distinctive break from the pop art and abstract minimalism that dominated the galleries at the time.

Rauschenberg continued to incorporate X-rays and transparencies in his 1984–85 series *Sling Shots* where he assembles skeletal images suspended in Plexiglas lightboxes against a lithographed background. In his use of layers of Plexiglas, Rauschenberg recalls Gabo and his brother Anton Pevsner who introduced plastics in their quest for transparency in the 1920s in Russia. The directly personal quality of the X-ray images in *Booster* and again in *Autobiography* haunts the works of many late twentieth-century artists.

The Imperfect Body

At about the same time that CT and ultrasound entered the clinic in the mid-1970s, the human body slipped back into the art world. There is no causal connection—none that can be spelled out—save that the body had become extremely interesting again as new views into the interior explained more about the exterior. Of course, the figure had never completely disappeared, as Bacon's very personal interpretations of the body illustrate.[18]

However, in contrast to Bacon, another group of artists began depicting the body—inside as well as out—in a new kind of self-portrait. Frida Kahlo's self-portraits from the early 1950s, showing her face like a snapshot atop her deformed body (painted with the internal organs exposed), foreshadowed the rage expressed by the next generation who railed against homogenized images of physical perfection.

Recording the presence of physical disease was a new kind of autobiography, different from that of Rauschenberg, who used X-rays as a snapshot of his healthy bones in the context of a snapshot of that moment in history. Capturing images of deteriorating internal organs opens a new perspective on the traditional depiction of aging as the accretion of lines and folds in the skin. Attracted by the natural beauty of the body's newly exposed deeper layers and inspired by what they could understand about the human body in general, artists now reached out to medical imagery, and did so in the very particular circumstances of their own lives. They sought to describe the nature of health, disease, and the space between them. The X-ray and especially digitized imagery enabled them to explore the connection between internal changes—even inside the brain—and the external expression those changes made in gait and posture.

The leaders of this new approach were energetic, assertive, and ambitious women who joined the ranks of professional artists in the 1970s. They had a profound effect on the way artists depicted the human form, as did the related movement to gain acceptance for people with disabilities. Women, and later men as well, began to question the media-hyped image of cosmetically "perfect" people. Women who were artists in the process of freeing themselves from externally defined standards began to find inspiration by looking inside their bodies. The new definition of autobiography expanded social conventions about just whose self-portraits should be seen. Women in general, as well as women and men in whom physical disability was both defining and, when confronted, liberating, were newly seen and heard.

New York painter Laura Ferguson, for instance, has scoliosis—a twisting of the skeleton that compresses her rib cage and makes breathing difficult. From her personal X-rays she created a one-of-a-kind artist's book in which she

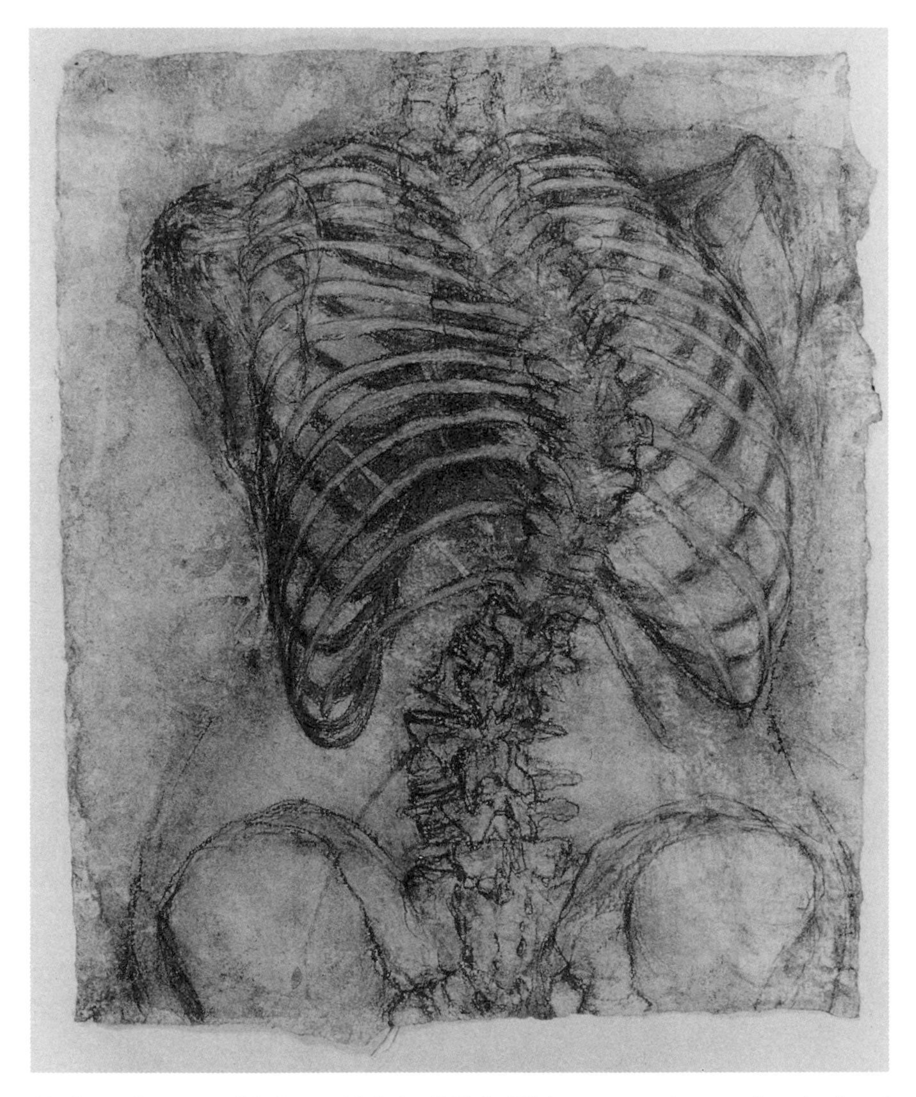

60. Laura Ferguson, *Rib Cage with Spine* (1994). Oil, bronze powder, pastel, and colored pencil on paper, 10" x 8 1/4". Courtesy of Laura Ferguson.

explores her experience. Blending oil paints with bronze powders, she created a layered look so that her images form bones, blood, and flesh, floating free from pain.

Ferguson's focus on her skeletal anomalies is part of the rejection by many women artists of the use of the female body to reflect a sexual ideal. These female artists used their own bodies, not as examples of some externally defined standard of beauty, but as works in progress. They frequently incorporate an X-ray or a CT scan to show their own interior structure, indications of deviations from anything like the Greek ideal proportions. Explaining the difference in her own source of inspiration from that of a character such as the title figure in Offenbach's *Tales of Hoffman,* a male poet who needed a female muse for inspiration, the Los Angeles artist Ruth Weisberg noted that for women, the muse is internal. It is themselves. As such, art is no longer a gift from the outside but a diary intended to be read.[19]

The distancing necessary to include personal X-ray imagery in art is explained by Tori Ellison, an artist working in mixed media in the 1980s and 1990s. "As to my use of X-ray images, I began working with them indirectly eight years ago. At that time I was in the midst of a series of abstract paintings, which concerned biomorphic forms. I conceived of each painting as a 'body,' a projection of self, at least metaphorically."[20] Then, after she obtained a set of radiographs of her spine following what she recalls as "a minor medical problem": "The X-ray plates began to fascinate me. I found them beautiful. To me the image was a point of physical origin, something I could study in terms of mapping a structure of growth." These resulted in sculptural works, including "one Plexiglas box piece of an abstract painting specifically of a spine, between sheets of Plexiglas and submerged in water."

Later, concerned with the idea of boundaries defining a 'self,' she used the image of an empty dress, and then emphasized "the spine, perhaps an essential self, a stronger source of self, and an interior, subjective sense of identity." While she was finishing these constructions, she experienced symptoms that would prove to be multiple sclerosis. "I can't say the fact that I have MS consciously informs the work, but it definitely puts me in touch with issues of the body, mortality. I hold the opinion that all artists' works of art are on some level self-portraits."

Shortly afterwards, following a spate of mysterious headaches, Ellison had MRI and sonograms of her head. She has these images of herself, and looks at them, but she had not yet used them in her work. "I found it too disturbing to work with the MRI when my diagnosis and prognosis were unclear." On balance, however, she has found the images an inspiration. "I find these records peculiarly fascinating. It is almost as though the X-rays, and other forms of imaging the body, are proof of my own existence, in a way that external images of me and the world are not. Or perhaps they signify a more personal sense of identity, beyond my outward appearance and experience."

The introduction of X-rays and computerized scans into late twentieth-century self-portraiture highlights the changed new sense of ownership. Art as autobiography displays what is intimate, the essentially private, but the choice

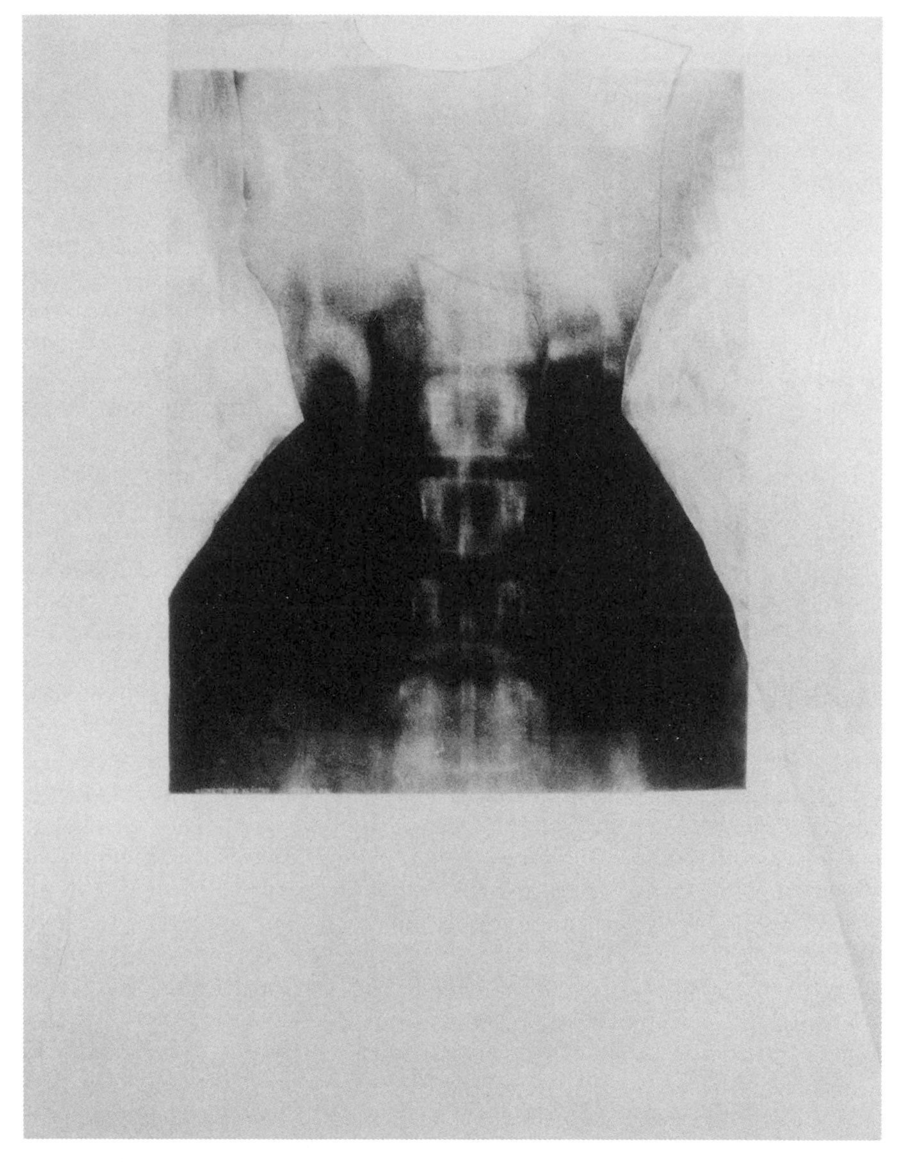

61. Tori Ellison, *X-Dress* (1993). Acrylic, charcoal, X-ray, paper, 50" x 38". Courtesy of Tori Ellison.

of what is revealed is the artist's. Newly confident female artists paint as if they are proclaiming: "I can undress myself, but you can't undress me." Women empowered by the feminist movement are among the strongest voices in the proliferation of body self-portraiture.

Participants in this movement include male artists, too. Ted Meyer, a victim of Gaucher's disease (an inherited enzyme deficiency that causes severe bone pain and deterioration, necessitating surgical implants) was inspired by his MRIs and X-rays to paint a series he calls *Structural Abnormalities.*

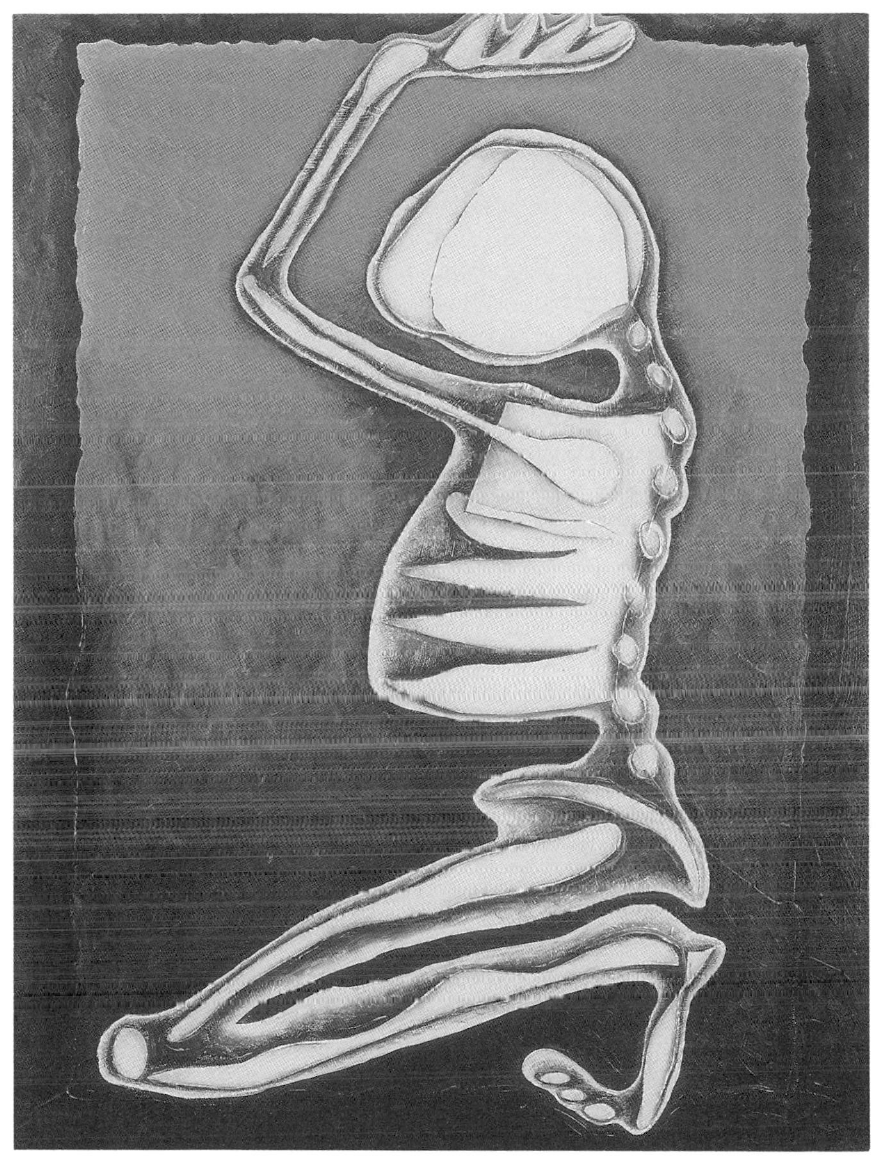

62. Ted Meyer, *Structural Abnormalities* (1992). Oil on canvas, 3' x 4'. Courtesy of Ted Meyer.

These haunting but surprisingly upbeat paintings are close-ups of bones clearly encased in a membrane that resembles the life-protecting placental sac.

Meyer's self-portraits exemplify both renewed interest among artists in the body as subject and a recognition by society of the need to appreciate human beings and their bodies on their own terms, as they are. The ability to see through the body has altered our sense of public and private and what the artist is entitled, even obliged, to portray. Artists have responded to the exposure of individual differences with a focus on the body—especially in the shadow of AIDS, which has heightened the sensibilities of sufferers to the entire range of ways to see and measure an inadequate immune system, as well as in response to the revelations of DNA sequencing, which enables us literally to see variations in the genome. This movement is also an assertion of individuality in a civilization threatened with visual homogeneity. Even as cosmetic surgery opened up opportunities for people to reconstruct their appearances, it has become a political statement to illustrate structural differences. The autobiographical artists who represent deformed bones or surgically amputated breasts in their work declare independence from societal norms. They demand acceptance on their own terms. What was once hidden is now displayed because the artists choose to display it. What was private is now deliberately public.

X-Rays as Palette Knife

Where artists like Ferguson, Ellison, and Meyer used X-rays to explore internal, personal truth, others used the technology of X-rays in the tradition of Gabo—to explore the world external to the human body. Shortly after the discovery of X-rays, a student of Roentgen's used them to discover the signature of Albrecht Dürer hidden beneath the paint on a disputed canvas, and in so doing established what would become an important forensic tool for authenticating works of art. By 1913 a system to use X-rays to analyze pigments and opacity of color had been patented by scientists in Germany and France. Scientists dominated the field: in 1932 thirty bogus Van Goghs were exposed, and a year later the idea of authentication by X-ray was reexamined and approved by an art historian.[21] The great galleries soon acquired their own X-ray machines and by the 1980s every museum of note included an X-ray facility in its conservation department.

However, when the Hungarian-American artist Agnes Denes won permission in 1972 from the Metropolitan Museum of Art in New York to X-ray several important paintings, she was not looking for forgeries or hidden underimages. Denes was interested in visualizing structure and in deconstructing a work of art, in much the same way literary critics in the 1970s analyzed poetry, wondered about the meaning of the "rough draft," and tried to trace the connection between the creator and the object created. Denes was concerned with the process of creation. Where a traditional self-portrait is the study of a face as a window into character, she was concerned with Rembrandt's own process as an artist making that interpretation. By tracking Rembrandt's brush-strokes and peeling away layer after layer to see how he had worked, changed his mind, painted, she could capture the rhythm of his paint strokes, moving back through time to the bare canvas. Her images of the stages of creation of the self-portrait are images never seen, even by Rembrandt. They are the creations of Denes, who, by slicing away X-rays of the painting process, created a new work of art. "What I am showing you with the X-ray is the process which you never see. Which even the artist himself or herself never sees." As much as

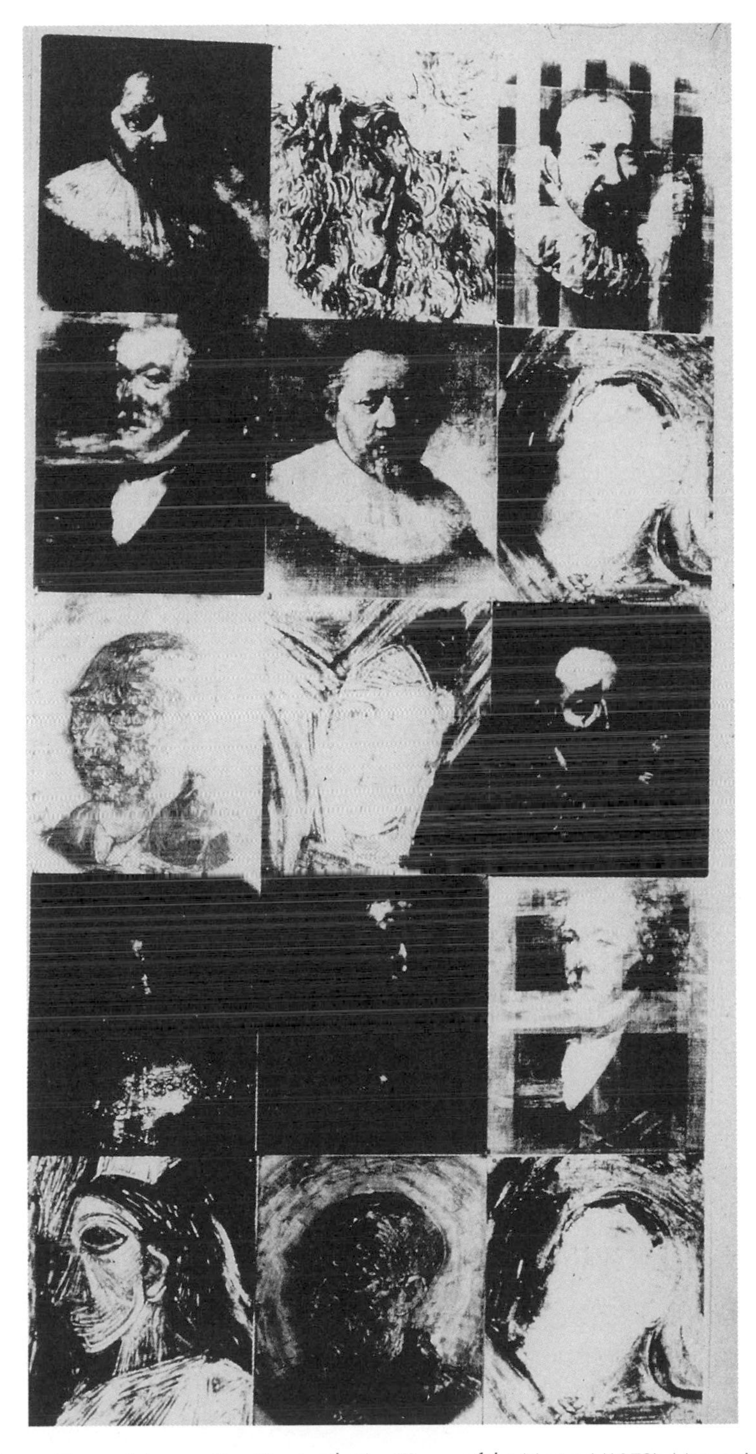

63. Agnes Denes, *Introspection III—Aesthetics (X-rays of the Masters)* (1972). Monoprint, 86" x 41". Copyright © 1972 Agnes Denes. Courtesy of Agnes Denes.

anyone else, Denes has made the X-ray her tool. "I have invented a painting process through the ray. But then I also found layers within the X-ray. By converting the positive to a negative, I found other layers inside it. I created other composite pieces."[22] Denes included Rembrandt's self-portrait in *Introspection III—Aesthetics (X-rays of the Masters)* (1972) along with

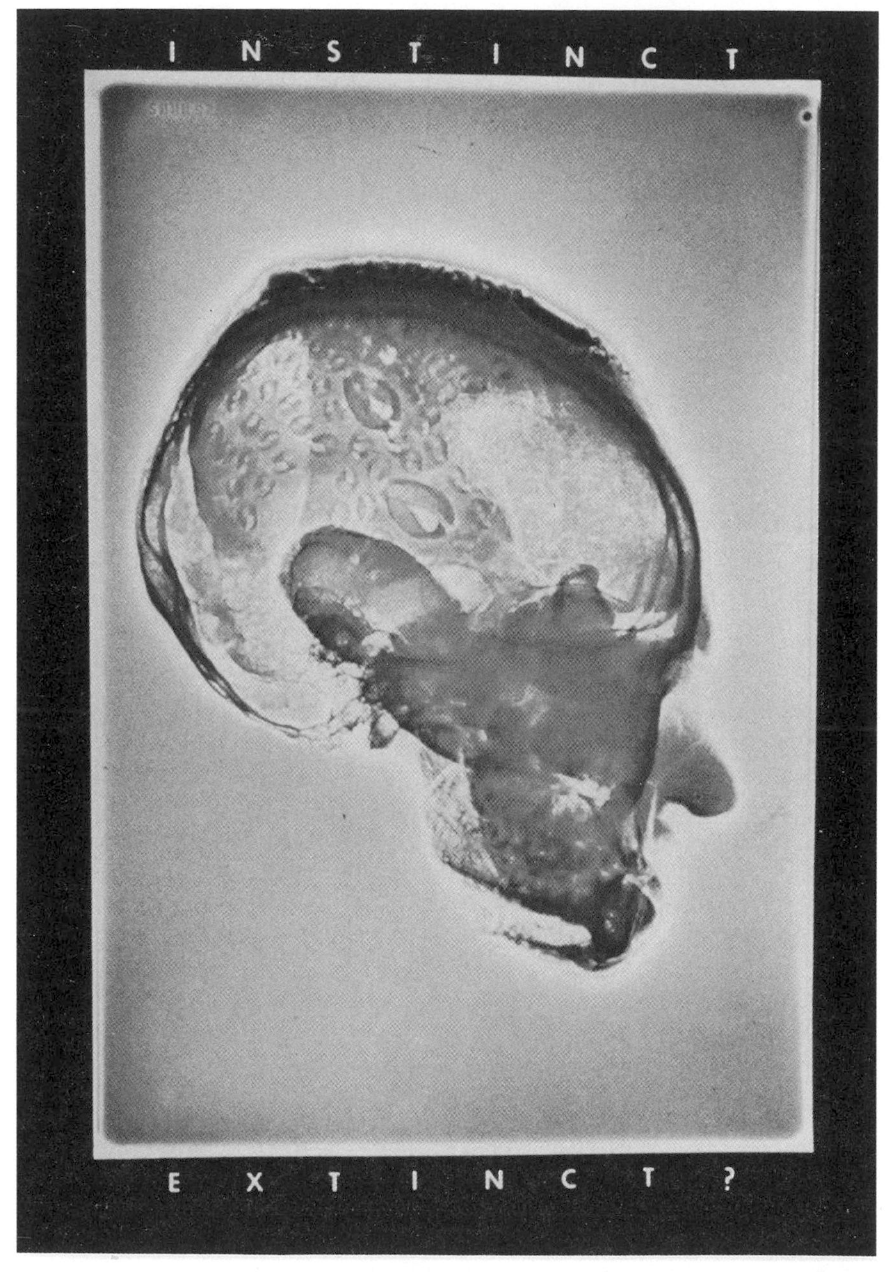

64. Sheila Pinkel, *Instinct Extinct?* Xeroradiograph/photoscan, 16" x 20". Courtesy of Sheila Pinkel.

X-rayed images of Picasso's *Les Demoiselles d'Avignon* and a Van Gogh self-portrait. "In this work, the finger points at the self, artist analyzes artist, and art is made of art."[23] The X-ray allowed her to reexplore Rembrandt, Picasso, and Van Gogh, but the new work of art is Denes's. It is part of an artistic tradition of alluding to, or quoting from, and then reinterpreting classical art.[24]

A different approach to using older art and artifacts to create new works of art was explored in the late 1970s by the California photographer Sheila Pinkel. With the cooperation of the xeroradiology laboratory at the Xerox Corporation in Pasadena, she explains how this new method of radiography caught her attention: "I had experimented with conventional X-rays and while I thought the results interesting, I was not moved to continue using X-rays because the results weren't sensitive enough." But the new xeroradiography was much more sensitive and she "fell in love with making visible forms in nature not normally seen." Fascinated "with the complexity and delicacy of nature when revealed by this process," she investigated the possibility of expressing how things have different "states of being," depending on imaging systems.[25]

She captured the xeroradiographic image of the skull of an extinct hominid embedded in a matrix of clay. The skull had been discovered centuries earlier in Africa by people who had sculpted and decorated it with cowry shells, then buried it again. Re-excavated and then photographed first in visible light and later by xeroradiography, Pinkel calls this work *Instinct Extinct?*, a title suggested by the hidden dimension of physical structure revealed by the X-ray functioning as an analogue for deeper levels in the persona. The process revealed to her that materials have a skin through which she was allowed to see all surfaces at one time. "It allowed me to have X-ray eyes."

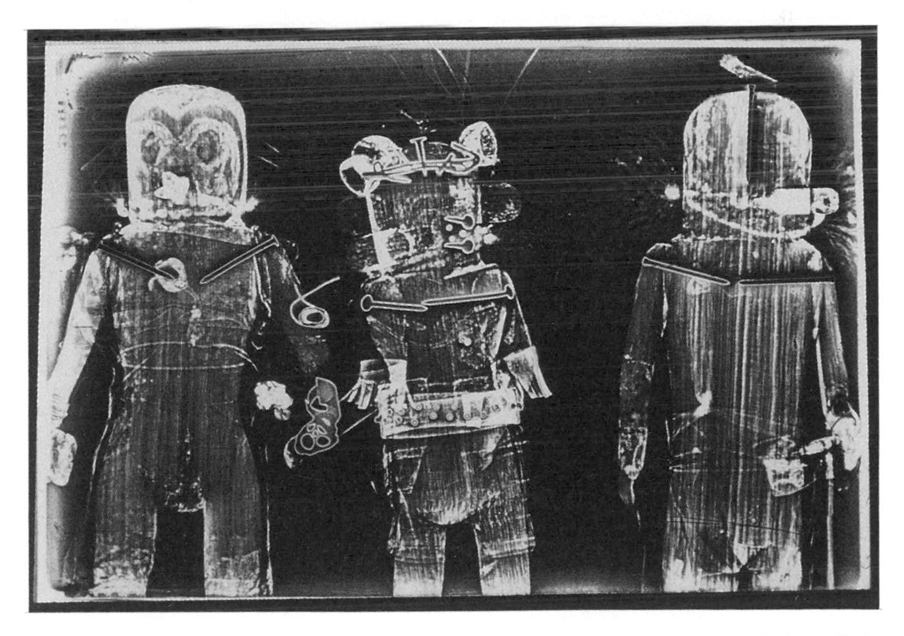

65. Sheila Pinkel, *Kachina Transform.* Xeroradiograph, 10" x 13". Courtesy of Sheila Pinkel.

In another project, Pinkel explored the paradox of examining an artificial humanoid figure through xeroradiology. With the help of the Southwest Museum in Los Angeles, she was able to image ancient Navaho kachina dolls whose construction had been a mystery. The xeroradiographs did not show anything like a human skeleton but, surprisingly, resembled figures in space suits like those worn by the Apollo astronauts. When a Native American saw the xeroradiography he noted that the gods were said to come from the heavens and in her images "the storm gods had come full circle." Pinkel and the Native American were surprised and delighted that technology could play a role in invigorating this fading legend.

The ranks of physicians have always included those attracted to the human body by its innate beauty. The Chicago photographer and plastic surgeon David Teplica has found X-rays a rich source of inspiration. Using leftover "discarded image heaps of contact prints from Roentgenograms" in 1988, Teplica arranged a selection of these prints as a photomontage.[26] In a series

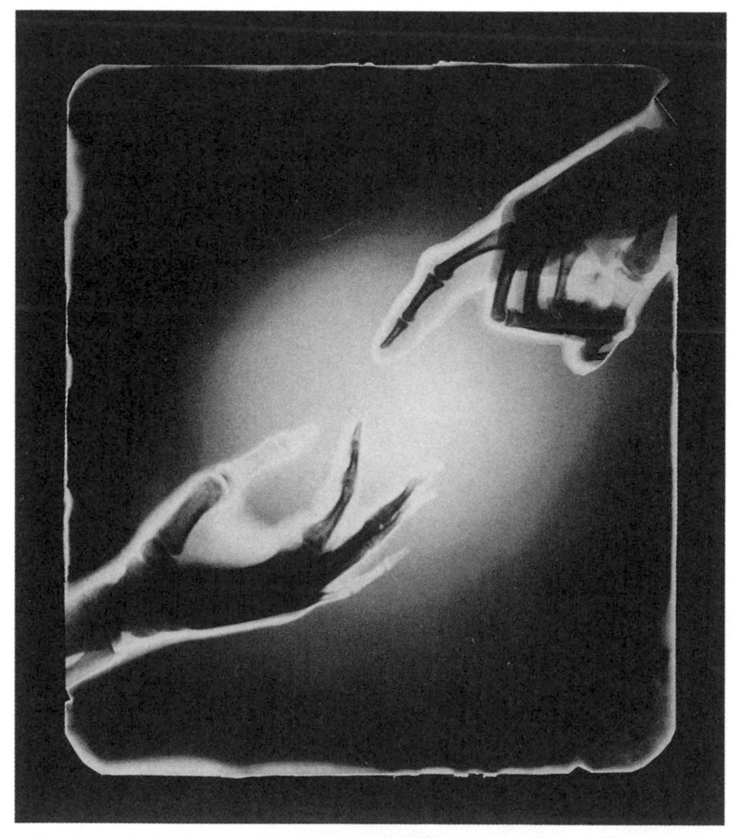

66. David Teplica, *Birth of Man with Homage to Michelangelo* (1987). Selenium-toned gelatin, silver roentgenogram, 16" x 20". The Collected Image, Evanston, Ill. Courtesy of David Teplica.

entitled *Archaeology in Eden*, Teplica, like Pinkel, plays on the idea of fossils and the layers of civilization that have to be excavated to unearth them. His X-ray images, which he has interlaced with layers of fabric, are enhanced by contact-printing, in the spirit of Man Ray and the early twentieth-century experimental photographers.[27] *Birth of Man with Homage to Michelangelo* echoes the fingertip-to-fingertip meeting on the ceiling of the Sistine Chapel with radiographs of hands that are printed by solarized light, leaving a halo behind them. Teplica gives the impression that he has simply X-rayed Michelangelo's original image, a kind of stylistic allusion that acknowledges art of the past while taking it out of context to be used in a new way. Teplica uses X-rays as an artist's tool, a combination scalpel-paintbrush.

X-Rays in Another Dimension

A completely different approach to X-ray photography has pervaded the expression of art since 1896. Excited by the concept of a dimension of reality that had heretofore been hidden, mystics turned to X-rays to validate their visions. Heirs of the old avant-garde accepted the reality of another dimension that could occasionally be visualized as fact. Not only did X-rays reveal structures invisible to the naked eye, their existence helped validate the mystics' claims by capturing "auras" on film, as in Kirlian photography (a process developed by Semyon and Valentina Kirlian in the Soviet Union in the early 1970s that supposedly trapped a living subject's inherent electrical emission when the subject was in direct contact with the photographic plate). The validity of these shadows is less important than the impression they made on artists. These "scientific" auras echo the frequently painted emanations of rays from holy figures that were revived in the work of the Russian mystic Pavel Tchelitchew who lived in New York during World War II.

The most visited painting in New York's Museum of Modern Art for four decades, Tchelitchew's *Hide-and-Seek* (completed and sold immediately to the museum in 1942) displays a chorus of X-ray images of children's see-through heads arranged in puzzle-like patterns as parts of a growing tree. The veins and bones of the children merge with the roots and bark of the tree in a now-you-see-it, now-you-don't puzzle pattern of arteries and landscape. Tchelitchew, like Sir William Crookes, saw the X-ray as a door to another dimension, not time, but a fourth dimension with echoes of spiritualism—ectoplasm and poltergeists. One biographer describes his work as "a sort of illusion: earthy bodies are everywhere qualified by wateriness, airiness or a kind of X-ray revelation of skeletonic structure that lightens its look."[28] The interiors of the bodies Tchelitchew paints include veins, muscle, and bone, superimposed on each other in transparent planes with physiological accuracy. In a sense Tchelitchew's calling children are a last cry for his kind of surrealism. This remarkable canvas was one of his last and arguably his most influential work.

A generation later the American multimedia artist Alex Grey found in

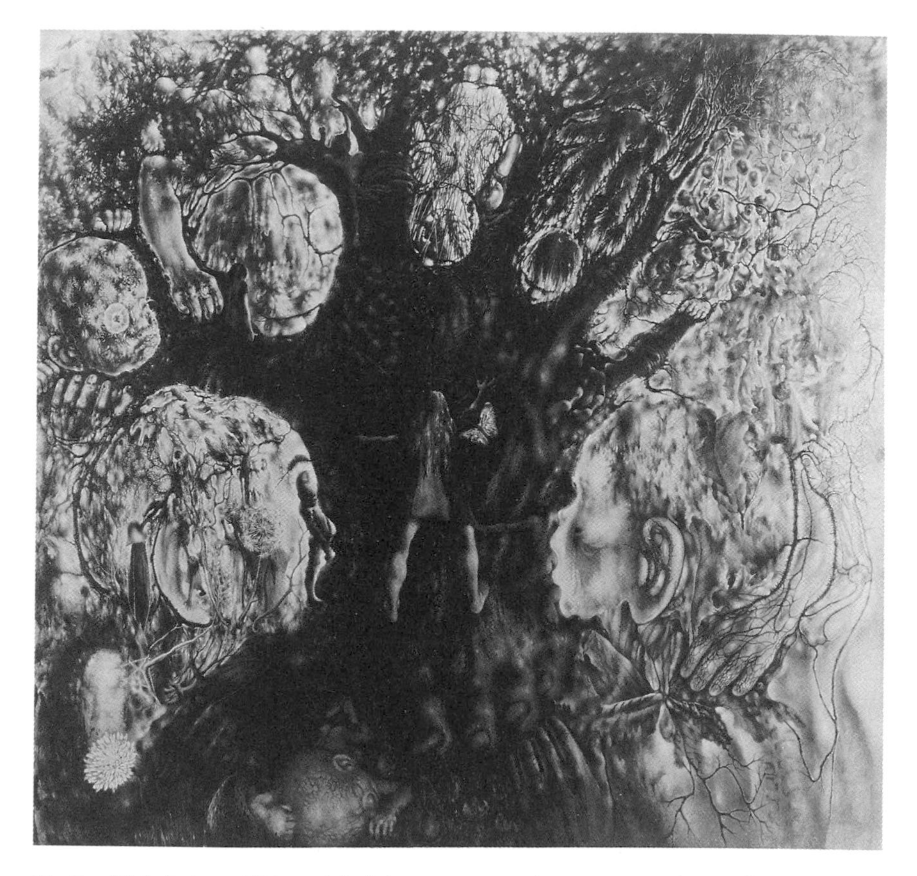

67. Pavel Tchelitchew, *Hide-and-Seek* (1940–1942). Oil on canvas, 6'6$^{1}/_{2}$" x 7'$^{13}/_{4}$" (199.3 cm x 215.3 cm). Copyright © 1996 Artists Rights Society (ARS), New York. Courtesy of The Museum of Modern Art: Mrs. Simon Guggenheim Fund. Photo copyright © 1996 The Museum of Modern Art.

Tchelitchew a sort of mentor and won a large personal following with similar mystic images. In *Sacred Mirrors,* initially an installation at the New Museum of Contemporary Art in New York in 1986 and later a book, the artist, who has studied medical imaging as well as Zen and mystic elements in Western religions, combines his knowledge of anatomy with mysticism. Grey explains: "The *Psychic Energy System* is the crux of the *Sacred Mirrors* because it presents an X-ray view of the physical body and interweaves the nonphysical or psycho-spiritual energy systems."[29] The series of twenty-one paintings includes references to all of human history. It begins with a shadow figure superimposed on the periodic chart of the elements and continues with a skeletal man and detailed representations of the interior of the body. In *Pregnancy,* one of his twenty-one paintings, Grey represents the embracing figures of a man and woman and the full-term fetus, surrounded by light and surrounded again by a frieze of representations of the sperm meeting the egg through ten stages of embryonic development as seen in ultrasound and X-ray. Grey's work enfolds medical imaging in a cacophony of mystical constructions.

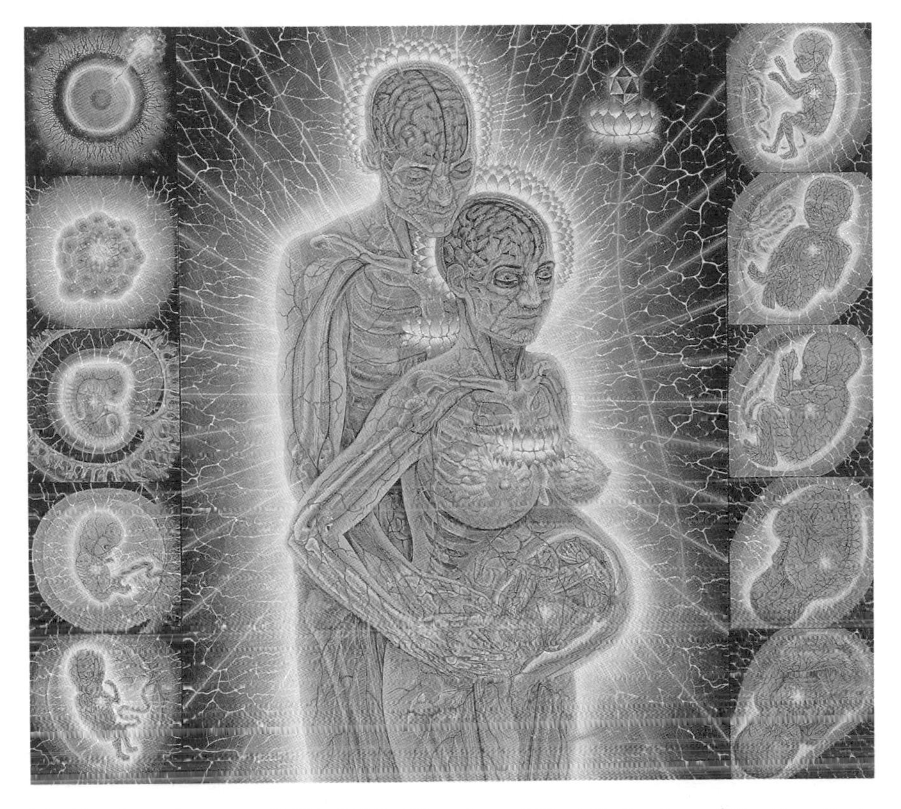

68. Alex Grey, *Pregnancy* (1988–1989). Oil on linen, 50" x 56". Courtesy of Alex Grey. Photo: D. James Dee.

False Impressions

The new photographic and computer images can be, and have been, manipulated to produce whatever message the artist intends. When Alex Grey presented his extraordinarily detailed anatomical interiors to express a very personal vision, his work was acknowledged to be interpretative because he used paint. Photographers, however, with the exception of photomontagists whose "tricks" were never meant to ape reality, have been accepted as recorders of truth. Moving beyond their appreciation of the beauty of organic life—inside and out—late twentieth-century photographers bent the X-rays to their creative wills, but somehow the public never appreciated how much creativity was involved.

The advent of miniaturized medical cameras in the 1960s and computerized imaging in the 1970s expanded the abilities of photographers beyond photomontage, enabling them to capture never-before-seen interiors of the body both at rest and in action. Going a step beyond X-rays, which deposit images on film from outside the body, new surgical procedures such as laparoscopies introduced miniature cameras directly into body cavities.

Beneficiaries of this new photography were readers of *Life* magazine and *National Geographic.* These magazines employed two remarkable photographers who played a major role in familiarizing the public with the new imaging technologies. Their work exposed the intricacy, beauty, and above all, the accessibility of the body's interior, and also carried subtle political messages about the nature of life, and the mission of doctors. But whether consciously or unconsciously, they conveyed an interior world of their own imagining and labeled it a reflection of reality.

Perhaps the most ingenious exploiter of this technology was Lennart Nilsson, a Swedish photographer. Famous for his *Family of Man* exhibition at the Museum of Modern Art in New York in 1955, he gained further renown with his remarkable cover story in *Life* magazine in April 1965. Using a camera with "a specially built, wide angle lens and a tiny flash beam at the end of a surgical scope," he produced what was described as the first portrait of a living fetus.[30] This was an exaggeration. The photographs' poor quality sent him to his laboratory at the Karolinska Institute in Stockholm. There he photographed fetuses removed from women who had suffered ectopic pregnancies. These images, of course, predate the wave of ultrasound pictures, but they were deployed later by right-to-life advocates because they looked as if they had been taken from ultrasound scans of live fetuses. Displayed to argue against abortion, these images had a powerful impact. When the same magazine ran another cover story in August 1990, Nilsson was able to use more sophisticated endoscopic equipment to capture what he describes as the sperm racing toward the yet-to-be fertilized egg.[31] Not only did Nilsson's work fuel anti-abortion sentiments, but its crisp, colored images created a psychological complement to the fuzzy black and white ultrasound images that were becoming commonplace. Prospective parents stared at their blurred black and white ultrasonographs and many mentally colored them in from recollections of *Life* illustrations.

At the same time that *Life* was publishing Nilsson, *National Geographic* was fostering the parallel career of the American photojournalist Howard Sochurek. A battlefront photographer in the Pacific during World War II, Sochurek developed an interest in medical photography and technical and computer image processing in the 1980s.

National Geographic's January 1987 issue features Sochurek's photo-essay in which, using himself as subject, he discovered that the CT scanner had revealed a glitch in his own system. The picture was a false alarm, though, and Sochurek continued experiencing and photographing images in every imaging mode. The high visual quality of Sochurek's photographic prints give the deceptive impression that the map of the brain is almost filled out, and that the interior of the brain exists in a vivid world of color, and that once seen, almost everything can be cured. The page describing CT includes the only black and white picture—the 1895 picture of Frau Roentgen's hand—of the whole story. Beside it is a digitized, mathematically enhanced colored X-ray of a modern hand, red bones glowing as if lit from within.

To purists in the imaging community, this colorized image is cheating. A spot visitor to nearly any emergency-care facility will find a radiologist peering at black and white radiographs stuck onto a lighted screen in a darkened room. CT and MRI scans are likewise displayed in black and white for clinical inspection. In Sochurek's two-page photograph of neurosurgeons inserting a brain shunt, the wall behind the surgeons is a gallery with CT and MRI scans of the patient, in blue and white, which may well have been black and white before they were photographed in "color." With few exceptions, black and white prevails in the clinic.

Yet the *National Geographic* story, as well as pages in the prestigious scientific journals *Science* and *Nature,* run illustrations in color, and not only for consumer appeal. Digitized scans offer an almost unlimited spectrum, and many researchers, including some who are physicians, find that the contrast color provides, as well as the ability to produce a variety of images from a single collection of data, argues for color images in almost every instance. It has been a long road for advocates of color. As far back as the 1960s, experimental efforts to produce colored X-rays were rejected by radiographers who, familiar with black and white, found the images difficult to read. After all, some reasoned, there is no color in the dark beneath the skin.

Whether in color or in shades of gray, CT images of the interior of the body are impressive. Going where no human eye has gone before, these images enable diagnosticians to see some diseases early enough to intervene successfully. To the dismay of many practitioners, the machines extract from patients a respect once reserved for the physician. As often as not, patients want to know what the pictures say, rather than what the doctor thinks.

Computers now merge images, allowing surgeons to operate from a single, remarkably detailed, often three-dimensional, and sometimes holographically represented, reconstruction of the area they will be excising. Patients, of course, are delighted by these advances, which they often credit with an accuracy in rendering their internal form that images do not yet possess. Medical consumers have begun to assume that such technological innovations are their birthright. They accept as an entitlement what was a shock of revelation for their great-grandparents in 1896. Since then the reality of seeing through and into the living body has continued to seep into the our cultural consciousness, transforming our sense of what can be and ought to be seen.

The exploration of the body by computerized scanners proceeded with unprecedented speed after 1973. These new images of the body's interior took about the same time to trickle into the imagination and work of graphic artists as X-rays had taken at the beginning of the century—about a decade. Just as cubist images of fractured planes of the internal body appeared in galleries after 1907, so embellished CT and MRI scans and ultrasound images appeared on museum walls and installations after the early 1980s.

Computerized imaging machines revolutionized diagnostic medicine, but they did not revolutionize the arts. Like a new telescope to astronomers, digitized scans expanded the artists' vision. Some artists undoubtedly responded to the innate beauty of the body's interior in its new forms, just as they had admired the images sent back from space, but they took them for granted. The original breakthrough, the paradigm shift in accepting the body as porous beyond ordinary vision, had occurred in 1896. By the time computerized scanners appeared, the art world and the general public for whom they spoke had grown used to visual innovation both in outer space, and inside the body. That these new images were something truly wonderful was apparent to physicians who sometimes saw more than they knew what to do with, and to artists who struggled to understand the physician's dilemma.

An indication of the ubiquity of CT scans by 1985 is Andy Warhol's series *Philip's Skull (CAT Scan).* This set of silk-screened scans of Philip Niarchos, the jet-setting son of the Greek shipping magnate, follows a logical progression in Warhol's career-long interest in representing parts of the human body.[32] In the 1950s, he sketched from life, and in the 1960s he was making silk screens of crude newspaper advertisements. Then in 1976 he silk-screened a series of skulls. In the 1985 CT scan, Warhol used synthetic polymer paint, silk screen, and urine on canvas, reflecting an interest in the chemistry, as well as the history, of the art process. (The use of urine as an oxidant is common with metallic paints, and has been used as far back as the Renaissance.) But *Philip's Skull* is everyman, as Warhol sets the two-dimensional scan of Niarchos's brain inside the traced outline of one of his 1976 silk-screened skulls.[33] This made the image familiar to the public and his client in 1985, whereas the scan by itself would not yet have been recognizable. The CT scan, a slice of the interior of the brain, is starkly two-dimensional and by itself gives no reference to any structure beneath it. By superimposing the outline, Warhol turned the personal CT scan into an anonymous image.

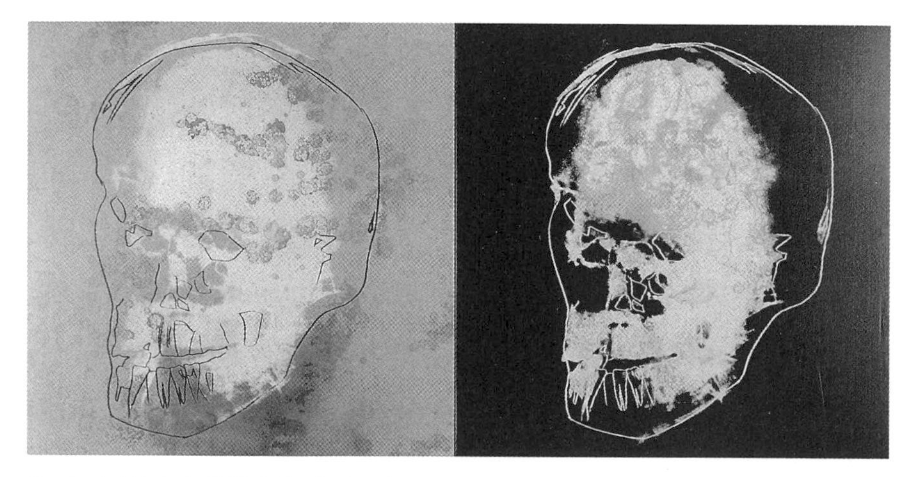

69. Andy Warhol, *Philip's Skull (CAT Scan)* (1985). Synthetic polymer paint, silkscreen, and urine on canvas. Copyright © 1997 Artist Rights Society (ARS), New York. Courtesy of the Andy Warhol Foundation for the Visual Arts, Inc. Photo by Richard Stoner.

A decade later, the New York Academy of Sciences celebrated the centennial of the discovery of X-rays with an exhibition entitled "Imaging the Body: An Artistic Diagnosis." Unlike Warhol, the four contributing artists used medical imaging to reflect intense and conflicted emotions. Representing three countries, each artist uses X-rays or scans to comment on our own fin du siècle civilization. Tina Potter and Christa Henn, two of the artists who proposed (and are included in) the exhibition explain: "As a scientific medium that transgressed the human skin, X-rays embody a central contradiction of modern life—that technology can be both complementary and invasive to human values."[34] Echoing the fragments into which the human body is seen in radiographs, Potter and Henn write about human overpopulation and the global economy and draw a parallel with these images: "The parts into which humanity has divided its environment do not function independently any more. A better understanding of what we are doing in particular and of the complexity of the world in general is needed." Potter, like Teplica, uses parts of discarded X-rays, but unlike Teplica's careful allusions to classic art, Potter's dense collage expresses confusion, blaming global conditions on the sins of technology.

Of the four artists in the exhibition, only Steven Miller, an American who exhibits frequently in France, responds directly to the challenge of incorporating images that devolve from medical procedures. He has made a series of portraits combining radiographs, MRIs, and sonograms. Miller has self-consciously hybridized art and medicine, overlapping in many instances almost all of the multiple forms of imaging. Whether doing a self-portrait, a portrait of a friend, a portrait alluding to another work of art, or in a single painting combining the three, Miller uses technologies meant to diagnose disease to enhance healthy people. In his double portrait of Jacques and Veronique Mauguin, Miller combines sonograms of two fetuses, which he has silk-screened and sandwiched between an acrylic background and beneath a radiograph of their father's hip. *L'Origine du Monde* echoes the fabled erotic portrait painted by Gustave Courbet for a rich Middle Eastern patron in 1866, a picture from nature of a model omitting her entire body except for the genitals. Miller's interpretation includes a silk-screened image of two ultrasounds of the subject's two daughters while in utero (dated in the picture) atop the mother's spread thighs as if in the process of childbirth. Beneath that image is a running chart of the mother's EKG. The picture was a birthday gift to the subject's husband and, indeed, represents maternity. From another angle, however, the spread thighs and frizzed hairs look like an explosion, a veritable "origin of the world." Elsewhere Miller has combined MRIs, chest X-rays, and mammograms with strokes of paint, removing all sense of medical instrumentation, reminding the viewer that the subject, as the portrait, is unique. Miller's portraits combine inner images of an individual with external, painted simulations of radar, or the semicircular strokes of a windshield wiper, personalizing the objective medical picture.[35]

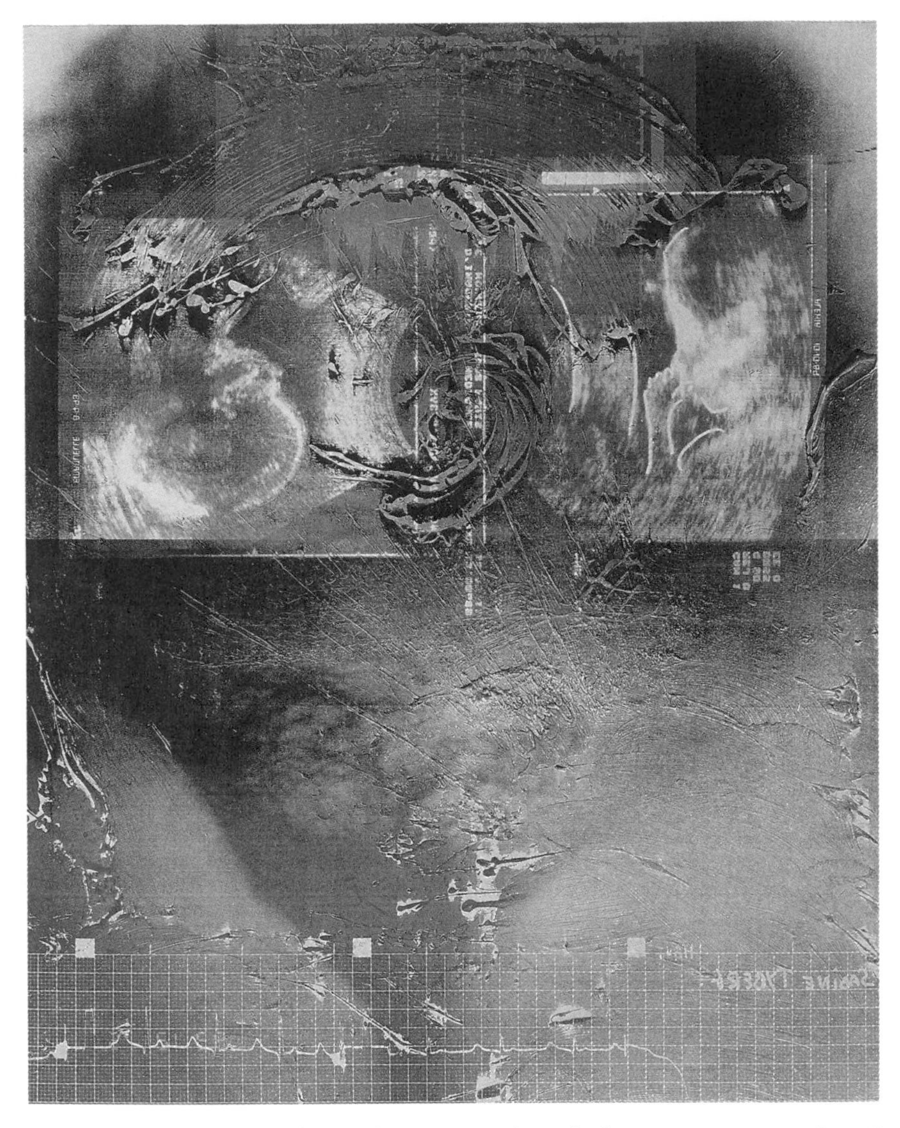

70. Steve Miller, *L'Origine du Monde* (1994). Acrylic and silkscreen on canvas, 79" x 60". Courtesy of Steve Miller.

The Bridge

Another way to personalize traditional images of the sick is from the inside of the hospital, from the perspective of those who spend their days examining the images of the internal organs of strangers. As technology grows more complex, separating physician from patient, some medical centers have turned to art and artists to bring the two back together. May Lesser is devoted to interpreting the emotions of both sides of the medical equation—healers and patients—in pen and ink and paint. She accompanied the class of 1971 through UCLA's medical school, beginning with the freshman year in 1967, and she continued to chronicle their journey through internships and residencies.

In a recent drawing she shows the doctor wincing as the patient looks at the image on the monitor even as he listens to her voice. If only the patient would look at her. In New Orleans, Lesser haunts the hospital where she sees herself,

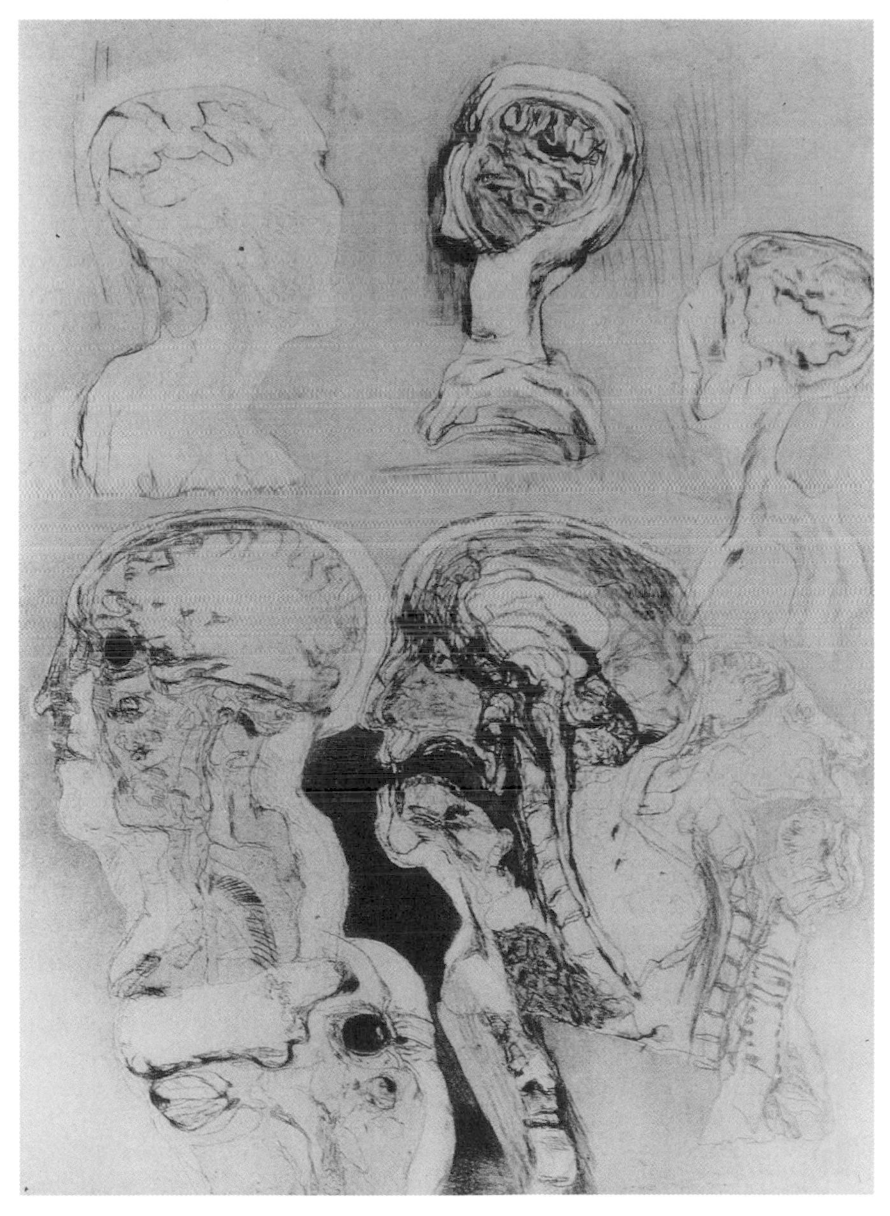

71. May H. Lesser, *Sagittal Series 1/10* (1994). Intaglio etching, 18" x 24". Courtesy of May H. Lesser.

metaphorically, binding patient to physician. In the shadow of formidable machines whose images reveal the depth of illness of patients eager for diagnoses and understanding, her pen and brush capture her belief that "underneath all the technical advances that have changed medicine in the last 40 years, the art of caring still is a part of medicine that is constant."[36]

Always concerned with showing "the intimacy between the student and his or her patients," that first year she etched views of the head as seen in introductory anatomy classes, which she titled *Sagittal Series 1/10.* She complemented these images with a companion copper plate engraving of MRI scans in 1993. Starting with black and white sketches, Lesser occasionally adds egg tempera. "It gives a vibrant color," she notes, content that the organic materials of egg yolk and water fit her subject. She sees herself as a "fly on the wall" in public hospital wards, carefully omitting faces to protect the privacy of the patients.[37] In the imaging center, Lesser acts as a translator between the person whose body is being analyzed on a monitor and the physician who must interpret the analysis. In *MRI Film of an AIDS Patient* she draws the neuroradiologist leaning away from the MRI screen. The virus had entered the brain and spinal column of the thirty-four-year-old patient. "When the physician can do something for a patient, he seems to move closer to that patient. Here the reverse appears. The young doctor kept his distance for emotional safety."[38]

Joyce Cutler Shaw did not know the medical world intimately before becoming the artist-in-residence at the Medical School of the University of California at San Diego in 1992. What she knew well were fossil bones, out of which she had already created several installations and a book devoted to her "Alphabet of Bones," a calligraphy of twenty-six characters based on the hollow bones of birds which has been laser-scanned from her original drawings and digitized into a font. Shaw approaches the sick and dying with a sense of awe, a feeling that she senses among the medical students she mingles with as well as among their seasoned instructors. With what amounts to a compulsion to draw, Shaw chronicles the experiences of the sick, the dying, and the dead. She has included these impressions in her book *The Anatomy Lesson.*[39] With a startling MRI image superimposed on the photograph of a face, her images move from X-rayed bones to computed reconstructions of slices of the brain.

She is at once fascinated and appalled by the power of these technologies. "In re-discovering the body, flesh, blood, and the tactile recede, as we are re-presented electronically by CT, and PET, and MRI. . . . We are holographically projected and sonically graphed by the wonders of ultrasound in a media based world. We are translated into minimalist tonal images which take highly developed skills of detailed visual reading to interpret. These skills are currently being nurtured in departments of radiology."

For instance, "a woman is about to give birth. But the nurse is not watching her. He is moving a metal mouse across her abdomen and watching a screen." She goes on to describe how medical training films fragment not only the body, but the event being described; that with new technologies "we are

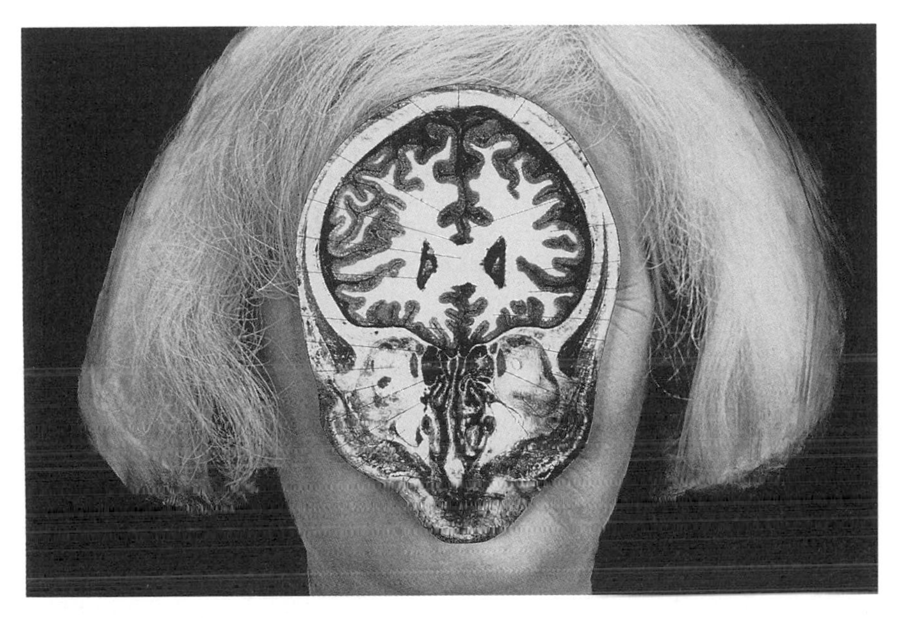

72. Joyce Cutler Shaw, *The Anatomy Lesson: Memory Picture with CT* (1992). Photo collage, 12" x 14". Courtesy of Joyce Cutler Shaw. Photo by Phel Steinmetz.

simultaneously dematerialized in an explosion of non-invasive imaging systems. We split our body from our sentient self."

She observes the newest techniques available to date in the medical school, and also sees mock-ups of techniques in progress that imply another leap of imagination. But she sees these in the company of medical students as well as the inventors. Her perspective is different from both groups. "As a visual artist I approach the body as the matrix of the human condition and its mysterious evolutionary history. . . . In an expanding technoculture, I embrace the diversity of our visual language, but insist on drawing by hand, on paper, as an essential, primary language. . . . Drawing is an act of empathy."[40] Shaw's posture on the tightrope between imaging technology and the hand of the physician differs from Lesser's in that Shaw senses the miraculousness of the developing technologies and feels that they do not have to alienate patient from healer.

As the century draws to an end, computers have infiltrated every corner of society and colored video monitors and the Internet compete to win the attention of our busy selves. Artists lost their wonder at the power of imaging technology as they mastered it. No longer limited to painting "as if" they have peered through fluoroscopes, they place their virtual selves before virtual fluoroscopes with a click of a mouse. Imaging machines and their images are now artists' tools. The media artist Nina Sobell is comfortable taming computers so that technology works for her. Using personal computers, with the accent on *personal,* Sobell welcomed computerized medical imaging systems into the art world. She realized in the early 1970s, when she lived in Los Angeles, that the only way people would pay attention to their own thoughts and feelings was to see them on television.[41] In *Interactive Electroencephalographic Brainwave Drawing* she used a television monitor and electroencephalographic equipment to track the visible brainwaves of volunteers as they watched. The installation took the mystery out of electronic medical equipment and introduced a personal, humanistic experience. Working with scientists at the Veterans Administration Neuropsychology lab in 1974, she developed a system of video camera, EEG hook-ups, and a television monitor that enabled pairs of participants to sit before a screen, watching their own faces and a readout of their brain activity in real time being superimposed on the video image of their faces, allowing them to

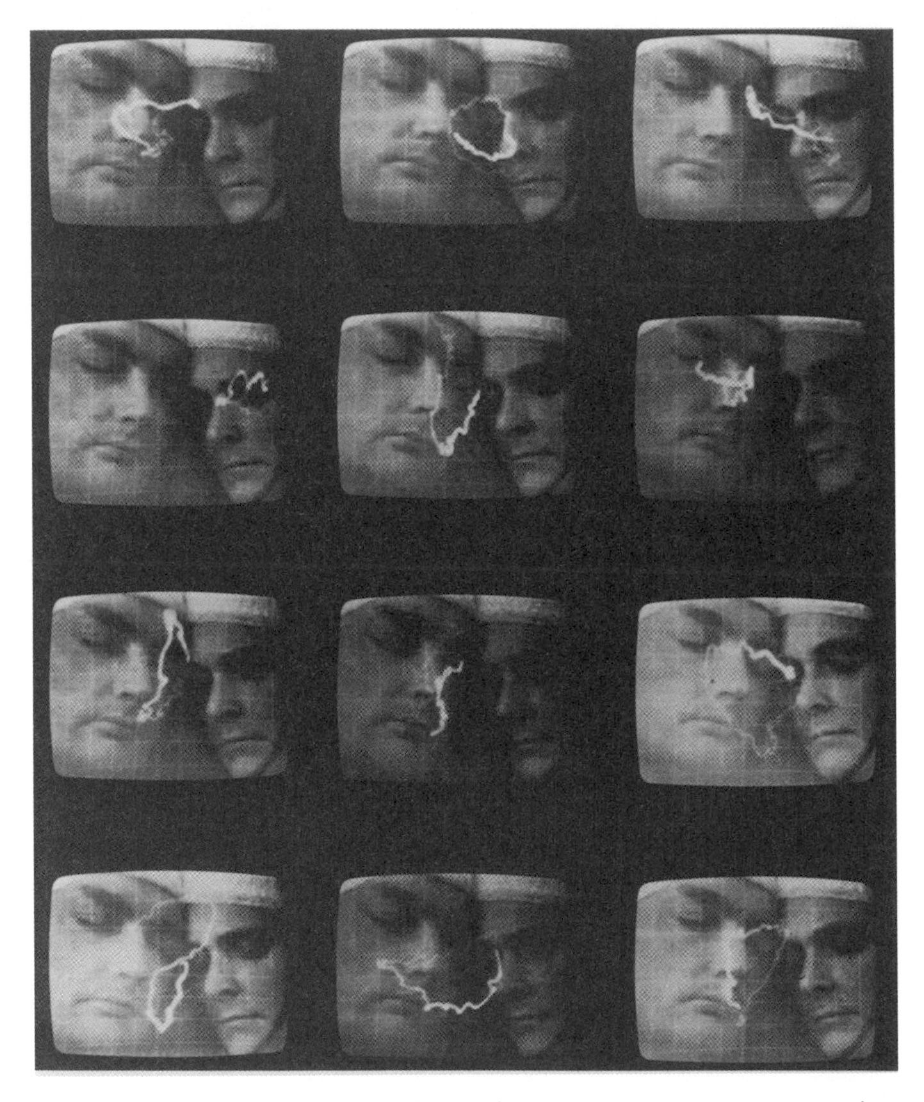

73. Nina Sobell, *Interactive Electroencephalographic Brainwave Drawing* (1974). From video. Courtesy of Nina Sobell.

see a composite of an internal and external portrait in a single, video image. Sobell invited strangers into street-front "shops" where, in pairs, she videotaped them, then wired their heads for EEG profiles of their brain waves.

In later installations she replaced the traditional EEG printout with an oscilloscope so that the jagged lines would move horizontally across a video screen. She discovered then that the participants' brainwave patterns sometimes merged into a single pattern. Then, at an installation in New York in 1992, Sobell discovered that the participants influenced each other's brainwave states. Where people got along, she captured a literal meeting of the minds, as the EEG's produced matching shapes in moments of rapport so that they were all part of a loop. By this time she was able to design a full-color graphics translation of the EEG signals so that participants could learn to control their waves. Sobell continues this kind of interactive art using medical imaging on the World Wide Web. Working with the cooperation of the medical imaging laboratory at New York University, she has perfected the use of telerobotics for interactive performances, inviting viewers from all over the world into her studio, via a robot and the Web.[42]

Digitized scans reflect a different interior from what can be seen by even the finest X-ray. At a 1995 retrospective of the photography of Annie Leibovitz, a single picture stood out. Amidst the full-body, posed portraits of celebrities and candid images of the artist's family there was a sheet of fifteen different colored MRI images of Laurie Anderson's brain. Anderson, a performance artist of remarkable versatility, delights in electronic innovations; Leibovitz's portrait looks at Anderson from the perspective of the kind of virtual images she likes to project—an apt metaphor for the soul of a performer immersed in computer technology. The carefully selected MRI slices, including an image of a single ear, unfailingly elicits nods and smiles from gallery-goers. A century

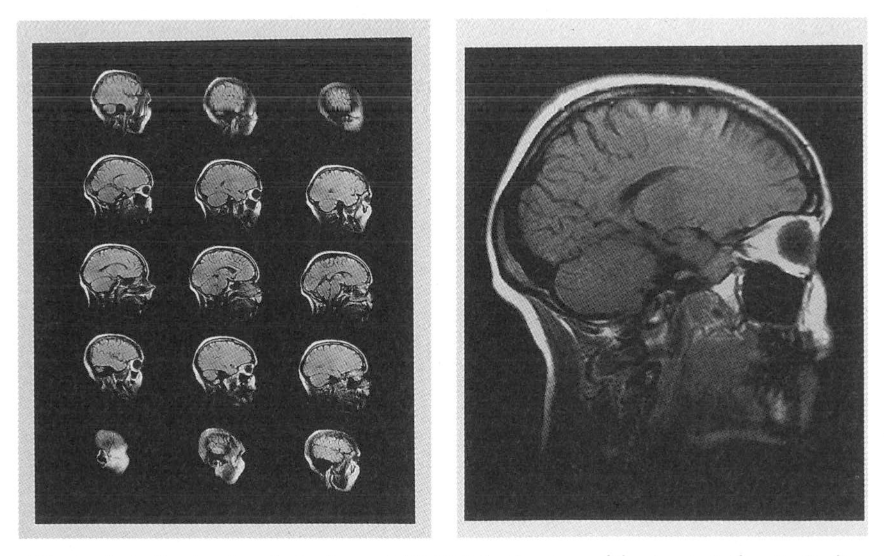

74. Annie Leibovitz, *Laurie Anderson MRI* (1994). Courtesy of the Annie Leibovitz Studio.

ago, it is reasonable to conjecture, no lay observer, seeing those images, would have been able to identify a brain. Annie Leibovitz's MRI is targeted at late twentieth-century eyes for whom the subject is at once recognizable but new enough to have special meaning.

Medical imagery attracts artists for a variety of reasons: the inherent beauty of natural structures; the very conflicted attitudes of our age towards technology in general and medical instruments in particular; and the effort to redefine the purpose of art even as they, as artists, reaffirm the value and possibility of portraiture. These images of the interiors of our bodies are redefining health, disease, and the space between them so that the technology that began as a kind of periscope in 1895—a device to peer through the skin to the skeleton beneath—has evolved into a series of mirrors. The new machines, equally accessible to artists and jurists as well as physicians, reflect what we want to know about what is happening inside each of us.

Epilogue

The dramatic entry of X-rays onto the historical stage altered instantly, and forever, the way people looked at each other and at themselves. The initial novelty vanished in less than a generation as X-rays became commonplace and its technology was incorporated into the machine-happy culture of the new century, enriching X-ray manufacturers as well as satellite industries from glass-blowers to film-makers to producers of lead-lined laboratory gear.

Excitement flared anew seventy-five years later as computer-generated imaging expanded the possibilities of seeing the interior of the human body. But by this time "miracle" and "medicine" had been linked so often that even detailed cross-sections of a living brain or the beating of a fetal heart did not elicit the kind of awe that greeted the image of the pale shadow of Frau Roentgen's bones in January 1896.

The discovery and exploitation of X-rays epitomizes the link between pure science and its technological applications. "Pure" research does not ring as true today as it did a century ago; even so, the benefits of X-rays are manifestly the result of basic research. In a speech in Newcastle-on-Tyne in September 1995, the Astronomer Royal, Sir Martin Rees, hailed the centennial of the X-ray, noting that the ways of science had so changed that if the bureaucracy of the 1990s had existed a century ago, "A proposal to make flesh appear transparent would not have got a research grant—even if it had, it surely would not have led to X-rays."[1] As much could be said for the idea of using a strong magnet to get a picture of the inside of the human brain.

A century ago, those startling X-rays undermined the validity of what it meant to see with the naked eye. Artists, among the first constituency to respond to the suddenly visible vital organs, combined images of age-old symbols—like the human heart—in an idiom appropriate to a mechanized, swift-paced, disposable, technological civilization. They pondered the new reality and realized that the distinctions between inside and outside, permanent and transient, translucent and opaque, depended upon who was looking at what, with what, and with what end in mind.

The giddiness of the first years after Roentgen's discovery gave way to a measured appraisal of the new technology. More slowly than seems reasonable in retrospect, the public became aware of the dangers of radiation. But there had never before been a technology with such a long fuse. Why doubt the word of great scientists like Rutherford and the Curies who worked with radiation and sang its praises? Three quarters of a century later the pendulum had swung so far that all technology was suspect: electromagnetic fields around power lines, cellular telephones, and microwave ovens were each singled out as possible carcinogens.

In medical practice, however, ultrasound and magnetic resonance slipped into use as easily as X-rays had, with some consideration paid to the possibility of eventual repercussions in the light of our experience with radiation, but without widespread testing. And despite occasional accidents, computerized imaging, like the overmaligned X-rays, has probably contributed far more to individual health than it has taken away.

The public has not complained about anything except cost, for in truth, our appetite for holographic reconstructions of the heart or brain is greater than our fear. At an annual conference extolling the link between medicine and virtual reality, a military physician projected images of an imaginary battlefield where robots, controlled by surgeons a continent away, performed stereotactic surgery as their puppet-masters manipulated three-dimensional images of the interior of the patient's skull.[2]

This enthusiasm led the American medical community to assume that new imaging technologies would keep reaching the market as soon as working prototypes demonstrated their benefits. As recently as 1994, doctors and hospitals invested generously in new instruments. They were blinded by success; a whole generation of doctors and patients already raised a collective eyebrow at the idea of "exploratory surgery," while lives once lost to a variety of tumors were being saved and people with MS, pituitary tumors, and Parkinson's disease were finding relief.

More frequently even than in the past, physicians are called on to repair the lowly gunshot wound. Bullets track our culture even as we track their lethal power. Chances of recovery from wounds like those that felled Presidents Garfield and McKinley have improved so that it is doubtful that either man would have died from similar injuries today. Emergency room personnel in America's cities today see bullets routinely on radiographs, and as often leave them where they came to rest (as they did with Teddy Roosevelt's). Today's physicians need to identify the *new* bullet in the torso of a young gang member whose body might already include five earlier slugs.[3]

As imaging technologies became increasingly refined, the window between proposed improvement and implementation narrowed. What was highly speculative yesterday—the ability to perform an operation with the patient and surgical team working within an MRI machine—is now reality. Teleradiology, long a goal to help underserved populations, is functioning all over North America. Florida hospitals send digitized CT, MRI, PET, and ultrasound images over telephone lines for diagnosis in Los Angeles, and patients on the island of Martha's Vineyard in Massachusetts have their scans read by the Teleradiology Center in North Carolina.[4]

What has remained constant since 1896 is the enthusiasm of scientists, physicians, lawyers, artists, and the general public for seeing the interior of the living body. The desire to peer through opaque flesh is seldom criticized, even by those fearful of radiation, dismayed by the mechanization of medicine and the associated distancing of doctor from patient, or by the overuse of expensive equipment by doctors and hospitals eager to recoup and profit from their investments. In truth, the abandon with which American medicine has invested in imaging technology has been rewarded by an enormous return in improved health.

Looking ahead, it is easier to imagine an exhibition in the Imaging Museum of the future than to foresee machines in future imaging centers. Radiographs on glass, the original X-ray technology, have already disappeared. Film is likely to follow soon, replaced by versions that have been digitized for easy storage and electronic telecommunication. The use of CT will probably diminish but not disappear; its speed guarantees it a place in emergency medicine. MRI has a clear path before it, for while machines are costly, they last a long time and the upgrades they need are largely a matter of software programs. Ultrasound, the cheapest method of all, offers excellent images of organs that defy other imaging approaches and will probably occupy more space in the future. PET is a different story: full of promise for over a generation, and excellent for specialized procedures, it continues to run into regulatory obstacles that arise like dragon's teeth even as others are overcome.

Whichever technologies survive will echo the priorities of society at least as much as those of the medical community. It is useful to recall that, at the time of their discovery, radiographs were limited to small glass plates that reflected the organizational deconstruction of medicine into specialties—each concentrating on the anatomical area covered by one small plate. Similarly, today's whole-body scans may reflect a reconceptualization of disease as systemic, rather than located in a single organ or brought into the body from outside, and a subsequent realignment of physicians. The face of medicine may look very different in twenty years.

It is likely that whatever medicine looks like, lawyers will remember the harm inflicted by radiation as well as the dangers of misdiagnoses. And they will continue to use medical images to convince juries, whatever the source of the image, of the peculiarities of the human body. What is unpredictable is whether there will be any new imaging devices.

For while the appearance of the CT scanner in 1972 set the pace for the development and marketing of all the modes that followed, the ingredients of CT, as we have seen, had been around for over a decade. The algorithms for reconstructing images from projections were available before the scanner was built, as were the techniques that were used in nuclear medicine. Whether individual strokes of genius in mathematics, the physical sciences, or engineering are credited with developing the first scanner, the computer-driven revolution that drove it did not emerge from any single imagination. It came from the unlikely collaboration of a British company flush with the unexpected earnings of four talented young men from Liverpool and their maverick engineer with a government newly committed to funding research in national health.

Once EMI demonstrated its machine and buyers appeared eager to spend unprecedented sums for a single instrument, the economic barrier collapsed. At that point innovative mathematical formulas and the hardware to put them to the test bounced like billiard balls from one technology to another, from CT to MRI to PET to ultrasound. After 1973 each technology gleaned something from its rivals' strengths in both image reconstruction and in marketing, and measured its own accomplishments against the others' images.

Looking back at the competition that accompanied the linkage of computers with imaging technologies, the timing suggests that, but for its few years' head start, CT could never have competed with MRI. But it is hard to see how, without CT as a precedent, the chemical laboratory's small-scale nuclear magnetic resonance technology would ever have, on its own, have become body-imaging MRI.

Medical care, which had been considered a luxury throughout most of recorded history, became an entitlement in parts of Europe in the nineteenth century, an entitlement which became almost universal there after World War II, and was instituted, at least for the elderly, in the United States with the inauguration of Medicare in 1976. But as early as 1975, high expenditures and an apparent oversupply of machines inspired some state legislatures to limit the purchase and distribution of imaging apparatus. After 1976 the effort to cut the medical budget moved to the national level. Since then physicians' groups, public health institutions, and investigative journalists have continued to expose the overuse of imaging machines, highlighting the ethically dubious practice that continues in some states of the acquisition by doctors of ownership in imaging centers to which they direct their patients.

The continuing on-screen revelation of vital organs only recently obscured from view has produced new dilemmas. One is the problem of the lag between the ability to diagnose and the ability to treat disease. The Tamaras of the world, people with inoperable brain tumors, may suffer more as they see their tumors grow with each successive scan. But the odds of a cure go up as surgery is refined in the wake of more precise identification of disorderly cells.[5] Ignorance is an analgesic only where there is no hope. Elsewhere it may signal tragically missed opportunities.

Another problem is the matter of who gets scanned. In a universe of selective insurance coverage, it becomes a question of cost-effectiveness to perform diagnostic screening.[6] Then there is the possibility that scans may reveal small tumors in the brains or breasts of people who have no symptoms and who may never suffer from cancer if left alone. Likewise, prostate cancers may sit quietly until stimulated by treatment. There is always the possibility that discovering hidden malignancies and treating them with chemicals or radiation may spread the condition, producing intense anxiety, if not worse, in previously symptom-free patients.

Fifty years ago science fiction writers dreamed of exploring the solar system. Of the dozens of projected scenarios, none predicted that a series of exploratory moon flights would be cut off midway and the rockets mothballed as the organization that built them fell apart. Medicine is, of course, different from space travel. There is no central organization and there has never been an acknowledged race for national supremacy. But the collapse of the space program demonstrates that there is no guarantee that increasingly expensive forms of technology will continue to emerge as they have in the twentieth century.

There is no technological imperative, no single path toward success, as CT's nursery at EMI's London laboratory demonstrates. The timing was right because computer development had stabilized, at least temporarily, and while the British health system could not support the purchase of expensive machines that would only benefit the few who happened to have brain tumors, American hospitals were willing to gamble on these machines because they could pass the bill on to public and private insurers. MRI's success also depended on the willingness of Americans to risk investing in new instruments, not all of which were successful. Less expensive or more specialized MRI machines did not sell even though there seemed to be a place for them.[7]

The imaging market was never a sure thing. With the exception of nuclear medicine, the United States left the greater part of early development to private investment. The seed projects, often imported, benefited from the British public's purse. The lesson, if there is one, suggests that basic research cannot count on private funding, but once a technology is developed, it thrives on the kind of consumer-driven economy that existed in the United States in the 1970s and 1980s. That market did not respond to the classic connection of supply and demand. Advertising directed at patients led many smaller hospitals to buy more powerful instruments than were really needed as they competed for patients by offering top-of-the-line machines on the cutting edge of medicine—medical status symbols—without regard to real cost. Middle-class Americans came to expect the best diagnostic imaging available.

The corporate world continues to invest in elaborations on established technologies while university laboratories look to new kinds of imaging. Still on the drawing board, and limited to the research arena, are computerized efforts to stimulate touch as well as sight. One approach combines MR with sound waves, allowing physicians to palpate tumors remotely, feeling the familiar stiff or hard cancer tissue on a computerized image with virtual reality tools before the cancer shows up visually.[8] Another promising technique is magnetoencephalography (MEG), which uses an array of superconducting sensors

(SQUID) to map sections of the brain invisible to other technologies. Mapping magnetic brainwaves, MEG can locate activities such as listening to music with millisecond resolutions. But MEG, which currently costs several million dollars to install, is still being developed and may not survive a changed economy.

The political upheaval in 1994 caught the imaging industry by surprise. Organized medicine had its forces aimed at government-controlled national health plans and failed to notice the threat to the status quo from profit-making, managed-care corporations touting cost-savings through preventive efforts. These promises ought to have boded well for diagnostic screening procedures, but the same cost-cutters also promised to eliminate the purchase and use of expensive technologies. Not surprisingly, sales of all imaging machines has flattened.

The majority of imaging machines in the United States are dispersed unevenly in medical centers and prosperous suburbs. In the past, some American physicians ordered too many diagnostic images as a defense against malpractice suits, or because their patients expected them, as well as in an effort to support their diagnoses with visual evidence.

The market, however, has changed, with rewards now going to the frugal. Researchers remain confident that the improved images they will soon get from all kinds of MRI and PET will be bought because the potentially ill who stand to benefit, is all of us. It is hard to see the medical consumer consciously giving up expectations of increasingly finer diagnostic images and their implications for better treatment, but it is even harder to see where new research fits into the emerging medical system. In its present form, research and development have been cut back, left to the invisible hand of the market, a hand that in the matter of long-term investment has closed into a tight fist.

Research continues, of course, on a more modest level, and the medical system, once stabilized in its new form, may elicit a resurgence of investment in imaging technologies. Or the history of medical imaging, from X-rays to functional PET scans, may turn out to have been a twentieth-century saga that begins with the miracle of Frau Roentgen's skeletal fingers and concludes in the specialized worlds of cancer treatment and brain mapping.

Artists will most likely continue to extrapolate and elaborate on the remarkable technologies already available. For as a civilization, perhaps even as a species, we like to look, like to look through, and like to look at and through ourselves. In black and white and in color, in two-dimensional slices or in three-dimensional volumes, in frozen instants or moving sequences, the X-ray and its daughter technologies seem to satisfy an innate curiosity to see ourselves naked to the bone.

Timeline

	X-Rays and radiation	Nuclear medicine, PET	MRI	Ultrasound	
1870s					
1873	William Crookes designs new cathode ray tube				
1877				Pierre and Jacques Curie discover piezo-electricity	
1881					
1895	Nov. 7: Wilhelm Roentgen discovers X-rays Dec. 28: Roentgen's paper published by Physico-Medical Society of Würzburg				
1896	GE and Siemens begin selling X-ray equipment Elihu Thomson conducts experiments on X-ray burns Mar.: Herbert Jackson invents the focus tube Apr.: Edison demonstrates his fluoroscope at the annual Electrical Exhibition in New York H. S. Ward publishes first text-book *Practical Radiography*				
1897					
1898					
1899					
1901					
1903					
1904	William Rollins describes hazards of radiation in "Notes on the X-Light"				
1905					
1907					
1910					
1911		George Hevesy uses radio-active isotope of lead as a tracer			

Arts	Legal landmarks	Historical and scientific events	
		Photography becomes commercial	1870s
			1873
		Edison invents phonograph Bell patents telephone	1877
		Assassination of President James Garfield	1881
		Dec. 28: Lumière brothers project first motion pictures to an audience	1895
	Tolman Cunnings introduces X-ray picture of his leg as evidence in a Canadian courtroom Apr.: *Smith v. Grant:* X-rays admitted into U.S. courtroom in Denver, Colorado Apr.: First forensic application of X-rays in the murder of Elizabeth Hartley in Nelson, England	Henri Becquerel discovers natural radioactivity May: X-rays used by Italy on battlefield in east Africa	1896
H. G. Wells's *The Invisible Man*	X-rays used to identify dead in Paris fire X-rays indicted in the murder case of George Orme in Elmira, New York X-rays enter French courtroom in Rouen		1897
		Pierre and Marie Curie discover Polonium and Radium U.S. Army uses X-rays in hospitals during Spanish-American War	1898
Jack London's "A Thousand Deaths"			1899
		Roentgen awarded first Nobel Prize in physics Sept.: Assassination of President William McKinley	1901
		Becquerel, Marie Curie, and Pierre Curie share Nobel Prize in physics	1903
		Death of Clarence Dally, first "martyr" to radiation	1904
		Death of Elizabeth Fleischmann, another "martyr"	1905
Pablo Picasso's *Les Demoiselles d'Avignon*			1907
The *Technical Manifesto of Futurist Painting*			1910
			1911

(continued)

	X-Rays and radiation	Nuclear medicine, PET	MRI	Ultrasound
1912	H. M. Luckett identifies "spontaneous pneumo-encephalography" in the case of a Manhattan trolley car victim			
1913	William Coolidge invents the Coolidge (hot cathode) tube Gustav Bucky invents the grid/diaphragm in Germany Albert Salomon studies breast cancer micro-calcifications with X-rays			
1914				Pierre Langevin constructs ultrasonic generator in effort to detect enemy submarines
1915	Hollis Potter in the U.S. augments Bucky's grid with movable element that eliminated the shadows of grid lines			
1916	Red goggles introduced for dark adaptation Marie Curie establishes mobile X-ray units and training programs in radiology for the military U.S. Army introduces portable X-ray units in Mexican campaign			
1917				
1918	Walter Dandy uses air as a contrast agent in first ventriculography			
1919	Dandy introduces pneumo-encephalography with injection of air into the brain via the lumbar region			
1920	Jan Athanase Sicard and Jacques Forestier use Lipiodol as a contrast agent			
1921	André Bocage, F. Portes, and M. Chausse apply for tomog-raphy patents			
1923				
1924	Arthur Mutscheller intro-duces the "tolerance dose" as a guide to limiting the exposure of an individual to radiation			
1925	First International Confer-ence of Radiology meets in London; Commission on X-ray Units set up to define units of radiation			

Arts	Legal landmarks	Historical and scientific events	
Duchamp's *Nude Descending a Staircase No. 1*		Max von Laue discovers X-ray crystallography Assassination attempt on ex-president Theodore Roosevelt: X-rays reveal bullet	1912
Francis Picabia's *Mechanical Expression seen through our own Mechanical Expression* and *New York through an X-ray*		H. G. J. Moseley discovers that X-ray spectra of elements are related to the charge on the atomic nucleus	1913
		Aug.: World War I begins in Europe	1914
			1915
			1916
		U.S. enters World War I; introduces routine X-ray screening of draftees Russian Revolution leads to establishment of the USSR	1917
	Runyan v. Goodrum: effects of X-rays on patients declared to be "idiosyncratic"		1918
		Armistice ends World War I	1919
The *Realist Manifesto* published			1920
			1921
Gertrude Atherton's *Black Oxen*		AMA approves a Section Council on Radiology limiting the practice to experts	1923
Thomas Mann's *The Magic Mountain* published in Germany			1924
Sinclair Lewis's *Arrowsmith*			1925

(continued)

	X-Rays and radiation	Nuclear medicine, PET	MRI	Ultrasound	
1926	Geiger-Muller counter detects and measures the intensity of radiation				
1927	Herman Muller's experiments with fruit flies indicates dangers of genetic mutations from radiation Egaz Moniz performs cerebral angiography using sodium iodide as a contrast agent				
1928	Second International Conference of Radiology meets in Stockholm: establishes *curie* and *roentgen* as units of radiation	Harvey Cushing notes correlation between blood flow and cerebral function		S. Y. Sokolov used ultrasound to detect discontinuities in metals	
1929	Jean Kieffer patents a method for tomography Werner Forssmann performs angiography by catheterization				
1930	Alessandro Vallebona builds model "stratigraph," a tomograph machine Eastman Kodak produces safety (nonflammable) X-ray film Charles Lauritsen develops high voltage X-ray machines for radiation therapy				
1931	Bernard Ziedes des Plantes develops "planigraph," a tomograph machine "Tolerance dose" adopted as the international standard				
1932	Alice Ettinger brings to the U.S. the spot-film device, which recorded fluoroscopic images on X-ray films				
1933		Positrons detected			
1934					
1935		Ernest Lawrence produces radioactive isotopes of sodium, which are harmless to the body			
1936		The Lawrence cyclotron in Berkeley, Calif., proves itself capable of making at least 18 radioisotopes of biologically significant elements			

Arts	Legal landmarks	Historical and scientific events	
			1926
			1927
			1928
			1929
Jean Cocteau's movie: *Blood of the Poet*			1930
		Ernest Lawrence invents the cyclotron	1931
Heartfield's *Hitler Swallows Gold and Spouts Junk*			1932
Picasso's *Girl before a Mirror*		Hitler elected Chancellor of Germany	1933
		Irène Curie and Frédéric Joliot receive Nobel Prize for producing artificial radioisotopes	1934
	Call v. City of Burley: Idaho court rules that X-rays are only useful when interpreted by experts	Committee for the Study of Sex Variants uses X-rays to study homosexuality	1935
		The Martyrs' Memorial erected in Hamburg, Germany, containing the names of (originally) 169 physicians and technicians who died from radiation-induced diseases	1936

(continued)

	X-Rays and radiation	Nuclear medicine, PET	MRI	Ultrasound	
1937	Jean Kieffer's "laminograph" (tomograph) built at the Mallinkrodt Institute		I. I. Rabi measures the magnetic moment of (or spin) of the nucleus of an atom	Karl and Friedreich Dussik obtain crude ultrasound image of the brain	
1938	Jacob Gershon-Cohen suggests studying normal breast as control for diagnosing diseased breast				
1939					
1941					
1942					
1943					
1944				Floyd Firestone patents the "Reflectoscope"	
1945					
1946	John Caffey uses X-rays as evidence of child abuse		Edward Purcell and Felix Bloch measure NMR in bulk matter		
1949	Raul Leborgne finds value of breast compression in mammography			Douglas Howry builds rudimentary ultrasound machine and obtains image of his own thigh John Wild applies ultrasound to distinguish malignant from healthy tissues	
1950				MIT laboratory builds unsuccessful ultrasonic brain scanner Howry builds "somascope" and obtains cross-sectional ultrasound images	
1950s				William Fry develops ultrasonic equipment for treatment not imaging Wild uses ultrasound in breast cancer research	
1951	Benedict Cassen invents "scintiscanner" Charles Gros develops first radiological unit designed specifically for the breast			Wild develops B-mode "contact" scanner	
1952					

Arts	Legal landmarks	Historical and scientific events	
			1937
			1938
Comic strip "Superman" is endowed with X-ray vision	Sterilization of criminals by X-rays legalized in Michigan	World War II begins in Europe	1939
		Germans plan to secretly irradiate reproductive organs of Jews Dec.: U.S. enters World War II	1941
Tchelitchew completes *Hide-and-Seek*		Manhattan Project begins	1942
		Hevesy receives Nobel Prize in chemistry	1943
Frida Kahlo's *The Broken Column*		I. I. Rabi receives Nobel Prize in physics	1944
		Aug.: Atomic bombs exploded over Hiroshima and Nagasaki Aug.: World War II ends	1945
		ENIAC (Electronic Numerical Integrator and Computer) put into operation. Computers enter worlds of research and commerce	1946
			1949
		Korean War begins	1950
		Television becomes commercially available	1950s
			1951
		Purcell and Bloch receive the Nobel Prize in physics	1952

(continued)

	X-Rays and radiation	Nuclear medicine, PET	MRI	Ultrasound	
1953				Lars Leksell uses ultrasound to successfully diagnose a hematoma in an infant's brain Inge Edler and Helmut Hertz develop M-mode ultrasound and launch echocardiography	
1954	David Kuhl invents the "photoscan"			Ian Donald applies ultrasound to obstetrics and gynecology	
1955		Louis Sokoloff uses radioisotopes to track local brain function in cats		Shigeo Satomura and Yasuharu Numura apply the Doppler effect to ultrasound to show the speed of blood in the heart	
1956	Ronald Bracewell publishes paper mapping sunspots using series of one-dimensional strips to reconstruct a two-dimensional image with Fourier transforms Alice Stewart correlates child deaths from cancer with prenatal X-ray exposures			Leksell uses ultrasound to identify the midline in the adult brain	
1957		Sokoloff uses 2-deoxyglucose as a tracer			
1958	William Oldendorf builds model CT scanner without a computer				
1959			Jay Singer measures the rates of blood flow in mice with NMR		
1960	Oldendorf applies for a patent for his model scanner Robert Egan adapts high-resolution film to mammography				
1963	Alan Cormack publishes results from experimental scanner using a computer to reconstruct images from data				
1965					
1966	David Kuhl publishes paper with the first transmission images of a subject's thorax				
1967	Bracewell reconstructs lunar images without using Fourier transforms Mammogram machines designed specifically for the breast commercially available				
1968	EMI patents Godfrey Hounsfield's method and apparatus for imaging the body by scanning with X-rays	First SPECT machines introduced			

Arts	Legal landmarks	Historical and scientific events	
		Korean War ends	1953
Francis Bacon's *Figure with Meats* Movie *Them*			1954
			1955
			1956
			1957
		USSR launches *Sputnik*	1958
			1959
			1960
		Nov. 22: Assassination of President John F. Kennedy	1963
		U.S. escalates role in Vietnam War Lennart Nilsson's photographs of a fetus appear on the cover of *Life* magazine	1965
Movie *Fantastic Voyage*			1966
Rauschenberg's *Booster*		Amniocentesis used to reveal the sex of the fetus and chromosomal evidence of Down's syndrome	1967
		Neil Armstrong becomes first man to walk on the moon	1968

(continued)

	X-Rays and radiation	Nuclear medicine, PET	MRI	Ultrasound
1971	The first CT scanner, limited to the head, demonstrated by EMI at Atkinson Morley's Hospital in London Xeroradiography becomes commercially available		Raymond Damadian publishes evidence that NMR can distinguish healthy from malignant tissues Paul Lauterbur extracts an image from NMR signals	
1972	First CT scanner demonstrated in the United States	Niels Lassen uses SPECT to track blood flow to map brain function	Damadian applies for a patent for an apparatus to detect cancer tissues	
1973	Robert Ledley markets ACTA, a whole-body CT scanner		Lauterbur publishes paper on NMR imaging in *Nature* Peter Mansfield describes NMR diffraction in solids	
1974				
1975	Second-generation Delta CT scanners are marketed GE's third-generation CT scanners are marketed	Michel Ter-Pogossian and Michael Phelps publish paper about PET machine	Richard Ernst introduces two-dimensional NMR	Ultrasound commercially successful with the improvements of gray-scale and real-time imaging
1976				
1977	Magnification mammography introduced		Damadian announces first whole-body NMR scanner: the "Indomitable" Mansfield introduces echoplanar MRI, which obtains data from a whole plane at a time	
1979		Kuhl, Wold, and Fowler develop the FDG tracer used in PET scanning		
1980s				
1980				
1981				
1982				
1983				

Arts	Legal landmarks	Historical and scientific events	
			1971
Agnes Denes exhibits *Intro-spection III—Aesthetics (X-Rays of the Masters)*			1972
			1973
Nina Sobell exhibits first *Brainwave Drawing*		Certificate of Need (CON) laws passed by U.S. federal government for approval of hospital purchases Betty Ford and Happy Rockefeller announce diagnoses of breast cancer and have mastectomies	1974
		Vietnam War ends	1975
		Medicare legislation passed by the U.S. federal government	1976
			1977
		Hounsfield and Cormack awarded the Nobel Prize for physiology or medicine	1979
		Personal computers alter homes and offices	1980s
Movie *Altered States*			1980
		Assassination attempt on President Reagan; CT scan used to save Press Secretary James Brady	1981
	CT introduced for first time in a U.S. trial by defense in case of John Hinckley, who shot Reagan and Brady		1982
	Swanson v. U.S. Government: CT scans deemed part of the standard medical care of 1976		1983

(continued)

	X-Rays and radiation	Nuclear medicine, PET	MRI	Ultrasound	
1985	Superfast CT is developed by Douglas Boyd				
1986					
1987					
1989	First spiral CT enters the market		Seiji Ogawa publishes paper introducing BOLD contrast agents in fMRI		
1991					
1992					
1993					
1994					
1995			High-field MRI reveals interior of a human tooth MRS used clinically fMR used in brain mapping		

Arts	Legal landmarks	Historical and scientific events	
Don DeLillo's *White Noise* Andy Warhol's *Philip's Skull: CAT Scan*		MRI receives FDA approval for clinical use	1985
Woody Allen's Movie *Hannah and Her Sisters*		American Cancer Society and ACR establish an accreditation program for mammography	1986
Howard Sochurek's photoessay on imaging technologies appears in the *National Geographic*			1987
Movie *Rampage*		Collapse of the USSR	1989
		Changes in cortical activity and other mental efforts recorded with MEG (Magnetic Encephalography)	1991
Movie *Memoirs of an Invisible Man* Joyce Cutler Shaw's *The Anatomy Lesson*		Teleradiology enables remote diagnoses of most imaging technologies	1992
	Los Angeles jury sees MR images of Rodney King's brain		1993
The Feld Ballet performs *MRI*			1994
Annie Leibovitz exhibits MRI image of Laurie Anderson's brain		PET approved for clinical use by the FDA	1995

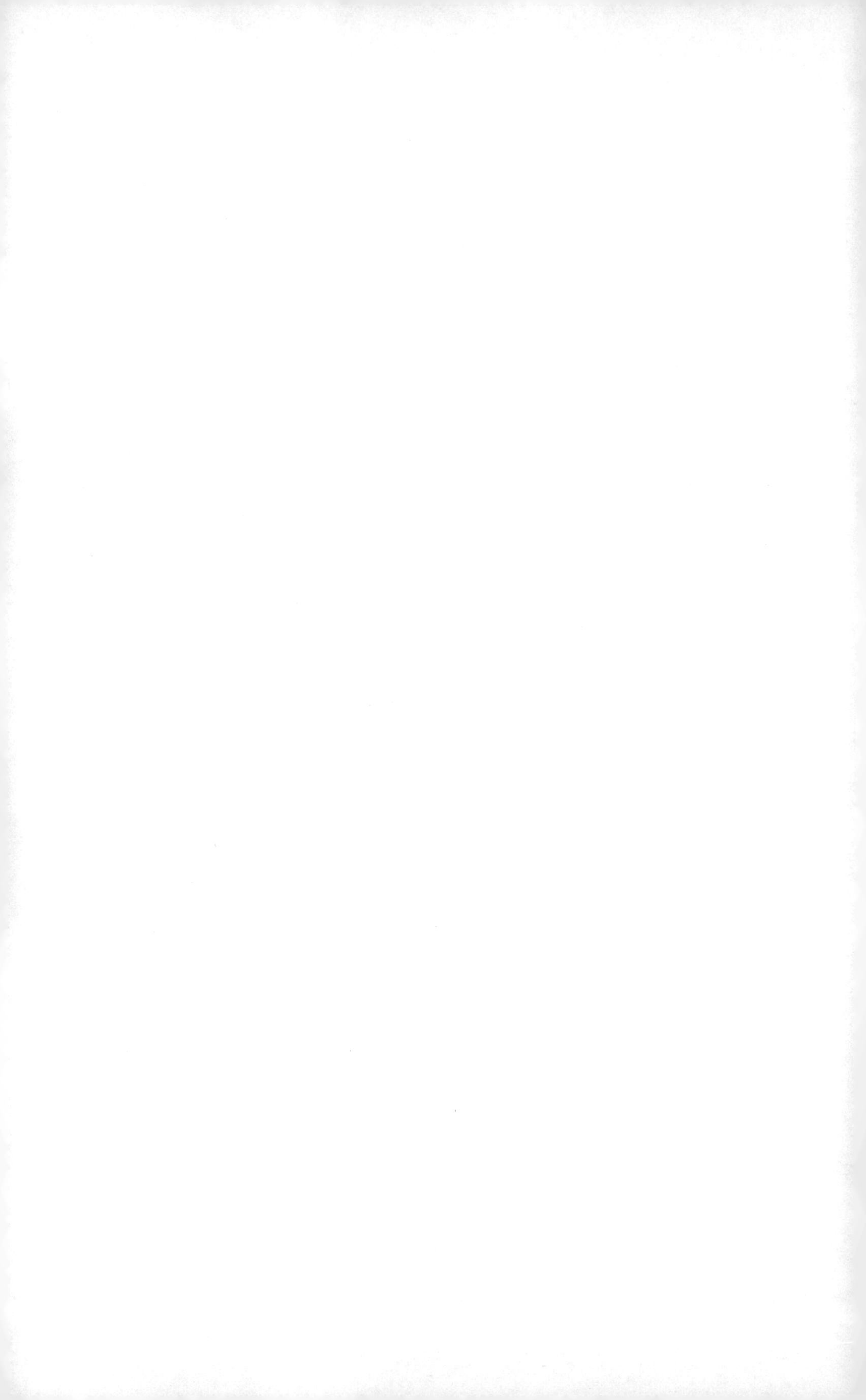

Acknowledgments

This book was inspired and subsequently supported by the Alfred P. Sloan Foundation, to which I am very grateful. I could not have mastered the century of events described without the generous cooperation, advice, and, in a number of instances, tutelage from many individuals, including physicians, scientists, engineers, artists, archivists, lawyers, and librarians in the United States, France, and Great Britain.

For consenting to interviews that provided information about their own careers or the groups in which they worked, I am grateful to Herbert Abrams, Richard Bing, Douglas Boyd, Ronald Bracewell, William Bradley, Thomas Brady, Barbara Carter, Peter Conti, Alan Cormack, Cynthia Corngold, Raymond Damadian, Agnes Denes, David Ellenbogen, Martin Harwit, Sir Godfrey Hounsfield, Everett James, Jr., John Jordan, Emanual Kanal, John Kassabian, Leon Kaufman, David Kramer, Niels Lassen, Paul Lauterbur, Robert Ledley, May Lesser, Sir Peter Mansfield, John Mazziotta, Steve Miller, Stella Oldendorf, William Oldendorf, Jr., Michael Phelps, Sheila Pinkel, Anne Roberts, John R. Roberts, Bruce Rosen, Rolf Schild, Joyce Cutler Shaw, Frank Shellock, Fred Silverman, Jay Singer, Robert Stanley, Jay Stein, Martin Weiss, and Samuel Williamson. For allowing me to shadow them during their work days as radiologists I wish to thank William Olmsted and William Bradley.

The Henry Huntington Library in San Marino, California, provided me with a second home, as well as invaluable research materials and assistance, for which I want to thank Robert C. Ritchie, Alan Jutzi, Linda Zoeckler, and Elsa Sink. The Millikan Library at the California Institute of Technology was indispensable, especially Tess Legaspi in Interlibrary Loan, and reference librarians

Janet Jencks and Judy Nollar. At Caltech I was fortunate to be able to learn from John Allman, the late William Fowler, Pratik Ghosh, Elizabeth Howard, Russell Jacobs, Bruce Murray, Christiane Orcel, and Paula Samazan. I am especially grateful to the Art Center College of Design in Pasadena, where Richard Hertz helped in every way possible, providing me with Hanna Hellsten, as a research assistant, and reference librarian Michelle Betty. My students Susan Aldrich, Daniel Chavkin, Joseph Essef, Suzanne Greenberg, Cameron Johann, Mary Kleinschmidt, Scharotte Storey, and Lise Tate helped with research.

I was encouraged from the start by Nancy Knight, archivist at the American College of Radiology, and later received indispensable help and advice from Otha Linton, a living encyclopedia of the recent history of medical imaging. Librarians at the American Roentgen Ray Society as well as those at the Smithsonian Museum of American History guided my search, and I was especially fortunate to have the help of Judy M. Chelnick. I was also helped at the Library of the National Institutes of Health in Bethesda, Maryland. Martin Harwit at the Smithsonian's Air and Space Museum and John Klineberg at the Goddard Space Center directed me to scientists and engineers involved with digital imaging. I was graciously welcomed at the Edison Archives in South Orange, New Jersey, the Countway Library at the Harvard Medical School, the library at the American Institute of Physics, and the California Museum of Photography in Riverside.

The papers presented at the University of Chicago in 1992 at the conference on "Imaging the Body: Art and Science in Modern Culture" were especially stimulating, and I thank Barbara Stafford and William Beck for allowing me to attend. I am grateful to the organizers of the first annual conference, "Medicine Meets Virtual Reality," which I attended in San Diego in 1994. The panoply of the annual RSNA (Radiological Society of North America) meeting in Chicago, which I attended in 1992, and the meeting of the SFR (Society of French Radiologists) in Paris in 1995, were tremendously helpful. It was at RSNA I met Peter Ogle, and then Philip Ward from *Diagnostic Imaging,* who provided me with much useful material.

I wish to thank Guy and Marie-José Pallardy, who offered me rich materials about the history of medical imaging in France; Heiner Brinnel, who allowed me to see the X-ray apparatus collected by Albert Renaud in Lyons; the archives at the École de Médicine; and Alain Renoux at the École de Radiologie in St. Germain en Laye, who provided me with a crucial volume on the history of neuroradiology in France. In England I was warmly welcomed by Sir Peter Mansfield in Nottingham, and conversed at length with Sir Godfrey Hounsfield in London, where I was fortunate to meet Rolf Schild, former board member at EMI.

For providing written accounts of their own work, and in some instances reading the appropriate chapters of mine, I wish to thank Larry Shepp and Seigi Ogawa at Bell Laboratories, Warwick Peacock and Robert Lufkin at the UCLA Medical School, Harry Chugani at the Children's Hospital of Michigan, Antonio Damazio, Alex Margulis, Richard H. Gold, Gerald D. Dodd, Roger Sanders, Barry Goldberg, and Robert Stanley. I am grateful to Juan del Regato and David di Santis for providing me with some of their own historical research. I am indebted to Ellen Koch for allowing me to see her dissertation.

I am grateful to Margaret Leighton for sharing information about her mother-in-law, Ingrid Lauritsen, and to Nicolas Tripodis for explaining the role of dental radiographs and for introducing me to Donald and Betty Parker. Milton Grimes kindly provided information about his client Rodney King.

For help in research in cultural history and the history of technology I am grateful to William S. Bartman, Rodney Sappington, Ruth Schwartz Cowan, Carl Maida, Aimée Brown Price, Linda Gerstein, Reyna Rapp, Rebecca Rothenberg, Christopher Whittick, John Sutherland, and for his considerable help with both cultural and technical aspects of PET scanning, Joseph Dumit.

Legal history was researched by Ruthie Pillar, Boyd Power, and Martin Brownstein, who supplemented Gilbert Whittemore's Ph.D. dissertation. Technical research was provided by Leonard Mlotinov and Allen Graubard, and last-minute research at the UCLA library was cheerfully performed by Jonathan Kevles.

It would have been daunting to cover so much different material without the help of those good enough to read specific chapters or the entire manuscript. I am grateful for the suggestions of John Kassabian, Sheila Pinkel, John Heilbron, and Susan Dimotakis who read selected chapters, and to Peter Conti, Sara Neustadtl, and Beth Kevles who critiqued the entire manuscript at different stages of completion, as did Otha Linton at the American College of Radiology and the Committee at the Sloan Foundation, all of whom contributed important advice.

I am grateful to the late Agatha Crowell for help setting up the file system, to Leona Kershaw for transcribing tapes, to Dan Rickels for computer assistance, to Mary Ellen Stote and William Bartlett for copyediting, and to Rudd Brown, Fran Yariv, Will Whittle, Emily Adelson, and Sasha Anawalt, who provided constant support. My editor Karen Reeds has had an uncanny ability to understand my vision. Anne Engle at the Jean Naggar Agency encouraged the project from the start, as did Jean Naggar.

Robert Merton played a special role with this book, guiding final revisions with awe-inspiring attention to thematic continuity. My research assistant, Magnolia Samadani, proved diligent, imaginative, and always optimistic throughout her two years with the project. The physicist David Salzman, who in the course of research became my son-in-law and then the father of my grandson, Michael, was an unanticipated source of technical information and a provocative and generous critic. My debt is immeasurable to my husband, Daniel Kevles, who graciously removed himself from the project until a full draft was ready to be read, and then added his critical talents to his constant moral support.

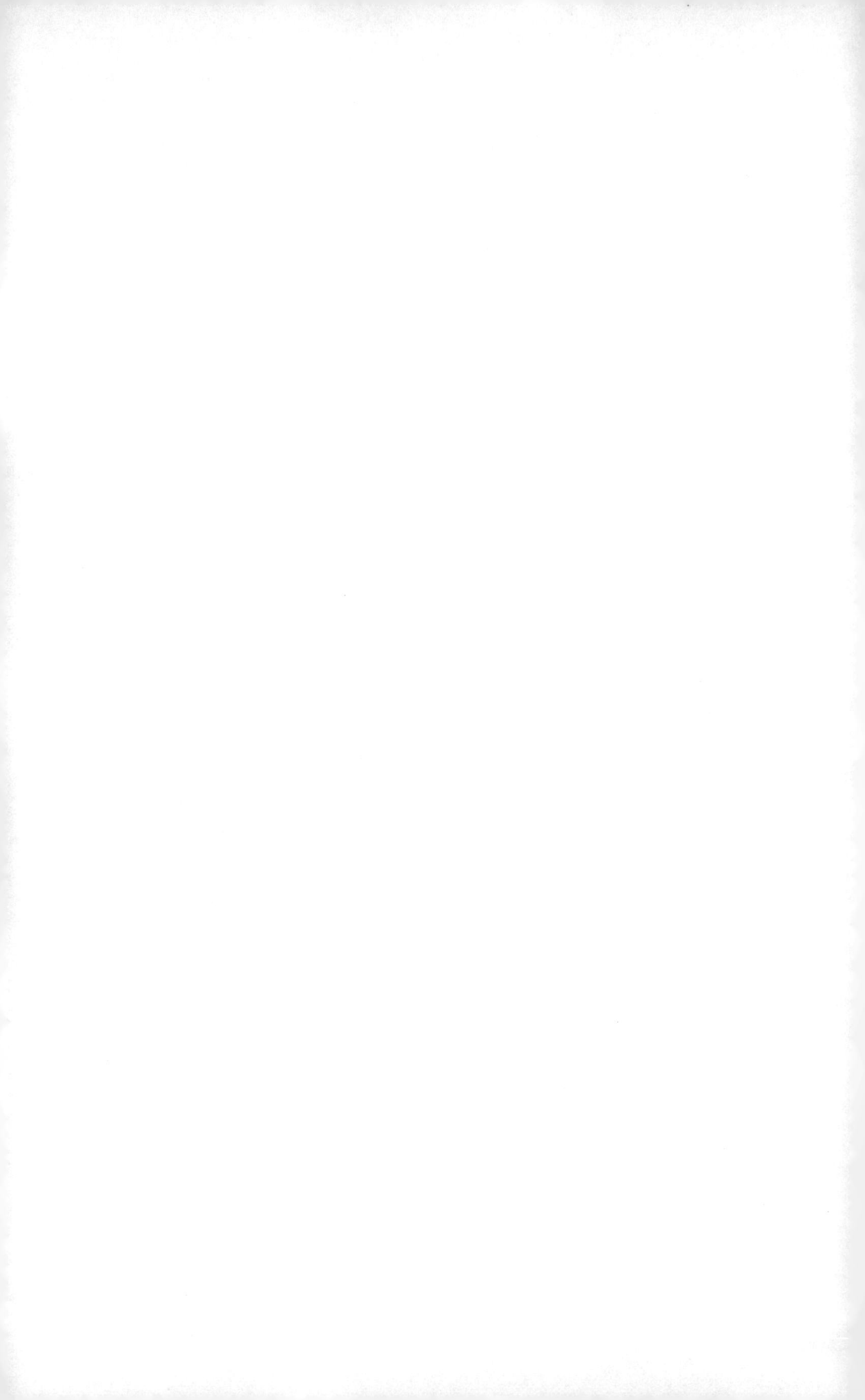

Notes

Introduction

1. Thomas P. Hughes, *American Genesis: A Century of Invention and Technological Enthusiasm, 1870–1970* (New York: Viking, 1989).

One The Discovery of X Rays

1. Catherine Mackenzie, *Alexander Graham Bell: The Man Who Contracted Space* (Boston: Houghton Mifflin, 1928).
2. Edward Bellamy, "With the Eyes Shut," in *The Blindman's World* (Boston: Houghton Mifflin, 1898), 362.
3. Quoted in Raymond A. Gagliardi, "Who Did It First?" *American Journal of Roentgenology* 158 (February 1992): 302.
4. James Da Costa, *Modern Medicine* (Philadelphia: J. B. Lippincott, 1872), 19.
5. Stephen Kern, *The Culture of Time and Space, 1880–1918* (Cambridge: Harvard University Press, 1983).
6. Graham Farmelo, "The Discovery of X-rays," *Scientific American* (November 1995): 87.
7. E. H. Burrows, *Pioneers and Early Years: A History of British Radiology* (Alderney, Channel Islands: Colophon Limited, 1986), 10.
8. Wallace was famous for his work on the theory of evolution through natural selection. In July 1858, he and Charles Darwin jointly presented the theory to the Linnean Society in London. His opinion on scientific matters was highly valued.
9. Wilhelm Conrad Roentgen, "On a New Kind of Rays," in Otto Glasser, *Wilhelm Conrad Roentgen and the Early History of the Roentgen Rays* (Springfield, Ill.: Charles C. Thomas, 1934), 19.
10. With the growth of the mystique surrounding the Nobel Prize, and the fact that the number of prizes remains the same while the number of practicing scientists has multiplied enormously, the prize itself has become both a carrot and a curse to scientific investigators.

11. Dennis D. Patton, "Roentgen and the 'New Light': Roentgen and Lenard," *Investigative Radiology* 27, no. 6 (June 1992): 413.
12. Joel D. Howell, *Technology in the Hospital: Transforming Patient Care in the Early Twentieth Century* (Baltimore: Johns Hopkins University Press, 1995), 136.
13. Today we know that the electron is also a photon—a particle of light—and that these photons, depending on their wavelength, may be both X-rays and gamma rays.
14. Howell, *Technology in the Hospital,* 142. Howell suggests this story is a myth. He searched the New Jersey state records and found no evidence of such legislation. However, Howell points out, the fact that so many people have repeated this story for so long reflects how reasonable it seemed in the light of the mood of the time.
15. Emily Culverhouse, "Photography Up to Date—And Beyond It," in *Elizabeth Fleischmann: Pioneer X Ray Photographer,* ed. Peter E. Palmquist (Berkeley: Judah L. Magnes Museum, 1990), 31–34.
16. Ruth and Edward Brecher, *The Rays: A History of Radiology in the United States and Canada* (Baltimore: Williams and Wilkins, 1969), 19.
17. Stafford Withers, "The Story of the First Roentgen Evidence," *Radiology* 17 (1931): 99–100.
18. Edward C. Halperin, "X-Rays at the Bar, 1896–1910," *Investigative Radiology* 23, no. 7 (July 1988): 640.

Two Medical Applications

1. Arthur Fuchs, "Edison and Roentgenology," *American Journal of Roentgenology* 57, no. 2 (February 1947): 146.
2. Ibid.
3. Ibid., 150.
4. Ibid.
5. Ibid.
6. Quoted in *American Journal of Photography* (April 1896): 159–162; or see ibid.
7. Fuchs, "Edison and Roentgenology," 152.
8. "Exhibition Notes—The Edison Fluoroscope Exhibit," *The Electrical Engineer* 21, no. 422 (April 26, 1896): 600.
9. Ibid.
10. Otto Glasser, *Dr. W. C. Roentgen* (Springfield, Ill.: Charles C. Thomas, 1945), 19.
11. Bernike Pasveer, "Knowledge of Shadows: The Introduction of X-Ray Images in Medicine," *Sociology of Health and Illness* 11 (December 1989), 360–381.
12. Germ theory had already made inroads on this approach, but a formidable old guard held on, and, indeed, idiosyncrasy remains a reputable way to explain the intensity of a disease and the fact that some people "catch" infections and others don't, because of what is beginning to be known about inherited genes.
13. Peter E. Palmquist, "Elizabeth Fleischmann: A Tribute," in *Elizabeth Fleischmann: Pioneer X Ray Photographer,* ed. Peter E. Palmquist (Berkeley: Judah L. Magnes Museum, 1990), 5–10.
14. Peter E. Palmquist, "The Woman Who Takes the Best Photographs," in *Elizabeth Fleischmann: Pioneer X Ray Photographer,* 11–17.
15. Joel D. Howell, "Early Use of X-ray Machines and Electrocardiographs at the Pennsylvania Hospital," *JAMA* 225, no. 17 (May 2, 1986): 2320.
16. Adele Pillitteri, "O.R. Nursing 100 Years Ago: Nursing Care of President McKinley," *Today's O.R. Nurse* (December 1991).
17. "President's Double Tested the X-Rays," unidentified newspaper (1901) from Edison Archives.
18. Ruth and Edward Brecher, *The Rays: A History of Radiology in the United States and Canada* (Baltimore: Williams and Wilkins, 1969), 67.
19. Ibid.
20. William G. Eckert, "The History of Forensic Applications in Forensic Radiology," *The*

American Journal of Forensic Medicine and Pathology 5, no. 1 (March 1984): 53–56.
21. Terry Ramsaye, *A Million and One Nights* (New York: Simon and Schuster, 1926); and also *London Times* (May 5, 1897): 1.
22. Vincent P. Collins, "Origins of Medico-Legal and Forensic Roentgenology," in *Classic Descriptions in Diagnostic Roentgenology,* ed. Andre Johannes Bruwer (Springfield, Ill.: Charles C. Thomas, 1964), 1578–1604.
23. Albert Perée, *Études des Rayons de Röntgen Appliqués Aux Expertises Médico-Légales* (Paris: G. Steinheil, 1897), 49.
24. Collins, "Origins," 1589, 1590.
25. W. C. Borden, *The Use of the Roentgen Ray by the Medical Department of the United States Army in the War with Spain (1898),* report prepared under the direction of Surgeon General George M. Sternberg, United States Army (Washington, D.C.: Government Printing Office, 1900), 96.
26. James D. Nauman quotes Leonard in "Pioneer Descriptions in the Story of X-ray Protection," in *Classic Descriptions in Diagnostic Roentgenology,* ed. Andre Johannes Bruwer (Springfield, Ill.: Charles C. Thomas, 1964), 311–344.
27. Edison did not mount an anti-X-ray campaign, but simply found the rays personally repugnant. His relatively low profile in this matter may well have been connected to the fact that his electrical company was successfully marketing a wide variety of X-ray apparatus.
28. "Blood Dried Up by X-Rays, Victim Died," from Edison Archives (October 4, 1904).
29. Neil Baldwin, *Edison: Inventing the Century* (New York: Hyperion, 1994), 406.
30. Dr. Fred Silverman, conversation with author, Palo Alto, California, October 29, 1993. Silverman repeated the anecdote but was unsure of its origin. Whether or not it is true, it has become part of the lore of early radiology.
31. "He Has Earned Rest," *The New Orleans States* (May 8, 1928); see also "Dr. C. E. Kells, Science Martyr, Ends Life by Gun," *The Times-Picayune,* New Orleans (May 8, 1928).
32. David J. DiSantis, "Wrong Turn on Radiology's Road of Progress," *Radiographics* 11 (1991): 1121–1138.
33. *Boston Globe* (January 25, 1904).
34. "X Ray to Turn Black Men White," *New York American* (December 28, 1903).
35. This suggests that before the era of I.Q. tests and African-American sports heroes, skin color was the only determinant of race. If science could remove this "stain," racial differences could be erased. The implications of medical "remedies" as addressed toward different races is a fascinating issue, but beyond the scope of this book.
36. Quoted in Ruth and Edward Brecher, *The Rays,* 89.
37. Percy Brown, M.D., *American Martyrs to Science through the Roentgen Rays* (Springfield, Ill.: Charles C. Thomas, 1936), 11.
38. Juan A. del Regato, "Francis Henry Williams," *International Journal of Radiation Oncology, Biology and Physics* 9 (1983): 740.
39. Quoted in Brown, *American Martyrs,* 17.
40. Daniel Paul Serwer, "The Rise of Radiation Protection: Science, Medicine and Technology in Society, 1896–1935" (Ph.D. diss., Princeton University, 1977), 43.
41. Susan Quinn, *Marie Curie: A Life* (New York: Simon and Schuster, 1995), 409.
42. David Walsh, "Deep Tissue Traumatization from Roentgen Rays Exposure," *British Medical Journal* (July 31, 1897): 272; reprinted in *Health Physics* 38, no. 6 (June 1980): 885–887.

Three Technological Innovation 1897–1918

1. Roentgen himself had demonstrated that the rays did not pass through lead. As radiation-induced burns, and worse, were increasingly reported, some kind of lead insulation was seen as a reasonable protection.
2. Machlett was bought by Raytheon, and sold again until, in 1993, after more corporate acquisitions, it became part of Fisher Industries.
3. Kenneth Nazinitsky and Burton M. Gold, "Radiology—Then and Now," *American Journal of Roentgenology* 151 (August 1988): 250.

4. Joel D. Howell, *Technology in the Hospital: Transforming Patient Care in the Early Twentieth Century* (Baltimore: Johns Hopkins University Press, 1995), 104.
5. George C. Johnston, "President's Address," *American Quarterly of Roentgenology* 2 (1909): 53–55.
6. Ruth and Edward Brecher, *The Rays: A History of Radiology in the United States and Canada* (Baltimore: Williams and Wilkins, 1969), 61.
7. Ibid., 196.
8. Ibid., 197.
9. Hollis E. Potter, "Diaphragming Roentgen Rays: Studies and Experiments," in *Classic Descriptions in Diagnostic Roentgenology,* ed. Andre Johannes Bruwer (Springfield, Ill.: Charles C. Thomas, 1964), 176.
10. Doctors especially did not identify with victims of radiation burns. Kassabian regularly waved his hand in front of the fluoroscope to reassure patients "as this tends to prevent the patient becoming emotional or excited." Although he recognized this habit as the source of his own skin lesions, described in a paper in 1900 on "X-ray as an Irritant," he did not worry about the danger. Kassabian died of this "irritant" before the decade was over.
11. Stanley Joel Reiser, ed. *Medicine and the Reign of Technology* (Cambridge: Cambridge University Press, 1978), 65. Reiser refers to, in particular, the report by G. E. Pfahler, "Physiologic and Clinical Observations on the Alimentary Canal by Means of the Roentgen Rays" (*JAMA* 49, 1907).
12. Juan A. del Regato, "Antoine Béclère," *International Journal of Radiation Oncology, Biology, and Physics* 4 (1978): 1069–1079.
13. *Van Boskirk v. Pinto,* No. 18330, Supreme Court of Nebraska, December 23, 1915.
14. Sinclair Lewis, *Arrowsmith* (New York: Harcourt, Brace & World, 1924. New American Library Edition, 1961).
15. G. Coury, *La Radiologie en France* (Paris: L'Expansion Scientifique Francais, 1943), 44.
16. Marie Curie, *Life of Pierre Curie* (Paris, 1922).
17. Marie Curie, *La Radiologie et La Guerre* (Paris: Librarie Felix Alcan, 1921), 111–112.

Four Medical Politics between the Wars

1. Screening apparently healthy people for incipient diseases that are often incurable remains a major dilemma of all medicine, from mammography for breast cancer to genetic tests for susceptibility to a large number of conditions including Huntington's and Alzheimer's diseases.
2. Published in German in 1924, it was translated and published in English a year later.
3. Thomas Mann, *The Magic Mountain* (New York: Knopf, 1925), 274, 275.
4. Sinclair Lewis, *Arrowsmith* (New York: Harcourt, Brace & World, 1924; reprint, New American Library, 1961), 259.
5. *Southwestern Reporter* 228 (Arkansas, 1921): 398.
6. Ibid., 403.
7. Joel D. Howell, *Technology in the Hospital: Transforming Patient Care in the Early Twentieth Century* (Baltimore: Johns Hopkins University Press, 1995), 155.
8. James Da Costa, *Modern Medicine* (Philadelphia: J. B. Lippincott, 1872), 18.
9. Joel D. Howell, "Early Use of X-Ray Machines and Electrocardiographs at the Pennsylvania Hospital," *JAMA* 255, no. 17 (May 2, 1986): 2320–2323; Joel D. Howell, "Machines and Medicine: Technology Transforms the American Hospital," in *The American General Hospital: Communities and Social Contexts,* ed. Diana Elizabeth Long and Janet Holden (Ithaca: Cornell University Press, 1989), 109–134. I am grateful to Dr. Howell for his articles, his books, and discussions about the early use of X-rays.
10. Joel D. Howell, *Technology in the Hospital,* 130. Howell also notes that these kinds of records tended to reduce patients to organs, symptoms, and diseases.
11. Donald Parker, conversations with author, December 18, 1992; January 2, 1994.
12. Ibid.

13. Daniel Paul Serwer, "The Rise of Radiation Protection" (Ph.D. diss., Princeton University, 1977), 13. Serwer's extraordinary thorough and clear dissertation covers French, German, Austrian, and British as well as American involvement in radiation issues through 1935. I am indebted to his research.
14. Arthur Goodspeed, a distinguished physicist, had an interest in photography that brought him to collaborate with the innovative photographer Eadweard Muybridge. An early interest in X-rays led him to find medical colleagues. He was a manager of the Franklin Institute in Philadelphia and a member of the American Philosophical Society.
15. Raymond A. Gagliardi, "Radiology: A Century of Achievement," *American Journal of Roentgenology* 165 (June 27, 1995): 2.
16. The Roentgen Ray Society demanded a medical degree, two years of X-ray work, and letters of recommendation from two active members of the society (exceptions were made for those few physicists and engineers who had made special contributions). Their geographical myopia discriminated against physicians west of the Alleghenies since recommendations from active members, who were concentrated in the East, were hard to get. By 1913 the Society had shrunk to 155 members, most of whom lived in New York, Pennsylvania, Ohio, and Massachusetts.
17. Serwer, "The Rise of Radiation Protection," 202.
18. Ibid., 175.
19. Susan Quinn, *Marie Curie: A Life* (New York: Simon and Schuster, 1995), 414.
20. Gilbert F. Whittemore, "The National Committee on Radiation Protection, 1928–1960: From Professional Guidelines to Government Regulation" (Ph.D. diss., Harvard University, 1986). This dissertation, with its emphasis on law, was extremely useful for the time period covered.
21. Radium emits gamma rays, which are similar to X-rays and adjacent to them on the electromagnetic spectrum. They penetrate the body but do not leave more than a blur on film; they are an important part of nuclear medicine.
22. A. Mutscheller, "Physical Standards of Protection Against Roentgen Ray Dangers," *American Journal of Roentgenology* 13 (1925): 67.
23. See chapter 7 for definitions of rem, rad, and roentgen, and chapter 10 for quantification of dosage.
24. Donald Parker, conversation with author, December 18, 1992.
25. Betty Parker, conversation with author, December 18, 1992.
26. Harvey R. Reed, "The X-rays from a Medico-legal Standpoint," *JAMA* 30 (1897): 1017–1019.
27. Quoted from Bernike Pasveer, "Knowledge of Shadows: The Introduction of X-Ray Images in Medicine," *Sociology of Health and Illness* 11, no. 4 (December 1989): 360–381.
28. Mihran Kassabian, *Roentgen Rays and Electro-Therapeutics*, ed. Francis Packard (Philadelphia: J. B. Lippincott, 1907).
29. Preston Hickey, "The First Decade of American Roentgenology," *American Journal of Roentgenology* 20 (1928): 152–153.
30. Reed, "The X-rays from a Medico-legal Standpoint," 1017–1019.
31. *Aaron Call and Samantha Call v. City of Burley, Idaho,* 6287ID (1936).
32. L. H. Garland, "The Interpretation of X-Rays in Court Hearings," *American Journal of Medical Jurisprudence* 1 (1938): 19–21.
33. Charles Waters, Whitmer Firor, and Ira I. Kaplan, eds., *The Year Book of Radiology* (Chicago: The Year Book Medical Publishers, 1940), 252.
34. Philip Mills Jones, "X-Rays and X-Ray Diagnosis," *JAMA* 29 (1897); quoted in Stanley Joel Reiser, *Medicine and the Reign of Technology* (Cambridge: Cambridge University Press, 1978).
35. A. L. Benedict, "The Art of Diagnosis," *Medical Age* 17 (1899): 604.

Five Technological Innovation 1918–1940

1. Ruth and Edward Brecher, *The Rays: A History of Radiology in the United States and Canada* (Baltimore: Williams and Wilkins, 1969), 221.

2. James W. Bull and Herman Fischgold, "A Short History of Neuroradiology," in *Contribution à L'Histoire de la Neuroradiologie Éuropéenne,* ed. Emmanuel Cabanis (Paris: Éditions Pradel, 1989), 14.
3. Bent Ljunggren, "The Case of George Gershwin," *Neurosurgery* 10, no. 6 (1982): 733–734.
4. Justine Sergent, "Music, the Brain and Ravel," *Trends in Neurosciences* 15, no. 5 (1993): 170; Madeleine Goss, *Bolero: The Life of Maurice Ravel* (New York: Tudor Publishing, 1945).
5. Bull and Fischgold, "A Short History of Neuroradiology," 17–18.
6. Ibid., 19–20.
7. Water-soluble organic salts were developed in the 1950s, just about the time that a follow-up study of patients treated with Thorotrast revealed an enormous number of malignancies in those who had used it. (A 1968 study followed twenty-seven patients of whom seventeen died of the disease for which they were being studied. Of the ten survivors, seven had developed lesions of the spinal cord, and six of them soon died. As late as 1995 victims of Thorotrast were seeking compensation for damages in a class action suit against a major teaching hospital in Philadelphia.)
8. Described in Richard J. Bing and D. Biam, "Cardiac Catheterization," in *Cardiology: The Evolution of the Science and the Art,* ed. Richard J. Bing (Switzerland: Harwood Academic Publishers, 1992.), 1–28.
9. Bing and Baim, "Cardiac Catheterization."
10. Forssmann shared the Nobel Prize for medicine in 1956 with the Americans André Cournand and Dickerson Richards for their pioneering work in diagnostic cardiac catheterization.
11. Ronald L. Eisenberg, *Radiology: An Illustrated History* (St. Louis: Mosby Year Book, 1992), chapter 31. Interventional radiology has grown to include procedures in the gall bladder and kidneys as well as the heart and other arteries. Some procedures use CT scans and ultrasound as well as traditional fluoroscopy. The performance of these procedures by radiologists has caused turf battles within medicine as cardiologists and other specialists vie for control. (Anne Roberts, M.D., electronic communication with author, October 15, 1995.)
12. Ruth and Edward Brecher, *The Rays,* 259–263.
13. Ibid.
14. Ibid.
15. "Beauty's Bones," *Time* (July 30, 1934).
16. I am grateful to Dr. Barbara Carter at the New England Medical Center for providing me with information about Alice Ettinger and the history of the Floating Hospital.
17. Ronald Eisenberg, Radiology, 154.
18. William A. Fowler, conversations with author, September 20, 1994.
19. Ruth and Edward Brecher, *The Rays,* 343.
20. David O. Woodbury, *Battlefronts of Industry: Westinghouse in World War II* (New York: John Wiley and Sons, 1948), 202–217.

Six X-Rays in the Imagination

1. Otto Glasser, ed., *The Science of Radiology* (Springfield, Ill.: Charles C. Thomas, 1933), 8.
2. H. G. Wells, *The Invisible Man,* in *Seven Science Fiction Novels of H. G. Wells* (New York: Dover Publications, 1934), 19.
3. Tuberculosis was to the late nineteenth century what cancer is today: the most dreaded disease, which seemed to be epidemic.
4. Albert Adams Merrill, *The Great Awakening* (Boston: George Book Publishing, 1899), 294.
5. Jack London, "A Thousand Deaths," in *Future Perfect,* ed. H. Bruce Franklin (New Brunswick, N.J.: Rutgers University Press, 1995), 211–219.
6. Jack Adams, *Nequa; or, The Problem of the Ages* (Topeka: Equity Publishing, 1900), 141–142.
7. W. S. Harris, *Life in a Thousand Worlds* (Atlanta: Column Book Company, 1905), 236–237.
8. Laurence Manning, "The Man Who Awoke," in *Before the Golden Age,* ed. Isaac Asimov (New York: Doubleday, 1974), 344–371.

9. John W. Campbell, Jr., "The Brain Stealers of Mars," in *Before the Golden Age,* ed. Isaac Asimov (New York: Doubleday, 1974), 835–850.
10. This painting is at the Yale museum in New Haven, Connecticut. It features a male doctor holding the hand of a woman, the rest of whose body is hidden behind what looks like a velvet curtain.
11. Joel Howell, *Technology in the Hospital: Transforming Patient Care in the Early Twentieth Century* (Baltimore: Johns Hopkins University Press, 1995), 147.
12. Robert Schmutzler, *Art Nouveau* (New York: H. N. Abrams, 1962), 10.
13. Spencer R. Weart, *Nuclear Fear: A History of Images* (Cambridge: Harvard University Press, 1988), 37.
14. Howell, *Technology in the Hospital,* 142. See chapter 1, n. 15.
15. Gertrude Atherton, *Black Oxen* (New York: Boni and Liveright, 1923), 138–139. The book is at the Huntington Library in San Marino, California. I thank John Sutherland for pointing it out.
16. Thomas Mann, *The Magic Mountain* (New York: Knopf, 1925), 236–237.
17. Robert Butler, *They Whisper* (New York: Henry Holt, 1994), 1–2.
18. Although this activity was not spelled out, it was implicit in procedures such as the lobotomies pioneered by Egaz Moniz. They were used to eliminate the embarrassing sexual behavior, as well as most other behaviors, among mentally ill or retarded persons by turning them into functional zombies.
19. Weart, *Nuclear Fear,* 48; see also Lawrence Badash, *Radioactivity in America: Growth and Decay of a Science* (Baltimore: Johns Hopkins University Press, 1979); J. B. S. Haldane, *Possible Worlds and Other Essays* (London: Chatto and Windus, 1927); U. V. Portman, "Roentgen Therapy," in *The Science of Radiology,* ed. Otto Glasser (Springfield: Charles C. Thomas, 1933).
20. George Chauncey, *Gay New York: Gender, Urban Culture, and the Making of the Gay Male World, 1890–1940* (New York: Basic Books, 1994), 360.
21. George Henry, M.D., *Sex Variants: A Study of Homosexual Patterns* (New York: Paul B. Hober, 1941).
22. Chauncey, *Gay New York,* 360.
23. Robert Proctor, *Racial Hygiene* (Cambridge: Harvard University Press, 1988), 205–207.
24. Weart, *Nuclear Fear,* 52.
25. There was a flurry of anxiety over the illness and death of radium dial painters, who were mostly young women. The clock companies were never found culpable as the victims were deemed to have an idiosyncratic susceptibility to necrosis.
26. Maria Gallagher, review of *Dizzy Dean* and *Baseball During the Depression,* in the *New York Times Book Review* (April 5, 1992), 21.
27. The first mention of a "superman" was Alfred Jarry's *Le Sûrmale* in 1902. Robert Hughes in *The Shock of the New* (Knopf, 1981) describes this hero winning a bicycle race from Paris to Siberia against a five-seater cycle and a locomotive, but in the act becoming more mechanical than human. No longer able to love a woman, this first Superman falls in love with an electric chair that gives him satisfying jolts (page 51).
28. Dennis Dooley and Gary Engle, eds., *Superman at Fifty: The Persistence of a Legend* (Cleveland: Octavia Press, 1987), 51, 134.
29. Although double-exposure photographs are also proposed as an influence on the cubists, they do not offer a different perspective or a sense of overlapping planes.
30. The groundwork for the impact of X-rays in the art of the avant-garde was done by Linda Dalrymple Henderson in two seminal articles: "X-Rays and the Quest for the Invisible Reality in the Art of Kupka, Duchamp, and the Cubists," *Art Journal* 47 (Winter 1988): 323–340; and "Francis Picabia, Radiometers, and X-Rays in 1913," *Art Bulletin* 71, no. 1 (March 1989): 114–123. Her examples, interpretation, and extensive bibliography were invaluable to me in this area.
31. Quoted in Henderson, "X-Rays and the Quest," 328.
32. Ibid., 323–340. Again in *Sonata,* another canvas Duchamp painted in 1911, the nose is a darkened triangle.

33. Linda Dalrymple Henderson, introduction to *Fourfield: Computers, Art and the 4th Dimension,* ed. Tony Robbin (Boston: Bulfinch Press, 1992), 18.
34. Henderson, "Francis Picabia, Radiometers, and X-Rays in 1913," 114–123.
35. Quoted in Robert Hughes, *The Shock of the New* (New York: Knopf, 1981), 51.
36. Christian Brinton, "Evolution Not Revolution in Art," *International Studio* 69, no. 194 (April 1913): 35.
37. Quoted in Marianne V. Martin, *Futurist Art and Theory, 1909–1915* (Oxford: Clarendon Press, 1968), 53–54.
38. Douglas Cooper, *The Cubist Epoch* (New York: Metropolitan Museum of Art and Phaidon Press, 1970), 158.
39. John E. Bowlt, "The Presence of Absence: The Aesthetic of Transparency in Russian Modernism," *The Structurist* 27, no. 8 (1987–1988): 15–22. I am indebted to this article as well as to the excellent translations Dr. Bowlt has made of the Russian avant-garde publications.
40. Pavel Florensky, "The Analysis of Perspective," quoted in Bowlt, "The Presence of Absence," 15–22.
41. John Willet, *Art and Politics in the Weimar Period* (New York: Pantheon, 1978), 23.
42. Naum Gabo and Anton Pevsner, *The Realist Manifesto,* in *Russian Art of the Avant-Garde: Theory and Criticism, 1902–1934,* ed. John E. Bowlt (New York: Viking Press, 1976), 208–215.
43. Bowlt, "The Presence of Absence," 21.
44. Both ideas and quotation from Bowlt, "The Presence of Absence," 15–22.
45. *Bauhaus,* German Exhibition, Pasadena, Calif.: Pasadena Art Museum (April 1970).
46. Davis Lomas, "Body Languages: Kahlo and Medical Imagery," in *The Body Imaged,* ed. Kathleen Adler and Marcia Pointon (Cambridge: Cambridge University Press, 1993), 5–19.
47. Jean-Claude Lemagny and Andre Rouille, eds., *A History of Photography: Social and Cultural Perspectives* (Cambridge: Cambridge University Press, 1986), 71.
48. Man Ray is the name adopted by this American Jew who grew up in New York and emigrated permanently, with the exception of the World War II years, to Paris. He was extremely successful as a fashion photographer but is remembered more for his experimental films and still images.
49. Dawn Ades, *Photomontage* (New York: Pantheon Books, 1976), 7.
50. Dawn Ades, *Photomontage,* rev. ed. (London: Thames and Hudson, 1986), 20.
51. Dain L. Tasker, "X-Raying Flowers," *Camera World* 54 (1938); Janet Tearnen, "The Photography of Will Connell: Reflections of Southern California, 1928–1950," Dept. of History, University of California, Riverside (1992), photocopy.
52. John Hersey, *Hiroshima* (New York: Knopf, 1946).

Seven The Story of CT Scanning

1. John Pekkanen, "The President," *The Washingtonian* (August 1981), 109–117; and Herbert Abrams, *"The President Has Been Shot"* (New York: W. W. Norton, 1992).
2. "Report, NIH Consensus Conference on Computed Tomography; November 6, 1981," quoted in the *American College of Radiology Bulletin* (December 1981).
3. David Davis, telephone interview with author, February 23, 1995.
4. An application devised by the nineteenth-century French mathematician Jean Baptiste Joseph Fourier to an infinite series whose terms are constants multiplied by sine and cosine functions that can, under the right conditions, approximate a wide variety of functions. *American Heritage Dictionary of the English Language,* Third Edition, 1992.
5. Ronald Bracewell, conversation with author, Palo Alto, California, November 3, 1993.
6. Ronald Bracewell, conversation with author in Palo Alto, California, October 29, 1993. See also Steve Webb, *From the Watching of Shadows: The Origins of Radiological Tomography* (Bristol, England: Adam Hilger, 1990). This is an extremely useful, highly technical book that emphasizes British contributions. It is absolutely necessary to anyone interested in the scientific origins of these technologies. And see also Stuart R. Blume, *Insight and Industry: On the Dynamics of Technological Change*

in Medicine (Cambridge: MIT Press, 1992).

7. At the Medical Research Council laboratory in Cambridge, England, in 1967, Aaron Klug, who would win the Nobel Prize in chemistry in 1983 for his work with the structure of viruses, was working with a graduate student, David DeRosier, exploring these incredibly small life forms. DeRosier and Klug also used Fourier transforms. Five years later, another of Klug's students, Peter Gilbert, worked out the specific structure of the tobacco mosaic virus protein—the first virus ever identified—and produced a model map for all viral research. Like Bracewell, whose work he references, Gilbert found a mathematical approach that was more efficient than Fourier transforms.
8. At UCLA Oldendorf joined the IEEE with Benedict Cassen, who was in the process of inventing the scintiscanner, an instrument crucial to the development of PET and discussed in chapter 9.
9. Unpublished memoir by Mrs. Stella Oldendorf, 1995. She goes on to explain:

   In the actual experiment, separating the information contributed by the internal nail from that contributed by the external ring of nails was possible because they contributed different frequency components to the signal output of the gamma ray detectors which measure the number of gamma rays deleted from the beam by absorption. The central nail, which absorbed gamma rays continuously, contributed a constant component to the signal. The external nails, which absorbed gamma rays transiently, contributed a fluctuating absorption at least twice the frequency of the rate of rotation of the gamma ray source, because each nail in the outer ring passed through the right twice during one rotation of the gamma ray source. . . . As the gamma source "circled" the model continuously, the gamma ray beam isolates one point in space at the center of rotation. . . . A more complete image of the interior of the object could be built up by moving this "flying spot" through the interior of the object. In Bill's experiment, this point was moved along a line connecting the location of these nails in the interior of the model. The experiment successfully showed that the location of these nails could be determined, and that their relative radiodensity (one was aluminum, one steel) could be measured.
10. Robert Beck, telephone conversation with author, spring 1993.
11. William H. Oldendorf, *The Quest for an Image of the Brain* (New York: Raven Press, 1980), 85.
12. Ibid., 85–86.
13. Alan Cormack, interview with author in Medford, Massachusetts, March 16, 1993.
14. What response there was came from William Sweet, a neurosurgeon who thought he saw a use for Cormack's methodology in treating certain conditions of the pituitary gland. Cormack was still thinking in terms of radiotherapy, as he had seen it done in Capetown. He conceived of CT as a way to limit the patient's exposure to radiation by hitting a target with a focused beam.
15. The letter was from Claude Jaccard. Author's personal communication with Alan Cormack.
16. David E. Kuhl, telephone interview with author, spring 1993.
17. There is some evidence that a decade earlier, in 1957 in the Soviet Union, Tetel'Baum and Korenblyum report that a scanner had been built in Kiev for medical imaging. There are drawings but no photographs to support this claim, and the authors' names vanish from the scientific literature at this time of purges and disappearances. Assuming a scanner was built, it seems to have led to a dead end. The right place is as important as the right time.
18. This is the Kenneth Burke rule, and was pointed out to me by Robert Merton. See David L. Sills and Robert K. Merton, eds., *International Encyclopedia of the Social Sciences*, vol. 19, "Social Science Quotations" (New York: Macmillan Publishing Company, 1991).
19. Quoted in David E. Kuhl, "Concerning the Role of David E. Kuhl, M.D., in the Evolution of Tomographic Imaging of Ionizing Radiation" (April 27, 1989).
20. A thorough discussion of the role of credit and prestige in science can be found in Sills and Merton, eds., *International Encyclopedia of the Social Sciences*, vol. 19, "Social Science Quotations."
21. Charles Suskind, "The Invention of Computed Tomography," in *History of Technology* 6, ed. A. Rupert Hall and Norman Smitz (Mansell Publishing, 1981); also Sir Godfrey Hounsfield, telephone conversation with author in London, England, May 20, 1994.

22. Sir Godfrey Hounsfield, telephone conversation with author in London, England, May 20, 1994.
23. Suskind, "The Invention of Computed Tomography," 47.
24. Personal conversation with Hounsfield in London, May 20, 1994.
25. David Davis, telephone conversation with author, February 23, 1995.
26. James Ambrose, "Computed Transverse Axial Scanning (Tomography) Pt. 2: Clinical Application," *British Journal of Radiology* 46 (1973): 1023.
27. Oddly enough, Kuhl says that he and his colleagues at the University of Michigan Medical School are now examining the numbers instead of the scans in a search for information. (Author's personal communication with Kuhl, January 1995.)
28. Robert Levis, M.D., telephone conversation with the author, May 1995.
29. Robert Stanley, conversation with author, November 15, 1995; J.K.T. Lee, S. S. Sagel, and R. J. Stanley, *Computed Body Tomography with MRI Correlation,* 1983.
30. Robert Ledley, interview with author in Washington, D.C., November 18, 1993.
31. This patent was eventually overturned, and Pfizer got out of the imaging business. It learned that medical machines needed constant updating as compared to pharmaceuticals, which once developed remained on the market unchanged.
32. Jay Stein and David Ellenbogen, conversation with author in Waltham, Massachusetts, June 16, 1994.
33. The scanner was not available in April 1972, but Shepp became involved because of his son's problem. The tumor turned out to be unremovable, but benign. Cobalt radiation treatments shrunk it and it never grew or caused a problem again. (Author's personal communication with Lawrence Shepp, August 18, 1994.)
34. Yost Michelsen was the neurosurgeon and Sadek Hilal the neuroradiologist at Columbia.
35. Personal communication with Larry Shepp, April and May 1994.
36. With algorithms that bumped the AS&E scanner into a higher level of image production, they added a filter function. AS&E eventually made the Shepp-Stein algorithm available to the industry in 1974, and some version of it produces the images now emblematic of standard fourth-generation CT.
37. Alan Cormack, interview with author, March 16, 1993.
38. *Federal Policies and the Medical Devices Industry,* Report of the Office of Technology Assessment, Congress of the United States, Washington, D.C. (New York: Pergamon Press, 1984), 194.
39. Interview with Rolf Shild, former member of the board of EMI, London, May 19, 1994.
40. Sir Godfrey Hounsfield, telephone conversation with author in London, May 20, 1994.
41. Interventional radiology is more than angioplasty or other vascular interventions. It is already used to deliver chemotherapeutic agents, drain fluids from blocked kidneys and livers, and open up Fallopian tubes to increase fertility.
42. Jordana Bieze, "CT Takes Roundabout Path to Faster Scanning," *Diagnostic Imaging* (November 1993).
43. Roger M. Lindahl, "Spiral Gives CTR Boost in Race Against MRI," *Diagnostic Imaging* (November, 1993).
44. The initial entry of the federal government into the funding of medicine was with the Hill-Burton Act in 1946, which in some way involved almost every hospital in the United States.
45. However, with Medicare, which was introduced at this time, hospitals were reimbursed the same amount, wherever their scans were made.
46. Stewart Wolf and Bedrock Bishop Belle, eds., *The Technological Imperative in Medicine* (New York: Plenum Press, 1981).
47. CT scans focus many highly collimated beams of X-rays on a single plane in the body. The best way to understand the radiation dosage from a typical scan is in relationship to dosages in other kinds of X-ray images.

    Dosage units have varied with increasing knowledge about radiation. The *roentgen* (R), the unit agreed upon in 1928, was based on the amount of ionization produced in the air. The problem with the roentgen was that it did not measure the amount of radiation absorbed by the human body. Thus it was necessary to introduce a new unit in the 1930s, the *rad,* which is defined in terms of the energy *absorbed* by a gram of tissue from a given beam of radiation. Following countless experiments, it was discovered that X-rays at higher voltages have a greater biological effect in some tissues than X-rays at lower voltages, so a new concept, "relative biological effectiveness" (RBE), was introduced. Then a new unit for comparing radiation effects emerged, called the *rem,* which is defined as the dose in rads multiplied by the RBE for humans. (From Ruth and Edward Brecher, *The Rays,* 356–357.)

The quantities of radiation are now given in international units called *sieverts* (sv), where 1 sv = 100 rem and 1 millisievert (mSv) = 100 mrem.

Examination	Dose in mSv
Skull	0.22
Chest	0.08
Upper GI series	2.44
Barium enema	4.06
Pelvis	0.44
Hip	0.83
Extremities	0.01
CT (head or body)	1.11

The GI and barium enema are fluoroscopic examinations.

From *Radiation Protection for Medical and Allied Health Personnel.* Recommendation of the National Council on Radiation Protection and Measurements (Bethesda, Md.: National Council on Radiation Protection and Measurements, 1989), 4–12.

48. Ronald Bracewell, conversation with author in Palo Alto, California, November 3, 1993.
49. Larry Shepp, conservation with author, August 18, 1994.
50. George Sarton, "The Discovery of X-rays," *Isis* 26 (1936): 362.
51. As quoted in Rolf L. Schapiro, "Opinions of an Editor," *Journal of Computed Axial Tomography* 1, no. 1 (1977): 3.
52. Harry Schwartz, "Cost Cuts Never Get a Nobel," *New York Times* (October 12, 1979): A31.
53. Lincoln Caplan, *The Insanity Defense and the Trial of John W. Hinckley, Jr.* (Boston: David R. Godine Publishers: 1984), 80.
54. Robert L. Jackson, "Witness Minimizes Brain Abnormality of Hinckley," *Los Angeles Times* (June 4, 1982).
55. *Swanson v. the United States of America,* Civ.No. 82–1029, U.S. District Court, D.Idaho, February 14, 1983.
56. Fredric Tusk, "Suit Alleges Psychic Lost Career," *Philadelphia Inquirer* (March 25, 1986): B1.
57. "Psychic's $986,000 Award Voided; Blamed X-Ray for Loss of Powers," *Los Angeles Times* (August 9, 1986).
58. Emanuel Kanal, telephone conversation with author, March 1994.
59. CT images appear in black and white except when used to illustrated advertisements or magazine stories. The colors are arbitrary, usually enhanced to exaggerate whatever the viewer is supposed to see.

Eight Magnetic Resonance Imaging

1. Today MR is the term used clinically to describe the procedure, and MRI to describe the picture obtained by the machine. The general public, however, persists in referring to both procedure and product as MRI, which is the term used most often in this book. The redundant "MRI image" is avoided whenever possible.
2. The medical evidence was made available to me by Milton Grimes, the attorney who represented King in the civil case and who arranged for much of the medical imaging.
3. This refers to a 1923 ruling in Washington, D.C., where James Alphonzo Frye, who had been convicted of murder, filed an appeal in order to submit evidence from a new scientific

instrument—a lie detector. The judge denied Frye's request, stating that expert opinions must be "deduced from a well-recognized scientific principle or discovery . . . sufficiently established to have gained general acceptance in the particular field to which it belongs." As recently as 1994 MRI had to pass the Frye test each time it was used in California, and prove its relevance to the particular question under consideration.

4. After immigrating to the United States in the 1930s, Pauli worked on the problem of atomic fission, for which he was awarded the Nobel Prize in 1945.
5. Paul Lauterbur, interview with author in Urbana, Illinois, December 2, 1992.
6. Ibid.
7. Ibid.
8. Ibid.
9. Paul Lauterbur, "Image Formation by Induced Local Interactions: Examples Employing Nuclear Magnetic Resonance," *Nature* 242 (1973): 190–1.
10. Ernst had collaborated in 1966 with Weston Anderson on developing pulse Fourier transforms that improved the speed in NMR spectroscopy by several orders of magnitude. Nine years later in Zurich, he introduced two-dimensional NMR, which was among his contributions to chemistry that earned him a Nobel Prize in 1991.
11. Sir Peter Mansfield, interview with author in Nottingham, England, May 18, 1994.
12. Ibid.
13. Ibid.
14. Ibid.
15. Ibid., and Leon Kaufman, interview with author in South San Francisco, September 11, 1992.
16. Alex Margulis, conversation with author, October 3, 1994.
17. Kaufman, interview with author.
18. Ian Young, "Industrial Responses to Academic Research in Imaging Technology," 1992 International Conference, San Francisco.
19. Leon Kaufman, interview with author.
20. Robert K. Merton, "Priorities in Scientific Discovery: A Chapter in the Sociology of Science," *American Sociological Review* 22, n. 6 (December 1957).
21. Alex Margulis, conversation with author.
22. David Kramer, interview with author in South San Francisco, September 15, 1992.
23. "Nuclear Magnetic Resonance (NMR): Medical Diagnostic Device that Produces Pictures Based on Response of Atomic Nuclei in Magnetic Field Is Expected to Perform Significantly Better and More Safely than CAT Scanners," *New York Times* (November 28, 1982): A1.
24. Paul Lauterbur, interview with author.
25. Leon Kaufman, interview with author.
26. This is a common complaint, yet MRI makes no claims to extending longevity. Its major contribution is toward early diagnosis and a better quality of life. This, of course, is much harder to measure.
27. As Damadian redesigned his machine, replacing the superconducting magnet with a permanent magnet, most of the other manufacturers began switching to higher power superconducting magnets.
28. Robert D. Boutin, Jonathan E. Briggs, and Michael R. Williamson, "Injuries Associated with MR Imaging: Survey of Safety Records and Methods Used to Screen Patients for Metallic Foreign Bodies before Imaging." *American Journal of Roentgenology* 162 (January 1994).
29. Leon Kaufman, interview with author.
30. Emanuel Kanal and Frank G. Shellock, "Safety Considerations in MR Imaging," *Radiology* 176 (1990): 593–606.
31. Emanuel Kanal and Frank G. Shellock, "MR Imaging of Patients with Intracranial Aneurysm Clips," *Radiology* 187 (1993): 612–614; also Frank G. Shellock, conversation with author in Los Angeles, February 25, 1993.
32. The GE system, which is in use at Boston's Brigham and Women's Hospital, works as an adjunct to therapy and is called MRT (Magnetic Resonance Therapy). In conjunction with CT, ultrasound, PET, SPECT, and angiography, it is used for diagnosis and as part of

surgical procedures. See F. A. Jolesz, "MRI-Guided Interventions," *The Coolidge Scientific Review* 2 (November 1994).

33. Interventional radiologists are now participating in neurosurgical procedures in open MRI machines.
34. John D. Roberts, interview with author in Pasadena, California, September 18, 1992; also see William Bradley and David Stark, "MRI Hemorrhage in the Brain," in *Magnetic Resonance Imaging* (St. Louis: The C. V. Mosby Co., 1988), 371–374.
35. Joseph Kirschvink, interview with author in Pasadena, California, February 19, 1993; also Joseph L. Kirschvink, et al., "Magnetite Biomineralization in the Human Brain," *Proceeding of the National Academy of Science* 89 (August 1992): 7683–7687.
36. CTs are relatively benign, except when applied to the head. There is a risk of damaging the eyes because they are especially vulnerable and close to many target areas in the brain.
37. Child abuse is a new concept. When early in the nineteenth century, Mr. Sadler, a member of Britain's Parliament, demanded that the House of Commons do something to protect child factory workers from being beaten (he displayed a special kind of whip) to keep them awake at the job, Parliament did nothing. It was only decades later, after animal protection laws were passed, that children's advocates approached the Society for the Prevention of Cruelty to Animals for help. They reasoned that human children are also animals and so won the animal care community's support in helping to reform child labor laws.
38. John Caffey, "The Parent-Infant Traumatic Stress Syndrome," *American Journal of Roentgenology* 114, no. 2 (February 19, 1972): 219.
39. John Caffey, "On the Theory and Practice of Shaking Infants," *Journal of Diseases of Children* 124, no. 2 (August 1972): 161–169.
40. William Bradley, conversation, January 5, 1993.
41. Louis J. Rosner and Shelley Ross, *Multiple Sclerosis* (New York: Simon and Schuster, 1992).
42. Seiji Ogawa, et al., "Functional Mapping by Blood-Oxygenation Level-Dependent Contrast Magnetic Resonance Imaging," *Biophysical Journal* 64 (March 1993): 803–812.
43. John Allman, conversation with author in Pasadena, California, March 1995.
44. Roland Krels, et al., "Proton MRS in Children Resuscitated After Near-Drowning: A Possible Prognostic Indicator?" *Review of Magnetic Resonance in Medicine Book of Abstracts* 1 (1992): 237.
45. S. Eleff, N. G. Kennaway, et al., "^{31}P NMR Study of Improvement in Oxidative Phosphorylation by Vitamins K_3 and C in a Patient with a Defect in Electron Transport at Complex III in Skeletal Muscle," *Proceedings of the National Academy of Sciences* 81 (June 1984): 3529–3533.
46. The team was led by Pratik Ghosh, and the paper, "Pure Phase-Encoded MRI and Classification of Solids," *IEEE Trans. Medical Imaging* 14, no. 3 (September 1995), is also credited to David H. Laidlaw, Kurt W. Fleischer, Alan H. Barr, and Russell E. Jacobs.
47. Ibid. The approach of the Ghosh team employs new algorithms for classifying volume data that avoids artifacts. It promises to be an elegant method for in vivo tests and may, one day, be applicable to body imaging.
48. Terry Trucco, "Eliot Feld's Middle Name? Inventive," *New York Times,* Arts and Entertainment Section (February 13, 1994): 28
49. Clive Barnes, "Ballet Meets the Big Top at the Joyce," *New York Post,* Post Plus Section (February 26, 1994): 25.
50. Anna Kisselgoff, "An Athletic New Feld Work," *New York Times* (February 25, 1994).
51. Janice Berman, "Feld Makes Images of 'MRI' Resonate," *New York Newsday* (February 25, 1994).

Nine PET in Nuclear Medicine

1. Samuel Glasstone, *Sourcebook on Atomic Energy* (Toronto: Van Nostrand, 1992), 666. Hevesy loved this story and repeated it often, changing the main course from a soufflé to goulash to hash. The point remained the same.

2. Peter Crane, "The Nuclear Stockpile America Needs," *New York Times,* April 5, 1996, A17. Crane argues that Poland's distribution of potassium iodide has shown, a decade after Chernobyl, that it has saved the Polish population from the epidemic of childhood thyroid cancers that marks the rest of the area affected by the same amount of fallout: Ukraine, western Russia, and Belarus.
3. Daniel J. Kevles, *The Physicists* (New York: Knopf, 1977).
4. Lawrence, John H. "Early Experiences in Nuclear Medicine." *Northwest Medicine* 55(1956): 527–533; rpt. in *The Journal of Nuclear Medicine* 20, n. 6 (June 1979): 561–564. Lawrence administered the first man-made radioactive treatment to a leukemic patient on Christmas Eve of 1936. Lawrence also described how in 1935 no one had any idea how much exposure to the cyclotron was dangerous, so they borrowed a rat and rigged up a small chamber where they exposed the rat for three minutes. When they retrieved the rat, it was dead. Everyone crowded around and had a great respect for the new radiation. A few days later they found that the rat had died of suffocation, not radiation, but they did not advertise the fact, "since a healthy fear was instilled which served to save the early workers from damage, especially radiation cataracts."
5. Marshall Brucer, "Nuclear Medicine Begins with a Boa Constrictor," *Heritage of Nuclear Medicine* (1979): 20.
6. Ibid.
7. But the PET signal changes constantly as the isotope loses its radioactivity, requiring the development of kinetic mathematical models that have to be tailored to each case.
8. Joseph Dumit, "Desiring a Beautiful Image of the Brain: A Cultural-Semiotics of Functional Imaging" (University of California, Santa Cruz, photocopy, 1994).
9. James G. Kereiakes, "The History and Development of Medical Physics Instrumentation: Nuclear Medicine," *Medical Physics* 14, no. 1 (January/February 1987): 146–155.
10. The "miracle" tubes were made from high-density, transparent crystals that absorb gamma rays, or photons, and vastly increase their intensity in a flash called a scintillation. The tube itself requires a lot of electricity which enables one light photon to become a cascade of light photons, intense enough to be detected. This way a minuscule amount of light is turned into an electrical signal, which can then be counted.
11. This is the radioimmunoassay process (RIA), which identifies minute quantities of radiolabeled antibodies. It was developed by Rosalyn Yalow to explore the pathology of tissue using radio-tagged insulin, measuring its retention in the bodies of diabetics, and for which she received the Nobel Prize in physiology or medicine in 1977.
12. Kuhl worked with Roy Edwards, who was the head of the engineering shop in the Department of Radiology at Penn until Edwards's death in 1975.
13. David E. Kuhl, "Concerning the Role of David E. Kuhl, M.D., in the Evolution of Tomographic Imaging of Ionizing Radiation" (unpublished, April 1989).
14. Other researchers developed SPECT at the Massachusetts General Hospital in Boston, at Washington University in St. Louis, and at the Donner Laboratory at the University of California at Berkeley.
15. Niels Lassen, "On the History of Measurement of Cerebral Blood Flow in Man by Radioactive Isotopes," in *New Trends in Nuclear Neurology and Psychiatry,* ed. D. C. Costa, C. F. Morgan, and N. Lassen (London: John Libbey & Co., 1993), 3–13.
16. SPECT most commonly uses iodine molecules, which have a half-life of thirteen hours, and go to the thyroid, or technetium-99m, which concentrates in the brain, heart, blood, lungs, liver, kidneys, thyroid, spleen, and bone, making it an almost universal tracer.
17. This resolution is adequate for many diagnostic needs. A 1994 study found no statistical difference in the sensitivity of SPECT and PET, at least when it concerned lesions that were larger than 1.6 centimeters and had also been found with CT and MRI.
18. Steve Webb, *From the Watching of Shadows* (Bristol: Adam Hilger, 1990).
19. This was carried out at Johns Hopkins in 1983 when Henry Wagner and Michael Kuhar manufactured a carbon molecule that binds preferentially to dopamine-2, a neuroreceptor in the base of the brain. A patient with Parkinson's has a declining level of dopamine that can be monitored.

20. H. Schelbert and R. J. Bing, "Isotopes in Cardiology," in *Cardiology: The Evolution of the Science and the Art,* ed. Richard J. Bing (Switzerland: Harwood Academic, 1992): 181–199.
21. Godfrey N. Hounsfield, "Computerized Transverse Axial Scanning (Tomography), Part I: Description of System," *British Journal of Radiology* 46 (1973): 1016–1022.
22. Peter S. Conti, "Introduction to Imaging Brain Tumor Metabolism with Positron Emission Tomography (PET)," *Cancer Investigation* 13, n. 2 (1995): 244–259.
23. Peter S. Conti, "Neuro-oncology," *Cancer Investigation* 13, n. 2 (1995): 244-259. This excellent account explains uses of PET in cancer and as a method for distinguishing lesions caused by cancer from lesions caused by infection in the brains of people with AIDS.
24. Henry N. Wagner and Peter S. Conti, "Advances in Medical Imaging for Cancer Diagnosis and Treatment," *Cancer* 67 (February 15, 1991, Supplement): 1126. Presented at the American Cancer Society National Conference on Advances in Cancer Imaging, New York, January 24-26, 1990.
25. Ibid., 1121–1128.
26. Joseph Dumit, "A Digital Image of the Category of the Person: PET Scanning and the Objective of Self-Fashioning" (Department of Cyborg Anthropology, School of American Research, October 1993, photocopy).
27. Ibid.
28. Nora D. Volkow and Laurence Tancredi, "Neural Substrates of Violent Behavior: A Preliminary Study with Positron Emission Tomography," *British Journal of Psychiatry* 151 (1987): 668–673.
29. John C. Mazziotta, "The Use of Positron Emission Technology (PET) in Medical-Legal Cases: The Position Against Its Use," for a 1992 course at UCLA directed by Vladimir Hachinsky, M.D., "Controversies in Neurology." Photocopy.
30. Dumit, "A Digital Image."
31. Electrocortography is a process of mapping the brain by removing the skull and attaching electrodes to the exposed tissue to take an EEG. This enables the neurologist to pinpoint exactly which cells are not functioning. This kind of map is very useful in deciding if and where to perform surgery. It is, however, a delicate procedure with a morbidity rate that makes the nonintrusive PET a preferable option.
32. Sandra Blakeslee, "Radical Surgery, the Earlier the Better, Offers Epileptics Hope," *New York Times,* Medical Sciences section (September 29, 1992): B6.
33. Harry T. Chugani, *Human Behavior and the Developing Brain,* ed. Geraldine Dawson and Kurt W. Fischer (New York: Guilford, 1994), chapter 5.
34. This has been identified as a problem with the neurotransmitter dopamine receptors that lie deep inside the *substantia nigra* in the basal ganglia. The reduction in number of these cells produces those clinical symptoms first described in 1817. From Greenfield's *Neuropathology,* fourth edition, ed. J. Hume Adams, J.A.N. Corsellis, and L. W. Dunchen (New York: John Wiley, 1987), 701–702.
35. Edwin W. Salzman, "Living with Parkinson's Disease," *New England Journal of Medicine* 334, no. 2 (January 1, 1996): 114–116.
36. June Kinoshita, "Mapping the Mind," *New York Times Magazine* (October 18, 1992): 44–54.
37. All of the information from Peter Conti, Jennifer S. Keppler, and James M. Hall, "Positron Emission Tomography: A Financial and Operational Analysis," *American Journal of Roentgenology* 162 (June 1994): 1279–1286.
38. Diane Gershon, "Is there a future for clinical PET?" *Nature Medicine* 1, no. 8, 1995.
39. "MRI Powerful But Complicated Machine to Detect Disease in Patients," RSNA news release (May 28, 1985).
40. Jack Clifford, Jr., et al., "Sensory Motor Cortex: Correlation of Presurgical Mapping with Functional MR Imaging and Invasive Cortical Mapping," *Radiology* 190 (November 1994): 85–92.
41. Conti et al., "Positron Emission Tomography."
42. One such new candidate is magnetic encephalography (MEG), which images the magnetic waves from the brain with an instrument that at the moment resembles an antique permanent-wave machine.

43. Anon., conversation with author at the University of Southern California Hospital in Los Angeles, April 1993.
44. Antonio Damasio, *Descartes' Error: Emotion, Reason, and the Human Brain* (New York: G. P. Putnam's Sons, 1994). This discussion of the intricate connection between the brain and the mind depends in large part on the results of research using PET.
45. There was an effort to remove all cyclotrons from the University of California campuses in the mid-1980s and early 1990s on the grounds that they could be used to manufacture nuclear weapons grade fuel. Their clinical usefulness was never made an explicit issue.

Ten Ultrasound and Mammography

1. Roger Cobban Sanders, "The Story of Cecil Jacobson" (unpublished paper).
2. The habit of photographing dead or dying fetuses continued. Lennart Nilsson's famous photographs of developing life, published in the April 1965 issue of *Life* magazine were, in fact, films of dying organisms.
3. Diagram from J. Hess, "The Diagnosis of the Age of the Fetus by Use of Roentgenograms," *American Journal of Diseases of Children* (1917): 399; reprinted in Ann Oakley, *The Captured Womb: A History of the Medical Care of Pregnant Women* (Oxford: Basil Blackwell, 1984), 99.
4. Spencer R. Weart, *Nuclear Fear: A History of Images* (Cambridge: Harvard University Press, 1988).
5. Alice Stewart, "Malignant Disease in Childhood and Diagnostic Irradiation in Utero," *Lancet* (September 1, 1956). Stewart remains an activist in the area of radiation diseases and in 1992 published data about the reduced life expectancies of people at the Hanford nuclear reservation in the state of Washington.
6. Barry B. Goldberg and Barbara A. Kimmelman, *Medical Diagnostic Ultrasound: A Retrospective on Its 40th Anniversary* (Eastman Kodak, 1988).
7. Elizabeth Kelly-Fry initiated a computer-based ultrasound program to detect breast cancer. Eventually she and her colleagues would explore the acoustic characteristics of malignant masses with the same fast Fourier transforms that were being used by the other imaging technologies.
8. Ellen B. Koch, "The Process of Innovation in Medical Technology: American Research on Ultrasound, 1947–1962" (Ph.D. diss., University of Pennsylvania, 1990).
9. B-mode scanning then depicted echoes returning from underlying tissues in a single plane—a cross-section of the plane of the body. This approach enabled the scanner to obtain information in depth and heralded the modern era of ultrasound. See Goldberg and Kimmelman, *Medical Diagnostic Ultrasound.*
10. Ellen B. Koch, "In the Image of Science? Negotiating the Development of Diagnostic Ultrasound in the Cultures of Radiology and Surgery" (unpublished paper).
11. Ibid., 24.
12. Wild was helped between 1953 and 1957 by John Reid, a young man with a fresh B.S. degree in engineering, who helped him build the B-mold echoscope. Reid left to continue his education and eventually worked on Doppler ultrasound.
13. Koch, "The Process of Innovation," 38.
14. Koch, "In the Image of Science?" 24. This use of "noise" is similar to Paul Lauterbur's attitude toward the NMR signal (see chapter 8).
15. This decision to exploit "noise" or "interference" is similar to Lauterbur's decision to organize the "noise" in early NMR by separating it into gradients. The pattern of deciding to eliminate unessential or confusing signals, or to try to make use of them, has been repeated, with different outcomes, in the evolution of imaging technologies.
16. Goldberg and Kimmelman, *Medical Diagnostic Ultrasound;* also Koch, "The Process of Innovation."
17. Annemarie Mol, "What Is New? Doppler and Its Others: An Empirical Philosophy of Innovations," in *Medicine and Change: Historical and Sociological Studies of Medical Innovation,* ed. Ilana Lowy (London: John Libbey Eurotext, 1992), 109.

18. Donald pointed out, in an address to the American Association of Obstetricians and Gynecologists in September 1968, that before their profession put ultrasound on the map, ob-gyns were in the forefront of the use of chloroform anesthesia, which opened the door to abdominal surgery.
19. Horace Thompson and Kenneth Gottesfeld at the University of Colorado Medical Center.
20. Ian Donald, "On Launching a New Diagnostic Science," *American Journal of Obstetrics and Gynecology* 103, no. 5 (1969).
21. This explains why President McKinley's aides asked a gynecologist to try to remove the bullet. They were the only surgeons then familiar with the abdominal area.
22. Donald, "On Launching a New Diagnostic Science."
23. George Leopold, "Seeing with Sound," *Radiology* 175 (April 1990): 23–27.
24. Kirk Beach, "1975–2000: A Quarter of a Century of Ultrasound Technology," *Ultrasound in Medicine and Biology* 18, no. 4 (1992): 377–388.
25. Stuart S. Blume, *Insight and Industry on the Dynamics of Technology Change in Medicine* (Cambridge: MIT Press, 1992), 107.
26. This was, and continues to be, a very controversial article. Stewart analyzed a third of the cases of 1,500 children in Britain who died of leukemia or malignant diseases between 1952 and 1955. Questionnaires included information about consanguinity, diet, and home background, and the cases were measured against a set of controls. She concludes, "So large a total difference . . . can hardly be fortuitous. . . . It could, however, be explained if children who are X-rayed before they are born are more prone to develop leukemia and other malignant diseases than children who have not been X-rayed in utero." She supports this conclusion by pointing out that radiation is more dangerous when the whole body is affected, and that it had already been known that therapeutic radiation to pregnant women is liable to cause microcephaly. Alice Stewart, "Malignant Disease in Childhood and Diagnostic Irradiation in Utero," *Lancet* (September 1, 1956): 447.

    Since then studies of major exposure to humans in utero from Hiroshima and Nagasaki have not demonstrated an increased incidence of leukemia or other cancers, which does not bear out Stewart's predictions. The other major category of studies comprises children whose mothers received pelvimetries during the third trimester. Some of the criticisms of Stewart's study are: the higher incidence of death in the X-rayed fetal sample may have been connected to the fact that other illnesses caused the mothers to be X-rayed, and the fact that the unexposed siblings of the children who received X-rays in utero had twice the probability of developing cancer as the control group. "The retrospective analysis by Stewart has not demonstrated a causal relationship, but rather an association between the frequency of X-rays and childhood malignancies." Fred A. Mettler, Jr., and Robert D. Moseley, Jr., *Medical Effects of Ionizing Radiation* (Orlando, Fla.: Grune & Stratton, 1985).
27. Oakley, *The Captured Womb,* 86.
28. Ibid., 159.
29. Barbara Duden, *Disembodying Women: Perspectives on Pregnancy and the Unborn* (Cambridge: Harvard University Press, 1991), 12–15.
30. Warren E. Leary, "Waste Is Found in the Use of Prenatal Ultrasound," *New York Times* (September 16, 1993): A16.
31. Heidi Evans, "When Should Pregnant Women Get a Sonogram?" *Wall Street Journal* (June 20, 1995) and "Womb with a View: Unborn Babies Star in Fetal Film Fest," *Wall Street Journal* (November 30, 1993).
32. Evans, "When Should Pregnant Women Get a Sonogram?"
33. *Planned Parenthood v. Casey,* 112 Supreme Court 2791 (1992).
34. This was the argument used against aborting the fetuses of the Muslim women raped in Bosnia, almost all of whom abandoned their babies upon delivery. The anticipated "bonding" never happened, and the babies were warehoused, adopted if possible, or died from neglect.
35. Salomon was discharged from the University of Berlin in 1933 and sent to a concentration camp; he fled to Holland in 1939, where he survived underground during World War II and continued as a leader in Dutch medicine during the postwar years.

36. Lawrence Bassett, Richard H. Gold, and Carolyn Kimme-Smith, "History of the Technical Development of Mammography" (RSNA Categorical Course in Physics, 1993), 10.
37. This was done under the leadership of Philip Strax, Louis Venet, and Sam Shapiro. Strax went on to develop and operate a self-contained mobile breast cancer screening unit. Richard Gold, Lawrence Bassett, and Bobbi Widoff, "Highlights from the History of Mammography," *Radiographics* 10, no. 6 (1990): 1111–1131.
38. Gros emphasized this, while H. Stephen Gallager and John E. Martin in Houston followed with studies identifying early lesions and introduced the concept of "minimal breast cancer," which they defined as highly curable when caught in time, and recognizable by citing "new density" in serial mammograms. They published their results in 1968.
39. The ACR had just responded to congressional legislation requiring help for coal miners with black lung disease who were newly eligible for benefits by teaching radiologists how to recognize black lung disease with X-rays. The ACR recognized that their members could also benefit from offering mammograms, and filled the role of quality controllers there, too.
40. Susan M. Love, *Dr. Susan Love's Breast Book* (Reading, Mass.: Addison-Wesley Publishing, 1991).
41. Ruth and Edward Brecher, *The Rays: A History of Radiology in the United States and Canada* (Baltimore: Williams and Wilkins, 1969), 415.
42. The "tolerance" dose gave way to the "safe" dose, and the prewar limit of 0.1 r per day for people in occupations that exposed them to radiation was cut to 0.3 r per week, and then to 5 r per year. In 1987 general public exposure was set at 0.1 r annually for those subjected frequently to radiation, and 0.5 r for infrequent exposure. By this time it was recognized that the effects of radiation are cumulative but not even on every organ of the body. They noted especially, however, the effect of radiation on genes; new X-ray machines have further reduced the amount of radiation for diagnostic imaging to a small fraction of the dosages of the 1930s and 1960s. The latest guidelines deem the least exposure as best.
43. Love, *Dr. Susan Love's Breast Book,* 163.
44. Otha Linton, American College of Radiology, telephone conversation with author, May 1995.
45. John J. Goldman, "Mrs. Rockefeller's Breast Is Removed in Cancer Surgery," *Los Angeles Times* (October 18, 1974): 1.
46. Otha Linton, draft document for the ACR.
47. In 1992 the FDA issued regulations to implement the Mammography Standards Act, which requires federal certification and an inspection program for mammography facilities. This followed the 1985 NEXT (Nationwide Evaluation of X-ray Trends) publication that found poor quality and no correlation between fees charged and the quality of machines and readings.
48. Carolyn Kimme-Smith, "New and Future Developments in Screening-Film Mammography Equipment and Techniques," *Radiological Clinics of North America* 30, n. 1 (January 1992): 55–66.
49. Gerald Dodd and Richard Gold report in "The History of Mammography" (in the Radiology Centennial volume, 1996) that a dose rate for screen-film systems varies between 100 and 300 millirads per image, a quantity with "negligible carcinogenic potential."
50. Dodd and Gold, "The History of Mammography," in the Radiology Centennial volume (1996).
51. Harold Kundel, a radiologist at the University of Pennsylvania, and his colleague Calvin Nodine. Letter to the editor from Calvin F. Nodine, *New York Times* (January 16, 1992). Computers that spot cancers on mammograms are already available. They are like a second opinion, although they err on the side of too many false positives. They also have a placebo effect, in that radiologists who know they are being second-guessed by computers tend to make fewer errors. *New York Times,* April 2, 1995.
52. Eliot Marshall, "Search for a Killer: Focus Shifts from Fat to Hormone," *Science* 259 (January 25, 1993): 618–621.
53. General practitioners and gynecologists were skeptical about the efficacy of the Papanicolaou smear, a way of detecting early cancer in a normal-appearing cervix with a laboratory cell test. Gerald Dodd and Richard Gold, in "The History of Mammography" they

have written for the Radiology Centennial volume published in 1996 by the American College of Radiology, point out that surgeons and oncologists were equally doubtful that an imaging technique could detect cancer in a clinically normal breast.

54. Eliot Marshall, "The Politics of Breast Cancer," *Science* 259 (January 29, 1993): 616–618.
55. Jane Brody, *New York Times,* May 3, 1995. This column refers to articles in *Cancer,* Gina Maranto's "Should Women in Their 40s Have Mammograms?" *Scientific American* (September 1996): 113, and especially to a report by Dr. Belinda N. Curpen in the *American Journal of Radiology.*

Eleven The Transparent Body

1. By this, as throughout the book, I am referring to life-size, rather than microscopic, images of the body's interior.
2. In Thomas Mann's 1924 novel, *The Magic Mountain,* discussed in chapter 6.
3. Spencer R. Weart, *Nuclear Fear: A History of Images* (Cambridge: Harvard University Press, 1988).
4. Ira Glasser, letter to the editor, *New York Times* (January 24, 1993).
5. The disputes have been settled out of court in the past, but the problem, according to Otha Linton at the American College of Radiology, has more or less been tabled, and with digitalization may become entirely moot. In the interim, he recalls that with the tendency of radiology departments in large, overcrowded hospitals to lose X-rays, young interns and residents took to hiding them from the radiologists under the patients' beds. That way, when they needed them, they always knew where to look. Most doctors run out of filing space, Linton recalls, and he suggests that most radiologists are happy to give patients their pictures, just to save space.
6. "Craft Appeal," *Metropolitan Home* (January/February 1994): 64–65.
7. Richard B. Gunderman and Mark Siegler, "One Hundred Years of Roentgen Rays: Radiology and the Changing Image of Man" (Department of Radiology, University of Chicago, photocopy), 13.
8. Don DeLillo, *White Noise* (New York: Viking, 1985), 141–142.
9. Gunderman and Siegler, "One Hundred Years of Roentgen Rays," 17.
10. Ibid.
11. Kay Redfield Jamison, *An Unquiet Mind: A Memoir of Moods and Madness* (New York: Knopf, 1995), 194.
12. Anne James, letter to author, June 17, 1993.
13. Quoted in Sir Lawrence Gowing, "La Position Dans La Representation: Réflexions sur Bacon et la Figuration du Passé et du Futur," *Cahiers du Musée National d'Art Moderne,* Paris, no. 19–22 (September 1987): 80, quoting from David Sylvester, *The Brutality of Fact: Interviews with Francis Bacon* (Thames and Hudson, 1956).
14. Gowing, "La Position Dans La Representation": 79–102.
15. Ibid.
16. The radiologist who carried out the request warned him to take care of himself as the experience would provide the artist with a decade full of radiation.
17. Rauschenberg printed *Autobiography* on three stones and ran it off on a billboard press (the first fine art print so treated) with a run of two thousand prints.
18. Of course, artists such as Lucien Freud and Picasso never stopped painting the body, but they made no reference to imaging technologies.
19. In a talk presented to Betty Friedan's think tank at the University of Southern California, March 1992. Weisberg was herself influenced by Mary D. Garrard's "Artemisia Gentilischi's Self-Portrait as the Allegory of Painting" (*Art Bulletin* 1977). Garrard spots Vasare in the sixteenth century as the first artist to use systematically female personifications of the arts. She goes on to show how the mannerist painters created a formula using female bodies to represent male minds, and then traces Gentilischi's role in reinterpreting this concept for a woman artist.
20. Tori Ellison, letter to author, March 11, 1995.

21. Alan Burroughs, *Art Criticism from a Laboratory* (Boston: Little Brown, 1938).
22. Agnes Denes, interview with author at her studio in New York, April 1994.
23. Agnes Denes, *Introspection III—Aesthetics* (1971-72).
24. Another approach to making X-rays from classic paintings was done in 1984 by the German artist Sigmar Polke. Polke noticed on a postcard of Goya's 1812 painting, *The Old Woman,* that something seemed to have been erased and painted over in the top left-hand corner. Using an X-ray, he discovered the ghostly image of an earlier image of the Resurrection, and blended the earlier effort in his own X-ray/photographic interpretation. Polke's photographs, like Denes's, render the invisible visible.
25. Sheila Pinkel, conversations with author, March 10 and 12, 1995.
26. David Teplica, telephone conversation with author, February 1995.
27. James R. Hugunin, "Archaeology in Eden: Eden in Extremis?" (unpublished paper).
28. Parker Tyler, *The Divine Comedy of Pavel Tchelitchew* (New York: Fleet Publishing, 1967), 131.
29. Alex Grey, *Sacred Mirrors: The Visionary Art of Alex Grey* (Rochester, Vermont: Inner Traditions International, 1990), 35; conversation with the artist, August 1995.
30. Joelle Bentley, "Photographing the Miracle of Life: The Work of Lennart Nilsson," *Technology Review* 95, n. 8 (November/December, 1992): 60.
31. Carol Stabile, "Shooting the Mother: Fetal Photography and the Politics of Disappearance," *Camera Obscura* 28 (January 1992): 179–205.
32. "The Andy Warhol Museum," inaugural publication of The Andy Warhol Museum, Carnegie Institute, Pittsburgh, 1994; and author's personal communication with Claudia Defendi, curator, Andy Warhol Foundation for the Visual Arts, Inc.
33. Kynaston McShine, *Andy Warhol: A Retrospective* (New York: The Museum of Modern Art, 1989), 343.
34. Quoted from the statement of purpose of the exhibition as set forth in a proposal written by Tina Potter and Christa Helm and sent to the author.
35. Personal communication with the author, as well as two catalogues: "Steve Miller Origine du Monde: A Retrospective, 1984–1994," Espace Art Brenne, 1994; "Le Revenu Français," A/B Galeries, Paris, 1993.
36. M. Theresa Southgate, "The Cover," *JAMA* 268, no. 9 (September 2, 1992).
37. "Artist's Works Mirror Moments in Medicine," *Clinical News Center,* New Orleans: Tulane University (January 1994).
38. May H. Lesser, *The Art of Medicine at the 21st Century* (National Institutes of Health: National Library of Medicine, January-March 1994).
39. Joyce Cutler Shaw, *"The Anatomy Lesson,"* from *Framework* 6, no. 2 (1993).
40. Joyce Cutler Shaw, *"The Anatomy Lesson"* (Panel Presentation for the Artist in Technoculture, College Art Association Conference, Seattle, February 1993).
41. Emily Hartzell, *Nina Sobell: The Years in Los Angeles 1971–1985,* from a television documentary.
42. Sobell has been artist in residence at NYU's Center for Advanced Technology in Digital Media since 1994 where, with Professors Richard Wallace and Naoko Tanese, she has pioneered the use of telerobotics for interactive performance over the Web. She uses the LabCam (a robotcamera developed for use on the World Wide Web by physicians for remote diagnosis) as an artist. The Media Research Laboratory is part of the Courant Computer Science Department Media Research Laboratory at New York University and is supported by the Center for Advanced Technology as well as the lab itself.

Epilogue

1. Tim Radford, "Basic Science Seen as 'Key,'" *Guardian Weekly,* September 24, 1995, 11.
2. Medicine Meets Virtual Reality conference, San Diego, California, January 20, 1994.
3. It may come to pass that bullets will be dated like milk cartons so that their place and year of manufacture will be decodeable from the inside out.
4. In the United States, teleradiology is located at university hospitals, such as UCLA's, and

through private groups such as Teleradiology Associates in Durham, North Carolina. This group has avoided jurisdictional problems by having its radiologists licensed in all the states with which it contracts. The ACR has established a set of standards, and new telecommunications technology permits high-speed transmission of images. Much of this information was supplied by David A. Forsberg in Durham and by Rachel Orr, "Long-Distance Radiology Is Saving Service," *Vineyard Gazette,* August 27, 1993.

5. PET scans combined with fused CT and MR images allow stereotaxic surgery in which individual cells are oblated in the treatment of Parkinson's disease.
6. It has been suggested by the radiologist Herbert Abrams in *"The President Has Been Shot"* that all presidential candidates routinely undergo brain scanning so the public is protected from a mentally impaired leader.
7. Interview with Leon Kaufman, UCSF, September 1992.
8. This research from the Mayo Clinic, dubbed "magnetic resonance elastrography," was described at the 1995 meetings of the RSNA.

Bibliography

History, Culture, and Society

Abbott, Francis C. "Surgery in the Greco-Turkish War." In *Classic Descriptions of Diagnostic Roentgenology,* ed. Andre Johannes Bruwer, 1325–1331. Springfield, Ill.: Charles C. Thomas, 1964.
Abrams, Herbert L. *"The President Has Been Shot."* New York: W. W. Norton, 1992.
———. "Introduction and Historical Notes." In *Angiography,* ed. Herbert Abrams, 3–13. Boston: Little Brown, 1983.
Adler, Kathleen, and Marcia Pointon, eds. *The Body Imaged.* New York: Cambridge University Press, 1993.
Ades, Dawn. *Photomontage.* London: Thames and Hudson, 1976.
Agnew, Harold M. "Early Recollections of the Manhattan Project—Day of Criticality." *The Journal of Nuclear Medicine* 22, no. 1 (January 1981).
Almond, Peter R. "The X-ray Centennial—Thomsons and Thomsons." *Medical Physics* 20, no. 2 (March/April 1993).
"The Andy Warhol Museum." Inaugural publication, The Andy Warhol Museum, Carnegie Institute, 1994.
Badash, Lawrence. "Radium, Radioactivity, and the Popularity of Scientific Discovery." *Proceedings of the American Philosophical Society* 122, no. 3 (June 1978).
Baldwin, Neil. *Edison: Inventing the Century.* New York: Hyperion, 1994.
Bassett, Lawrence, Richard H. Gold, and Carolyn Kimme-Smith. "History of the Technical Development of Mammography." RSNA Catagorical Course in Physics, 1993.
Bauhaus. German Exhibition. Pasadena, Calif.: Pasadena Art Museum, April 1970.
Beach, Kirk. "1975–2000: A Quarter of a Century of Ultrasound Technology." *Ultrasound in Medicine and Biology* 18, no. 4 (1992).
Béclère, Antoine. "A Physiologic Study of Physics in Fluoroscopic Examinations." In *Classic Descriptions in Diagnostic Roentgenology,* ed. Andre Johannes Bruwer. Springfield, Ill.: Charles C. Thomas, 1964.
Béclère, Antoinette. *Antoine Béclère.* Paris: J. B. Baillière, 1972.

Benedict, A. L., "The Art of Diagnosis." *Medical Age* 17 (1899).

Bentley, Joelle. "Photographing the Miracle of Life: The Work of Lennart Nilsson." *Technology Review* 95, no. 8 (November/December 1992).

Billeter, Erika, and José Pierre, eds. *La Femme et La Surréalisme.* Lausanne, Switzerland: Musée Cantonal des Beaux-Arts Lausanne, 1987.

Bing, Richard, ed. *Cardiology: The Evolution of the Science and the Art.* Switzerland: Harwood Academic Publishers, 1992.

Bishop, Joseph Bucklin. *Theodore Roosevelt and His Time.* New York: Charles Scribner's Sons, 1920.

Bleich, Alan Ralph. *The Story of X-Rays from Roentgen to Isotopes.* New York: Dover Publications, 1960.

Bloomer, Carolyn M. *Principles of Visual Perception.* New York: Van Nostrand Reinhold, 1976.

Blume, Stuart S. *Insight and Industry: On the Dynamics of Technological Change in Medicine.* Cambridge, Mass.: MIT Press, 1992.

Borden, W. C. *The Use of the Roentgen Ray by the Medical Department of the United States Army in the War with Spain (1898).* Prepared under the direction of Surgeon General George M. Sternberg. Washington, D. C.: Government Printing Office, 1900.

Bowlt, John E. "The Presence of Absence: The Aesthetic of Transparency in Russian Modernism." *The Structuralist* 27/28 (1987–1988).

———. *The Silver Age: Russian Art of the Early Twentieth Century and the "World of Art" Group.* Newtonville, Mass.: Oriental Research Partners, 1982.

———. ed. *Russian Art of the Avant-Garde: Theory and Criticism, 1902–1934.* New York: Viking Press, 1976.

Braun, Marta. *Picturing Time: The Work of Étienne-Jules Marey.* Chicago: University of Chicago Press, 1992.

Brecher, Ruth, and Edward Brecher. *The Rays: A History of Radiology in the United States and Canada.* Baltimore: Williams and Wilkins, 1969.

Brinton, Christian. "Evolution Not Revolution in Art." *The International Studio* 54, no. 194 (April 1913).

Brown, E. Richard. *Rockefeller Medicine Men: Medicine and Capitalism in America.* Berkeley: University of California Press, 1960.

Brown, Lawrason. *The Story of Clinical Pulmonary Tuberculosis.* Baltimore: Williams and Wilkins, 1941.

Brown, Percy. *American Martyrs to Science through the Roentgen Rays.* Springfield, Ill.: Charles C. Thomas, 1936.

Brucer, Marshall. "Nuclear Medicine Begins with a Boa Constrictor." In *The Heritage of Nuclear Medicine.* New York: Society of Nuclear Medicine, 1979.

Bruwer, Andre Johannes, ed. *Classical Descriptions of Diagnostic Radiology.* Springfield, Ill.: Charles C. Thomas, 1964.

Bull, James W., and Herman Fischgold. "A Short History of Neuroradiology." In *Contribution a l'Histoire de la Neuroradiologie Européenne,* ed. Emmanuel Cabanis. Paris: Editions Pradel, 1989.

Burger, G. "Blood Tests among Workers in X-Ray Factories." In *X-Ray Research and Development.* Eindhoven: N. V. Philip's Gloeilampenfabrieken, 1939.

Burroughs, Alan. *Art Criticism from a Laboratory.* Boston: Little Brown, 1938.

Burrows, E. H. *Pioneers and Early Years: A History of British Radiology.* Alderney, Channel Islands: Colophon Limited, 1986.

Cabanis, Emmanuel A., ed. *Contribution a L'Histoire de la Neuroradiologie Européenne.* Paris: Editions Pradel, 1989.

Camfield, William A. *Francis Picabia: His Art, Life and Times.* Princeton: Princeton University Press, 1979.

Cartwright, Lisa. "Women, X-rays, and the Public Culture of the Prophylactic Imaging." *Camera Obscura* 29 (May 1992).

Caton, Joseph Harris. *The Utopian Vision of Moholy-Nagy.* Ann Arbor, Mich.: UMI Research Press, 1980.

Caulfield, Catherine. *Multiple Exposures: Chronicles of the Radiation Age.* New York: Harper & Row, 1989.

Chamberlain, Edward. "Radiology as a Medical Specialty." *JAMA* 92, no. 13 (March 1929).

Chauncy, George. *Gay New York: Gender, Culture, and the Making of the Gay Male World, 1890–1940.* New York: Basic Books, 1994.

Chew, Felix S. "*AJR:* The 50 Most Frequently Cited Papers in the Past 50 Years." *American Journal of Roentgenology* 150 (February 1989).

Clapesattle, Helen. *Doctors Mayo.* Garden City, N.Y.: Garden City Publishing, 1943.

Coke, Van Deren. *The Painter and the Photograph from Delacroix to Warhol.* Albuquerque: University of New Mexico Press, 1964.

Coleman, William, and Frederic L. Holmes, eds. *The Investigative Enterprise.* Berkeley: University of California Press, 1988.

Collinas, Graham P. "Nobel Chemistry Prize Recognizes the Importance of Ernst's NMR Work." *Physics Today* 44 (December 1991).

Collins, Vincent P. "Origins of Medico-Legal and Forensic Roentgenology." In *Classic Descriptions of Diagnostic Roentgenology,* ed. Andre Johannes Bruwer. Springfield,Ill.: Charles C. Thomas, 1964.

Cooper, Douglas. *The Cubist Epoch.* New York: Metropolitan Museum of Art and Phaidon Press, 1970.

Cormack, Alan M. "Computed Tomography: Some History and Recent Developments." *Proceedings of Symposia in Applied Mathematics* 27 (1982).

———. "Reminisences to Steve Webb." 1992. Photocopy.

Coury, G. *La Radiologie en France.* Paris: L'Epansion Scientifique Francais, 1943.

Crary, Jonathan. *On Vision and Modernity in the Nineteenth Century.* Cambridge, Mass.: MIT Press, 1990.

Culverhouse, Emily. "Photography Up to Date—And Beyond It." In *Elizabeth Fleischmann: Pioneer X Ray Photographer,* ed. Peter E. Palmquist. Berkeley, Calif.: Judah L. Magnes Museum, 1990.

Curie, Irène, and F. Joliot. "Artificial Production of a New Kind of Element." *Nature* (February 10, 1934).

Curie, Marie. *La Radiologie et La Guerre.* Paris: Librarie Felix Alcan, 1921.

———. *Pierre Curie.* Paris, 1922; New York: Macmillan, 1923.

Da Costa, J. M. *Modern Medicine.* Philadelphia: J. B. Lippincott, 1872.

Dall'ava-Santucci, Josette. *Des Sorcières Aux Mandarines: Histoires des Femmes Médecins.* France: Callmann-Levy, 1989.

Damasio, Antonio. *Descarte's Error: Emotion, Reason, and the Human Brain.* New York: G. P. Putnam's Sons, 1994.

Darius, John. *Beyond Vision.* Oxford: Oxford University Press, 1984.

Daston, Lorraine, and Peter Galison. "The Image of Objectivity." *Representations* 40 (fall 1992).

Davis, Audrey B. *Medicine and Its Technology: An Introduction to the History of Medical Instrumentation.* Westport, Conn.: Greenwood Press, 1981.

Del Regato, Juan A. "Antoine Béclère." *International Journal of Radiation Oncology, Biology, and Physics* 4 (1978).

———. "Francis Henry Williams." *International Journal of Radiation Oncology, Biology, and Physics* 9 (1983).

———. "The Unfolding of Therapeutic Radiology." *JAMA* 262, no. 14 (October 1989).

Dervan, Peter B. "John D. Roberts." *Aldrichimca Acta* 21, no. 3 (1988).

Desjardins, Arthur. "The Status of Radiology in America." *JAMA* 92, no. 13, (March 1929).

Di Chiro, Giovanni, and Rodney A. Brooks. "The 1979 Nobel Prize in Medicine." *Science* 206, no. 30 (November 1979).

Dibner, Bern. *The New Rays of Professor Roentgen.* Norwalk, Conn.: Burndy Library, 1963.

DiSantis, David J. "Early American Radiology: The Pioneer Years." *American Journal of Roentgenology* 147 (October 1986).

DiSantis, David J., and Denise M. DiSantis. "Wrong Turns on Radiology's Road of Progress." *RadioGraphics* 11 (1991).
Dodd, Gerald D., and Richard H. Gold. "The History of Mammography." In Radiology Centennial Volume, American College of Radiology, 1996.
Donald, Ian. "On Launching a New Diagnostic Science." *American Journal of Obstetrics and Gynecology* 193, no. 5 (1969).
Donaldson, S. W. "Roentgenogram as Evidence." *American Journal of Medical Jurisprudence* 1, no. 4 (December 1938).
Dooley, Dennis, and Gary Engle, eds. *Superman at Fifty: The Persistence of a Legend.* Cleveland: Octavia Press, 1987.
Doub, Howard P. "The Radiological Society of North America." *Radiology* 83 (November 1964).
Dreyfuss, Jack R. "Tufts and New England Radiology." *Tufts Medical Alumni Bulletin* 28, no. 1 (March 1969).
Duden, Barbara. *Disembodying Women: Perspectives on Pregnancy and the Unborn.* Cambridge, Mass.: Harvard University Press, 1993.
———. *The Woman Beneath the Skin.* Cambridge, Mass.: Harvard University Press, 1991.
Dumit, Joseph. "Desiring a Beautiful Image of the Brain: A Cultural-Semiotic of Functional Imaging." University of California, Santa Cruz, 1994. Photocopy.
———. "A Digital Image of the Category of the Person: PET Scanning and Objective Self-Fashioning." Department of Cyborg Anthropology, School of American Research, October 1993. Photocopy.
Eckert, William G. "The History of the Forensic Applications in Radiology." *The American Journal of Forensic Medicine* 5, no. 1 (1984).
Eisenberg, Ronald L. *Radiology: An Illustrated History.* St. Louis: Mosby Year Book, 1992.
Evens, Ronald G. "The History of the Mallinckrodt Institute of Radiology." *American Journal of Roentgenology* 160 (1993).
"Exhibition Notes—The Edison Fluoroscope Exhibit." *The Electrical Engineer* 21, no. 422 (April 26, 1896).
Fabricant, Noah. *Thirteen Famous Patients.* Philadelphia: Chilton Company Publishers, 1960.
Farmelo, Graham. "The Discovery of X-rays," *Scientific American* (November 1995).
Feinstein, Roni. *Robert Rauschenberg: The Silkscreen Paintings, 1962–64.* New York: Whitney Museum of American Art, 1990.
Fletcher, Estelle. "A Review of 'Imaging Techniques in Reproductive Medicine.'" *Camera Obscura* 29 (May 1992).
Freidel, Robert, and Paul Israel. *Edison's Electric Light.* New Brunswick, N.J.: Rutgers University Press, 1986.
Fuchs, Arthur W. "Edison and Roentgenology." *American Journal of Roentgenology* 57, no. 2 (February 1947).
The Fundamentals of Radiography, 5th ed. New York: Medical Division, Eastman Kodak Company, 1942.
Gabo, Naum. *Of Divers Art.* Princeton: Princeton University Press, 1962.
Gagliardi, Raymond. "Clarence Dally: All American Pioneer." *American Journal of Roentgenology* 157 (November 1991).
———. "Radiology: A Century of Achievement." *American Journal of Roentgenology* 165 (September 1995).
———. "Who Did It First?" *American Journal of Roentgenology* 158 (February 1992).
Galison, Peter, and Bruce Hevly. *Big Science: The Growth of Large-Scale Research.* Stanford: Stanford University Press, 1992.
Gallagher, Catherine, and Thomas Laquer, eds. *The Making of the Modern Body.* Berkeley: University of California Press, 1987.
Gardiner, J. H. "The Origins, History and Development of the X-ray Tube." In *Classic Descriptions in Diagnostic Roentgenology,* ed. Andre Johannes Bruwer. Springfield, Ill.: Charles C. Thomas, 1964.

Garrels, Gary. *Photography in Contemporary German Art: 1960 to the Present.* Minneapolis: Walker Art Center, 1992.

Gilchrist, T. C. "A Case of Dermatitis Due to the X-Rays." *Bulletin of the Johns Hopkins Hospital* 8, no. 71 (February 1897).

Glasser, Otto. *Dr. W. C. Roentgen.* Springfield, Ill.: Charles C. Thomas, 1945.

———. *Wilhelm Conrad Roentgen and the Early History of the Roentgen Rays.* Springfield, Ill.: Charles C. Thomas, 1934.

Glasser, Otto, ed. *The Science of Radiology.* Springfield, Ill: Charles C. Thomas, 1933.

Glasstone, Samuel. *The Sourcebook on Atomic Energy,* 3rd ed. Princeton: D. Van Nostrand, 1967.

Goldberg, Barry, and Barbara Kimmelman. *Medical Diagnostic Ultrasound: A Retrospective on Its 40th Anniversary.* Eastman Kodak, 1988.

Goodstein, Judith R. *Millikan's School.* New York: W. W. Norton, 1991.

Goss, Madeleine. *Bolero: The Life of Maurice Ravel.* New York: Henry Holt, 1940.

Gowing, Lawrence. "La Position Dans La Représentation: Réflexions sur Bacon et la Figuration du Passé et du Futur." *Cahiers du Musée National d'Art Moderne,* no. 19–22, Paris (September 1987).

Grey, Alex. *Sacred Mirrors: The Visonary Art of Alex Grey.* Rochester, Vermont: Inner Traditions International, 1990.

Grigg, E. R. N. *The Trail of the Invisible Light.* Springfield, Ill.: Charles C. Thomas, 1965.

Gunderman, Richard B., and Mark Siegler, "One Hundred Years of Roentgen Rays: Radiology and the Changing Image of Man." Department of Radiology, University of Chicago. Photocopy.

Gutiérrez, C. "The Birth and Growth of Neuroradiology in the USA." In *Contribution a L'Histoire de la Neuroradiologie Européenne,* ed. Emmanuel A. Cabanis. Paris: Editions Pradel, 1989.

Gwinn, John L. *Western Radiology Then and Now.* California Radiological Society, 1980.

Hacker, Barton C. *The Dragon's Tail.* Berkeley: University of California Press, 1987.

Hagland, William D., and Corinne L. Fligner. "Confirmation of Human Identification Using Computerized Tomography (CT)." *Journal of Forensic Sciences* 38, no. 3 (May 1993).

Hall, Stephen S. *Mapping the Next Millennium.* New York: Random House, 1992.

Halperin, Edward C. "X-rays and the Bar, 1896–1910." *Investigative Radiology* 23 (August 1988).

Harder, Dietrich. "Roentgen's Discovery: How and Why It Happened." *British Journal of Radiology* 59 (1986).

Hartouni, Valerie. "Fetal Exposures: Abortion Politics and the Optics of Allusion." *Camera Obscura* 29 (May 1992).

Hartz, Jill, ed. *Agnes Denes.* Ithaca, New York: Herbert F. Johnson Museum of Art, Cornell University, 1992.

Heilbron, J. L., and Robert W. Seidel. *Lawrence and His Laboratory: A History of the Lawrence Berkeley Laboratory,* vol. 1. Berkeley: University of California Press, 1989.

Helman, Cecil. *The Body of Frankenstein's Monster.* New York: W. W. Norton, 1991.

Henderson, Linda Dalrymple. "Francis Picabia, Radiometers and X-Rays in 1913." *Art Bulletin* 71, no. 1 (March 1989).

———. Introduction to Tony Robbin, *Fourfield: Computers, Art and the 4th Dimension.* Boston: Bullfinch Press, 1992.

———. "X-Rays and the Quest for Invisible Reality in the Art of Kupka, Duchamp, and the Cubists." *Art Journal* 47 (winter 1988).

Henry, George. *Sex Variants: A Study of Homosexual Patterns.* New York: Paul B. Hober, 1941.

Herrera, Hayden. *Frida: A Biography of Frida Kahlo.* New York: Harper and Row, 1983.

Hersey, John. *Hiroshima.* New York: Knopf, 1946.

Herzog, Alfred W. *Medical Jurisprudence.* Indianapolis: Bobbs-Merrill Company Publishers, 1931.

Hevesy, George. "A Scientific Career." *Perspectives in Biology and Medicine* 1, no. 4 (summer 1958).
Hickey, Preston. "The First Decade of American Roentgenology," *American Journal of Roentgenology* 20 (1928).
Hollis, Donald P. *Abusing Cancer Science.* Chehalis, Wash.: The Strawberry Fields Press, 1987.
Howell, Joel. "Early Perceptions of the Electrocardiogram: From Arrhythmia to Infraction." *Bulletin of History of Medicine* 58 (1984).
———. "Early Use of X-ray Machines and Electro-Cardiographs at the Pennsylvania Hospital." *JAMA* 255, no. 17 (May 1986).
———. "Machines and Medicine: Technology Transforms the American Hospital." In *The American General Hospital: Communities and Social Context,* ed. Diana Elizabeth Long and Janet Golden. Ithaca, New York: Cornell University Press, 1989.
———. "Regional Variation on 1917 Health Care Expenditures." *Medical Care* 27, no. 8 (August 1989).
———. *Technology in the Hospital.* Baltimore: Johns Hopkins University Press, 1995.
———, ed. *Technology and American Medical Practice, 1880–1930.* New York: Garland Publishing, 1988.
Hughes, Robert. *The Shock of the New.* New York: Knopf, 1981.
Hughes, Thomas P. *American Genesis: A Century of Invention and Technological Enthusiasm, 1870–1970.* New York: The Viking Press, 1989.
"The Importance of X-ray in the Diagnosis and Treatment of Cancer." *Cancer News* (June 1947).
Isherwood, Ian. "The Golden Age: A Shifting Spectrum." *British Journal of Radiology* 59, no. 703 (1986).
Jablonski, Edward. *Gershwin Remembered.* Portland, Ore.: Amadeus Press, 1992.
Jamison, Kay Redfield. *An Unquiet Mind: A Memoir of Moods and Madness.* New York: Knopf, 1995.
Jarre, Hans. "Roentgen Cinematography." In *The Science of Radiology,* ed. Otto Glasser. Springfield, Ill.: Charles C. Thomas, 1933.
Jelavich, Peter. *Berlin Cabaret.* Cambridge, Mass.: Harvard University Press, 1993.
Johnston, George C. "President's Address," *American Quarterly of Roentgenology* 2 (1909).
Kahmen, Volker. *Art History of Photography.* New York: The Viking Press, 1973.
Karshan, Donald. *Archipenko: Sculpture, Drawings and Prints, 1908–1963.* Danville, Ky.: Centre College, Bloomington, Ind., Indiana University Press, 1985.
Kassabian, Mihran Krikor. *Roentgen Rays and Electro-Therapeutics.* Philadelphia: J. B. Lippincott Company, 1907.
Kaufman, Leon. "Taking a Close Look at MRI on Its 10th Anniversary." *Diagnostic Imaging* (December 1987).
Keats, Theodore. "Origins of Stereoscopy in Diagnostic Roentgenology." In *Classic Descriptions in Diagnostic Roentgenology,* ed. Andre Johannes Bruwer. Springfield, Ill.: Charles C. Thomas, 1964.
Kelvin, Patricia. "Alice Ettinger, M.D. 'The Complete Radiologist.' " *Tufts Health Science Review* (fall 1970).
Kennedy, Charles. "Louis Sokoloff at Three Score and Ten." *Journal of Cerebral Blood Flow and Metabolism* 11 (1991).
Kereiakes, James. "The History and Development of Medical Physics Instrumentation: Nuclear Medicine." *Medical Physics* 14, no. 1 (January/February 1987).
Kern, Stephen. *The Culture of Time and Space: 1880–1918.* Cambridge, Mass.: Harvard University Press, 1983.
Kevles, Daniel J. *The Physicists: The History of a Scientific Community in Modern America.* Cambridge, Mass.: Harvard University Press, 1985.
Kieffer, Jean. "The Laminograph and Its Variations." *American Journal of Roentgenology* 39, no. 4 (April 1938).
Kirk, Edward C., ed. *The American Text-Book of Operative Dentistry.* Philadelphia: Lea & Febiger, 1911.
Kleinfield, Sonny. *A Machine Called Indomitable.* New York: Times Books, 1985.

Knight, Nancy. "How Radiography Aids Forensic Medicine." *Radiography* 50, no. 589 (January 1984).

———. " 'The New Light': X Rays and Medical Futurism." In *Imaging Tomorrow: History, Technology, and the American Future,* ed. Joseph J. Corn, 10–34. Cambridge, Mass.: MIT Press, 1986.

———. " 'The Soothing Beam': Early Anesthetic Applications of the X-Ray." Presented at the American Association of the History of Medicine annual meeting, May 1983.

Koch, Ellen B. "In the Image of Science? Negotiating the Development of Diagnostic Ultrasound in the Cultures of Radiology and Surgery." Photocopy.

———. "The Process of Innovation in Medical Technology: American Research on Ultrasound, 1947–1962." Ph.D. diss., University of Pennsylvania, 1990.

Kraft, Ernest. "W. C. Roentgen: His Friendship with Zehnder." *New York State Journal of Medicine* (April 1973).

Kuhl, David. "Concerning the Role of David E. Kuhl, M.D. in the Evolution of Tomographic Imaging of Ionizing Radiation." University of Michigan, April 27, 1989. Photocopy.

Lassen, Niels. "On the History of Measurement of Cerebral Blood Flow in Man by Radioactive Isotopes." In *New Trends in Nuclear Neurology and Psychiatry,* ed. D. C. Costa, C. F. Morgan, and N. Lassen. London: John Libbey & Company, 1993.

Lauterbur, Paul C. "NMR in Medicine: A Brief Historical and Prospectus." Paper presented at the 4th Annual Conference in Integrated Body Imaging, Tokyo, Japan, August 7–8, 1981.

Lawrence, John H. "Early Experiences in Nuclear Medicine." *The Journal of Nuclear Medicine* 20, no. 6 (June 1979).

Leech, Margaret. *In the Days of McKinley.* New York: Harper & Brothers Publishers, 1959.

Lemagny, Jean-Claude, and André Rouille, eds. Trans. Janet Lloyd. *A History of Photography: Social and Cultural Perspectives.* Cambridge: Cambridge University Press, 1987.

Leonard, Charles Lester. "The Past, Present, and Future of the Roentgen Ray." *American Medicine* 10, no. 25 (December 1905).

Leopold, George. "Seeing With Sound," *Radiology* 175 (April 1990).

Lerner, Barron H. "The Perils of 'X-ray Vision': How Radiation Images Have Historically Influenced Perception." *Perspectives in Biology and Medicine* 35, no. 3 (spring 1992).

Les Prix Nobel, 1979. Stockholm: The Nobel Foundation, 1980.

Lesser, May H. *The Art of Medicine at the 21st Century.* National Library of Medicine, National Institutes of Health, January-March 1994.

———. *An Artist in the University Medical Center.* New Orleans: Tulane University Press, 1989.

Levi, Hilde. *George de Hevesy: Life and Work.* Bristol: Adam Hilger Ltd., 1985.

Lindahl, Robert M. "Spiral Gives CTR Boost in Race Against MRI." *Diagnostic Imaging* (November 1993).

Lindegaard-Anderson, Asger, and Leig Gerward. "Roentgen Centenary—100 Years of X-rays." *Radiation, Physics, and Chemistry* 46, no. 3 (1995).

Ljunggren, Bengt. "The Case of George Gershwin." *Neurosurgery* 10, no. 6 (1982).

Love, Susan M. *Dr. Susan Love's Breast Book.* Reading, Mass.: Addison-Wesley, 1991.

Lowe, Sarah M. *Frida Kahlo.* New York: Universe Publishing, 1991.

Luckett, W. H. "Air in the Ventricles of the Brain Following a Fracture of the Skull." In *Classic Descriptions in Diagnostic Roentgenology,* ed. Andre Johannes Bruwer. Springfield, Ill.: Charles C. Thomas, 1964.

Mackenzie, Catherine. *Alexander Graham Bell, The Man Who Contracted Space.* Boston: Houghton Mifflin, 1928.

MacMeal, Harry B. *The Story of Independent Telephony.* Chicago: Independent Pioneer Telephone Association, [1934?].

McShine, Kynaston, ed. *Andy Warhol: A Retrospective.* New York: The Museum of Modern Art, 1989.

Manges, Willis F. "Military Roentgenology." In *The Science of Radiology,* ed. Otto Glasser. Springfield, Ill.: Charles C. Thomas, 1933.

Margulis, Alexander, and Ronald Eisenberg. "Gastrointestinal Radiology from the Time of Walter B. Cannon to the 21st Century." *Radiology* 178 (1991).
Martin, Emily. *Flexible Bodies.* Boston: Beacon Press, 1994.
Martin, Marianne W. *Futurist Art and Theory, 1909–1915.* Oxford: Clarendon Press, 1968.
Mees, C. E. Kenneth. *Dry Plates, Ektachrome Film: The Story of Photographic Research.* New York: Ziff-Davis, 1961.
Merton, Robert K. "Priorities in Scientific Discovery." *American Sociological Review* 22, no. 6 (December 1957).
Millard, Andre. *Edison and the Business of Innovation.* Baltimore: Johns Hopkins University Press, 1990.
Mitchell, Lisa M. "Making Babies: Routine Ultrasound Imaging and the Cultural Construction of the Fetus in Montreal, Canada." Ph.D. diss., Case Western Reserve University, 1993.
Morgan, Russel H. "The Emergence of Radiology as a Major Influence in American Medicine." *American Journal of Roentgenology* 111, no. 3 (March 1971).
Morton, William J. *The X ray or the Photography of the Invisible and Its Value in Surgery.* New York: American Technical Book Co., 1896.
Mould, Richard. F. *A Century of X-rays and Radioactivity in Medicine.* Bristol: Institute of Physics, 1993.
Murphy, William A., Jr. "Radiologic History Exhibit." *Radiographics* 10 (1990).
Mutscheller, A. "Physical Standards of Protection Against Roentgen Ray Dangers," *American Journal of Roentgenology* 13 (1925).
Myers, William G. "The Anger Scintillation Camera." *The Journal of Nuclear Medicine* 20, no. 6 (June 1979).
———. "Bequerel's Discovery of Radioactivity in 1896." *The Journal of Nuclear Medicine* 17, no. 7 (July 1976).
———. "Hevesy Nuclear Medicine Pioneer Lecture." *The Journal of Nuclear Medicine* 22, no. 6 (June 1981).
———. "Hevesy Nuclear Medicine Pioneer Lecture—1979: George Charles de Hevesy: The Father of Nuclear Medicine." *The Journal of Nuclear Medicine* 20, no. 6 (June 1979).
Myers, William G., and Henry N. Wagner. "Nuclear Medicine: How It Began." In *Nuclear Medicine,* ed. Henry N. Wagner. H. P. Publishing Company, 1975.
Nash, Steven A., and Jorn Merkert, eds. *Naum Gabo: Sixty Years of Constructivism.* Munich: Prestel Verlag, 1985.
Nauman, James. "Pioneer Descriptions in the Story of X-ray Protection." In *Classic Descriptions in Diagnostic Roentgenology,* ed. Andre Johannes Bruwer. Springfield, Ill.: Charles C. Thomas, 1964.
Nazinitsky, Kenneth J., and Burton M. Gold. "Radiology—Then and Now." *American Journal of Roentgenology* 151 (August 1988).
Newhall, Beaumont. *Latent Image: The Discovery of Photography.* Garden City, N.Y.: Doubleday & Doubleday, 1967.
Nienaber, Christopher, et al. "The Diagnosis of Thoracic Aortic Dissection by Non-invasive Imaging Procedures." *The New England Journal of Medicine* 328, no. 1 (January 1993).
Nobel Lectures: Chemistry, 1942–1962. Amsterdam: Elsevier Publishing Company, 1964.
Numbers, Ronald L. "The Third Party: Health Insurance in America." In *Sickness and Health in America,* ed. Judith Walzer Leavitt and Ronald L. Numbers. Madison: University of Wisconsin Press, 1985.
Oakley, Ann. *The Captured Womb: A History of the Medical Care of Pregnant Women.* Oxford: Basil Blackwell Publishers, 1984.
O'Hara, F. S. "Looking Backward." *Radiography and Clinical Photography* 8 (1932).
Olby, Robert C. "Constitutional and Hereditary Disorders." In *Companion Encyclopedia of the History of Medicine,* vol. 1, ed. W. F. Bynum and Roy Porter. London: Routledge, 1993.
Opfell, Olga. *The Lady Laureates: Women Who Have Won the Nobel Prize.* Metuchen, N. J.: Scarecrow Press, 1978.
Pachnike, Peter, and Klaus Honnef, eds. *John Heartfield.* New York: Harry N. Abrams, 1991.
Pallardy, Guy. "Laboratoires Guerbet." *Journal de la Radiologie* 71, no. 4 (1990).

———. "Massiot." *Journal de la Radiologie* 70, nos. 6-7 (1989).

———. "A Propos de L'Histoire." *Journal de la Radiologie* 74 (1993).

Pallardy, Guy, Marie-José Pallardy, and Auguste Wackenheim. *Histoire Illustrée de la Radiologie.* Paris: Les Editions Roger Dacosta, 1989.

Palmquist, Peter E. "Elizabeth Fleischmann: A Tribute." In *Elizabeth Fleischmann: Pioneer X-Ray Photographer,* ed. Peter E. Palmquist. Berkeley, Calif.: Judah L. Magnes Museum, 1990.

———. "The Woman Who Takes the Best Photographs." In *Elizabeth Fleischmann: Pioneer X-Ray Photographer,* ed. Peter E. Palmquist. Berkeley, Calif.: Judah L. Magnes Museum, 1990.

Pancoast, Henry. "The Future of Radiology as a Medical Specialty." *The American Journal of Roentgenology and Radium Therapy* 30, no. 6 (December 1933).

Pasveer, Bernike. "Depiction in Medicine as a Two-way Affair: X-ray Pictures and Pulmonary Tuberculosis in the Early Twentieth Century." In *Medicine and Change: Historical and Sociological Studies of Medical Innovation,* ed. Ilana Lowy. Paris: John Libbey Eurotext, 1993.

———. "Knowledge of Shadows: The Introduction of X-Ray Images in Medicine." *Sociology of Health and Illness* 11 (December 1989).

Patton, Dennis D. "Roentgen and the 'New Light': Roentgen and Lenard." *Investigative Radiology* 27, no. 6 (June 1992).

Peabody, Dr. "Some Experiments and Conclusions in the Exact Measurement of X-Ray." *The American Quarterly of Roentgenology* 11, no. 3 (September 1910).

Perée, Albert. *Etude des Rayons Roentgen Appliqués Aux Expertises Medico-Legales.* Paris: G. Steinheil, 1897.

Peskin, Alan. *Garfield.* Kent, Ohio: Kent State University Press, 1978.

Pfahler, G. E. "Physiologic and Clinical Observations on the Alimentary Canal by Means of the Roentgen Rays." *JAMA* 49 (November 25, 1907).

Pflaum, Rosalynd. *Grand Obsession: Madame Curie and Her World.* New York: Doubleday & Doubleday, 1989.

Pillitteri, Adel. "OR Nursing 100 Years Ago: Nursing Care of President McKinley." *Today's O.R. Nurse* (December 1991).

Pizon, Pierre. *La Radiologie en France, 1896–1904.* Paris: L'Expansion Scientifique Française, 1943.

Plum, George E., Jr. "Ventriculography and Encephalography." In *Classic Descriptions in Diagnostic Roentgenology,* ed. Andre Johannes Bruwer. Springfield, Ill.: Charles C. Thomas, 1964.

Pollia, Joseph A. *Fundamental Principles of Alveoli-Dental Radiology.* New York: Dental Items of Interest Publishing Co., 1930.

Potter, Hollis E. "Diaphragming Roentgen Rays: Studies and Experiments." In *Classic Descriptions in Diagnostic Roentgenology,* ed. Andre Johannes Bruwer. Springfield, Ill.: Charles C. Thomas, 1964.

Proctor, Robert. *Racial Hygiene: Medicine Under the Nazis.* Cambridge, Mass.: Harvard University Press, 1988.

Proger, Samuel and Robert E. Paul. "Doctor Alice Ettinger: 'Grande Dame Extraordinaire' of Radiology." *Tufts Medical Alumni Bulletin* 43, no. 1 (winter 1982).

Quinn, Susan. *Marie Curie: A Life.* New York: Simon and Schuster, 1995.

Raeburn, Michael, ed. *Salvador Dali: The Early Years.* London: South Bank Center, 1994.

Ramsay, Norman F. "Early Magnetic Resonance Experiments: Roots and Offshoots." *Physics Today* (October 1993).

Ramsey, George H., and William Cornwell. "Cineroentgenology." In *Classic Descriptions in Diagnostic Roentgenology,* ed. Andre Johannes Bruwer. Springfield, Ill.: Charles C. Thomas, 1964.

Rauschenberg Overseas Culture Interchange. Washington, D.C.: National Gallery of Art, Prestel, 1991.

Ray, Man. *Self Portrait.* Boston: Little, Brown, 1963.

Reed, Harvey. "The X-Ray from a Medico-Legal Standpoint." *JAMA* (April 30, 1898).
Reiser, Stanley Joel, ed. *Medicine and the Reign of Technology.* Cambridge: Cambridge University Press, 1978.
Reiser, Stanley Joel, and Michael Anbar, eds. *Medicine at the Bedside: Strategies for Using Technology in Patient Care.* Cambridge: Cambridge University Press, 1984.
Robert Rauschenberg. Washington, D.C.: National Collection of Fine Arts, Smithsonian Institute, 1976.
Robert Rauschenberg: Boooster and 7 Studies. Los Angeles: Gemini G.E.L., 1967.
Roberts, John D. *The Right Place at the Right Time.* Washington, D.C.: American Chemical Society, 1990.
———. "Useful Knowledge about the Application of Nuclear Magnetic Resonance to Medicine." *Proceedings of the American Philosophical Society* 133, no. 4 (1989).
Rogers, Emory, Martin Packard, and James Shoolery. "The Origins of NMR Spectroscopy." Papers presented at the 25th Annual Meeting of the Industrial Research Institute, Inc., May 16, 1963.
Rojas-Burke, J. "Practical Matters with Henry N. Wagner, Jr., M.D." *The Journal of Nuclear Medicine* 32, no. 10 (October 1991).
Rosenberg, Charles E. *The Care of Strangers: The Rise of America's Hospital System.* New York: Basic Books, 1987.
———. *The Trial of the Assassin Guiteau.* Chicago: University of Chicago Press, 1968.
Rutkow, Ira M. "How American Surgeons Introduced Radiology into U.S. Medicine." *The American Journal of Surgery* 165 (February 1993).
Sanders, Roger Cobban. "The Story of Cecil Jacobson." Unpublished paper.
Sarton, George. "The Discovery of X-rays." *Isis* 26 (1936).
Schapiro, Rolf L. "Opinions of an Editor." *Journal of Computed Axial Tomography* 1, no. 1 (1977).
Schiebinger, Londa. *The Mind Has No Sex.* Cambridge, Mass.: Harvard University Press, 1989.
Schmutzler, Robert. *Art Nouveau.* New York: Harry N. Abrams, 1962.
Sergent, Justine. "Music, the Brain and Ravel." *Trends in Neurosciences* 15, no. 5 (1993).
Serwer, Daniel Paul. "The Rise of Radiation Protection: Science, Medicine and Technology in Society." Ph.D. diss., Princeton University, 1977.
Shapiro, Stuart H., and Stanley M. Wyman. "CAT Fever." *The New England Journal of Medicine* 294, no. 17 (April 1976).
Shaw, Joyce Cutter. *The Anatomy Lesson from Framework* 6, no. 2, 1993.
Shryock, Richard H. *American Medical Research: Past and Present.* New York: Commonwealth Fund, 1947.
Siegel, Ronald. *Whispers: The Voices of Paranoia.* New York: Crown Publishers, 1994.
Skinner, Edward H. "Accidents in Radiology." *American Journal of Medical Jurisprudence* 1, no. 2 (October 1938).
Smith, Francis. "NMR—Historical Aspects." In *Contributions a L'Historie de la Neuroradiologie Européenne,* ed. Emmanual Cabanis. Paris: Editions Pradel, 1989.
Sochurek, Howard. *Medicine's New Vision.* Easton, Pa.: Mack Publishing Company, 1988.
Speigel, Peter K. "The First Clinical X-Ray Made in America." *American Journal of Roentgenology* 165 (1995).
Stabile, Carol. "Shooting the Mother." *Camera Obscura* 28 (January 1992).
Stafford, Barbara Maria. *Body Criticism: Imaging the Unseen in Enlightenment Art and Medicine.* Cambridge, Mass.: MIT Press, 1993.
Starr, Paul. *The Social Transformation of American Medicine.* New York: Basic Books, 1982.
Stevens, Rosemary. *American Medicine and the Public Interest.* New Haven: Yale University Press, 1971.
Stewart, Alice. "Malignant Disease in Childhood and Diagnostic Radiation." *Lancet* (September 1, 1956).
The Story of X-Ray. General Electric Company, 1963.

Suits, C. G. "William David Coolidge." In *National Academy of Sciences Biographical Memoirs,* vol. 53. Washington, D.C.: National Academy Press, 1982.

Susskind, Charles. "The Invention of Computed Tomography." In *History of Technology,* ed. A. Rupert Hall and Norman Smith. London: Mansell Publishing, 1981.

Taylor, John. *Garfield of Ohio: The Available Man.* New York: Norton Publishing, 1970.

Taylor, Lauritson S. "Roentgen-Ray Protection." In *The Science of Radiology,* ed. Otto Glasser. Springfield, Ill.: Charles C. Thomas, 1933.

Teich, Mikulas, and Roy Porter, eds. *Fin de Siècle and Its Legacy.* Cambridge: Cambridge University Press, 1990.

Terry, Jennifer. "Lesbians Under the Medical Gaze: Scientists Search for Remarkable Differences." *The Journal of Sex Research* 27, no. 3 (August 1990).

Tibol, Raquel. *Frida Kahlo: An Open Life.* Albuquerque: University of New Mexico Press, 1993.

Tomkins, Calvin. *The Bride and the Bachelors: Five Masters of the Avant Garde.* New York: The Viking Press, 1962.

Trout, E. Dale. "Tubes and Generators." In *Classic Descriptions in Diagnostic Roentgenology,* ed. Andre Johannes Bruwer. Springfield, Ill.: Charles C. Thomas, 1964.

Trucchi, Lorenza. *Francis Bacon.* New York: Harry N. Abrams, 1975.

Tuddenham, William J. "Dark Adaptations." In *Classic Descriptions in Diagnostic Roentgenology,* ed. Andre Johannes Bruwer. Springfield, Ill.: Charles C. Thomas, 1964.

Tyler, Parker. *The Divine Comedy of Pavel Tchelitchew.* New York: Fleet Publishing Corp., 1967.

Valenstein, Elliot S. *Great and Desperate Cures.* New York: Basic Books, 1986.

Vallebona, Alessandro. "Three Dimensional Stratigraphic Examination, Part I." *American Journal of Roentgenology* 74, no. 5 (November 1955).

Vogel, Morris J., and Charles E. Rosenberg, eds. *The Therapeutic Revolution: Essays in the Social History of American Medicine.* Pennsylvania: University of Pennsylvania Press, 1979.

Wallace, Alfred Russel. *The Wonderful Century.* New York: Dodd, Mead and Co., 1899.

Waters, Charles A., Whitmer Firor, and Ira I. Kaplan, eds. *The Year Book of Radiology.* Chicago: The Year Book Medical Publishers, 1940.

Watkins, W. Warner. "Errors in X-ray Diagnosis of Industrial Injuries." *Radiology* 28 (1937).

Wayne, Cynthia. *Dreams, Lies and Exaggerations: Photomontage in America.* College Park, Md.: The Art Gallery, University of Maryland at College Park, 1991.

Weart, Spencer R. *Nuclear Fear.* Cambridge, Mass.: Harvard University Press, 1988.

Webb, Steve. *From the Watching of Shadows: The Origins of Radiological Tomography.* Bristol and New York: Adam Hilger, 1992.

———. "Historical Experiments Predating Commercially Available Computed Tomography." *British Journal of Radiology* 65 (1992).

Wehrli, Felix. "The Origins and Future of Nuclear Magnetic Resonance Imaging." *Physics Today* (June 1992).

White, Robert I., Jr. "Interventional Radiology: Reflections and Expectations." *Radiology* 162 (1987).

Whittemore, Gilbert F. "The National Committee on Radiation Protection, 1928–1960: From Professional Guidelines to Government Regulation." Ph.D. diss., Harvard University, 1986.

Willet, John. *Art and Politics in the Weimar Period: The New Sobriety, 1917–1933.* New York: Pantheon Books, 1978.

Wise, George. *Willis R. Whitney, General Electric, and the Origins of U.S. Industrial Research.* New York: Columbia University Press, 1985.

Withers, Stanford. "The Story of the First Roentgen Evidence." *Radiology* 17 (July-December 1931).

Wolf, Reinhart, and Jan Visscher. "Elvis Revisited." *American Journal of Roentgenology* 165 (1995).

Woodbury, David O. *Battlefronts of Industry: Westinghouse in World War II.* New York: John Wiley and Sons, 1948.

Young, I. R., et al. "Initial Clinical Evaluation of a Whole Body Nuclear Magnetic Resonance (NMR) Tomograph." *Journal of Computer Assisted Tomography* 6, no. 1 (February 1982).

Law and Policy

Anderson, Cerisse. "Brain Scan Deemed Admissible at Trial." *New York Law Journal* 208, no. 77 (October 1992).

Barley, Stephen Richard. "The Professional, The Semi-Professional, and the Machine: Computer Based Imaging Modalities in Radiology." Ph.D. diss., Alfred P. Sloan School of Management, 1984.

Bijker, Wiebe E., Thomas P. Hughes, and Trevor F. Pinch. *The Social Construction of Technological Systems: New Directions in the Sociology and History of Technology.* Cambridge, Mass.: The MIT Press, 1987.

Caplan, Lincoln. *The Insanity Defense and the Trial of John W. Hinckley, Jr.* Boston: David R. Godine Publishers, 1984.

Cho, Paul. "U.S. Department of Energy Program of Support for PET and Nuclear Medicine." In *Clinical Positron Emission Tomography,* ed. Karl L. Hubner. St. Louis: Mosby Year Book, 1992.

Convert, Babette. "The Construction of the 'Battered-Child Syndrome'. A Comparison Between Two Analytical Frameworks." In *Medicine and Change: Historical and Sociological Studies of Medical Innovation,* ed. Ilana Lowy. Paris: John Libbey Eurotext, 1993.

Cormack, Alan M. "EMI Patent Litigation in the U.S." Department of Physics and Astronomy, Tufts University.

Danzon, Patricia M. *Medical Malpractice: Theory, Evidence, and Public Policy.* Cambridge, Mass.: Harvard University Press, 1985.

Evans, K. T., and B. Knight. *Forensic Radiology.* Oxford: Blackwell Scientific Publications, 1981.

Evans, Ronald, and Ronald Evans, Jr. "Analysis of Economics and the Use of MR Imaging in the United States." *American Journal of Roentgenology* 157 (September 1991).

Figley, Melvin M., and Alexander R. Margulis. "The Impact of New Imaging Technology on Health Care, Research, and Teaching: An International Symposium." *American Journal of Roentgenology* 149 (December 1987).

Fitzpatrick, John J. "The Role of Radiology in Human Rights Abuse." *The American Journal of Forensic Medicine and Pathology* 5, no. 4 (December 1984).

Foote, Susan Bartlett. *Managing the Medical Arms Race.* Berkeley: University of California Press, 1992.

Freidson, Eliot. *Profession of Medicine: A Study of the Sociology of Applied Knowledge.* New York: Harper and Row, 1970.

Freiherr, Greg. "Vendors Formalize Case for Cost-Effectiveness." *Supplement to Diagnostic Imaging* (November 1994).

Garland, L. H. "The Interpretations of X-Rays in Court Hearings." *American Journal of Medical Jurisprudence* 1, no. 1 (September 1938).

Green, Jeffrey. "Combatting the High Cost of High-Tech." *Trustee* (August 1990).

Hagland, William D., and Corinne L. Fligner. "Confirmation of Human Identification Using Computerized Tomography (CT)." *Journal of Forensic Sciences* 38, no. 3 (May 1993).

James, A. Everette, Jr., ed. *Medical/Legal Issues for Radiologists.* Chicago: Precept Press and American College of Radiology, 1987.

Jennett, Bryan. *High Technology Medicine: Benefits and Burdens.* Oxford: Oxford University Press, 1986.

Linton, Otha, et al. "Education Programs of the American College of Radiology: Task Force on Pneumoconiosis." American College of Radiology, Reston, Virginia. Photocopy of talk to the 16th International Congress of Radiology, Singapore, 1994.

Marshall, Eliot. "The Politics of Breast Cancer," *Science* 259 (January 29, 1993).

———. "Search for a Killer: Focus Shifts from Fat to Hormone." *Science* 259 (January 29, 1993).

Mazziotta, John C. "The Use of Positron Emission Tomography (PET) in Medical-Legal Cases:

The Position Against Its Use." For a course directed by Vladimir Hachinsky, Controversies in Neurology, UCLA. Photocopy.
Mock, Harry E. "Medical Testimony." *American Journal of Medical Jurisprudence* 1, no. 2 (October 1938).
Moeller, Dade W. *Environmental Health.* Cambridge, Mass.: Harvard University Press, 1992.
Mohr, James C. *Doctors and the Law.* New York: Oxford University Press, 1993.
Mol, Annemarie. "What Is New? Doppler and Its Others. An Empirical Philosophy of Innovations." In *Medicine and Change: Historical and Sociological Studies of Medical Innovation,* ed. Ilana Lowy. Paris: John Libbey Eurotext, 1993.
Roberts, Edward B., et al, eds. *Biomedical Innovation.* Cambridge, Mass.: The MIT Press, 1981.
Solomon, Alisa. "The Politics of Breast Cancer." *Camera Obscura* 28 (January 1992).
Stark, David D. "Standards of Quality in Medical Research: Who Decides?" *American Journal of Roentgenology* 151 (November 1988).
Steinberg, Earl P., and Alan B. Cohen. *Nuclear Magnetic Resonance Imaging Technology: A Clinical, Industrial, and Policy Analysis.* Office of Technology Assessment, Health Technology Case Study 27. Washington, D.C.: Government Printing Office, 1984.
Stocking, Barbara, and Stuart L. Morrison. *The Image and the Reality: A Case Study of the Impacts of Medical Technology.* Oxford: Oxford University Press, 1978.
Thomas, William A., ed. *Symposium on Science and the Rules of Evidence.* Arlic, Va.: Arlic House, 1983.
United States Congress. Report of the Office of Technology Assessment, *Federal Policies and the Medical Devices Industry.* New York: Pergamon Press, 1984.
Wagner, Mary. "Medicare Payments for MRIs Promote Proliferation—GAO." *Modern Healthcare* (July 20, 1992).
Wilkinson, Richard. "MR: Profits Climb, Bad Debt Drops." *Hospitals* (November 5, 1987).
Wolf, Stewart, and Bedrock Bishop Bell, eds. *The Technological Imperative in Medicine.* New York: Plenum Press, 1981.

Fiction

Adams, Jack. *Nequa, or, The Problem of the Ages.* Topeka, Kans.: Equity Publishing Company, 1900.
Asimov, Isaac, ed. *Before the Golden Age.* Garden City, N.Y.: Doubleday, 1974.
Atherton, Gertrude. *Black Oxen.* New York: Boni and Liveright Publishers, 1923.
Bellamy, Edward. "With the Eyes Shut." In *The Blindman's World.* Boston: Houghton Mifflin, 1898.
Butler, Robert Olen. *They Whisper.* New York: Henry Holt, 1994.
Campbell, John W., Jr. "The Brain Stealers of Mars." In *Before the Golden Age,* ed. Isaac Asimov. New York: Doubleday, 1974.
DeLillo, Don. *White Noise.* New York: Viking, 1995.
Haldane, J.B.S. *Possible Worlds.* London: Chatto and Windus, 1927.
Harris, W. S. *Life in a Thousand Worlds.* Atlanta: The Columbian Book Company, 1905.
Lewis, Sinclair. *Arrowsmith.* New York: Harcourt, Brace, & World, 1924.
Mann, Thomas. *The Magic Mountain.* New York: Knopf, 1925.
Manning, Laurence, "The Man Who Awoke." In *Before The Golden Age,* ed. Isaac Asimov. New York: Doubleday, 1974.
Merrill, Albert Adams. *The Great Awakening.* Boston: George Book Publishing Company, 1899.
Ramsaye, Terry. *A Million and One Nights.* New York: Simon and Schuster, 1926.
Sprague de Camp, L. *The Wheels of If and Other Science-Fiction.* New York: Berkley Publishing Corp., 1949.

Medicine, Science, and Technology

Ackerman, Sandra. *Discovering the Brain.* Institute of Medicine. Washington, D.C.: National Academy Press, 1992.

Adams, J. Hume, J. Corsellis, and L. Dunchen, eds. *Greenfield's Neuropathology.* New York: John Wiley & Sons, 1984.
Alexander, Randall, et al. "Incidence of Impact Trauma with Cranial Injuries Ascribed to Shaking." *American Journal of Diseases of Children* 144, no. 6 (June 1990).
Alker, George J. "Computed Tomography in Neuroradiology." *New York State Journal of Medicine* (April 1978).
Amisano, Pietro. "Three Dimensional Stratigraphic Examination, Part II." *American Journal of Roentgenology* 74, no. 5 (November 1955).
Andreasen, Nancy. "Brain Imaging: Applications in Psychiatry." *Science* 239 (March 1988).
Anger, Hal. "Gamma-Ray and Positron Scintillation Camera." *Nucleonics* 21, no. 10 (October 1963).
Belliveau, J. W., et al. "Functional Mapping of the Human Visual Cortex by Magnetic Resonance Imaging." *Science* 254 (November 1991).
Bernardi, Bruno, et al. "Neuroradiologic Evaluation of Pediatric Craniocerebral Trauma." *Topics in Magnetic Resonance Imaging* 5, no. 3 (1993).
Bieze, Jordana. "CT Takes Roundabout Path to Faster Scanning." *Diagnostic Imaging* (November 1993).
Boutin, Robert D., Jonathan E. Briggs, and Michael R. Williamson. "Injuries Associated with MR Imaging: Survey of Safety Records and Methods Used to Screen Patients for Metallic Foreign Bodies Before Imaging." *American Journal of Roentgenology* 162 (January 1994).
Bracewell, Ronald N. "Image Reconstruction in Radio Astronomy." In *Image Construction from Projections,* ed. G. T. Herman, 81-104. *Topics in Applied Physics* 32 (July 1979).
Bradley, William G., Jr., ed. *Magnetic Resonance Test and Syllabus.* Reston: American College of Radiology, 1991.
Bradley, William G., Jr., and Graeme Bydder. *MRI Atlas of the Brain.* London: Martin Dunitz, 1990.
Brady, Thomas J., et al. "Future of MR Imaging Is Linked to Functional Imaging." *Journal of Magnetic Resonance Imaging* 2 (1992).
Brownell, Gordon, et al. "Positron Tomography and Nuclear Magnetic Resonance Imaging." *Science* 215 (February 1982).
Budinger, Thomas F., et al. "High Resolution PET for Medical Science Studies." Lawrence Berkeley Laboratory, University of California, September 1989. Photocopy.
Budinger, Thomas F., and Paul C. Lauterbur. "Nuclear Magnetic Resonance Technology for Medical Studies." *Science* 226 (October 1984).
Caffey, John. "On the Theory and Practice of Shaking Infants." *American Journal of Diseases of Children* 124, no. 1 (June 1972).
———. "The Parent-Infant Syndrome (Caffey-Kempe Syndrome); Battered Baby Syndrome." *American Journal of Roentgenology* 114, no. 2 (February 1972).
Chugani, Harry T. "The Application of PET and SPECT Imaging in Pediatric Neurology." In *New Trends in Pediatric Neurology,* ed. N. Fejerman and N. A. Chamoles. Proceedings of the 6th Congress of the International Child Neurology Association, Buenos Aires, Argentina, November 1992. Amsterdam: Excerpta Medica, 1993.
———. "Development of Regional Brain Glucose Metabolism in Relation to Behavior and Plasticity." In *Human Behavior and the Developing Brain,* ed. Geraldine Dawson and Kurt Fischer. New York: Guilford Publications, 1994.
———. "Metabolic Recovery in Caudate Nucleus of Children Following Cerebral Hemispherectomy." *Annals of Neurology* 36, no. 5 (1994).
———. "Positron Emission Tomography Study of Human Brain Functional Development." *Annals of Neurology* 22, no. 4 (October 1987).
———. "The Role of PET in Childhood Epilepsy." *Journal of Child Neurology* 9, supplement no. 1 (October 1994).
Chugani, Harry T., Michael E. Phelps, and John C. Mazziotta. "Metabolic Assessment of Functional Maturation and Neuronal Plasticity in the Human Brain." In *Neurology of Early Infant Behavior,* ed. Curt von Euler, Hans Forssberg, and Hugo Lagercrantz. Wenner-

Gren International Symposium Series vol. 55. New York: Stockton Press, 1989.

Conti, Peter. "Introduction to Imaging Brain Tumor Metabolism with Positron Emission Tomography (PET)." *Cancer Investigation* 132, no. 2 (1995).

———. "Synthesis of Carbon-11 Labeled Biological Molecules for the in Vivo Study of Biochemical Processes and Structure-Activity Relationships in Normal and Malignant Tissues." Ph.D. diss., Cornell University, 1985.

Conti, Peter, Jennifer J. Keppler, and James M. Hall. "Positron Emission Tomography: A Financial and Operational Analysis." *American Journal of Roentgenology* 162 (1992).

Convert, Babette. "The Construction of the 'Battered-Child Syndrome.' A Comparison Between Two Analytical Frameworks." In *Medicine and Change: Historical and Sociological Studies of Medical Innovation,* ed. Ilana Lowy. Paris: John Libbey Eurotext, 1993.

Cormack, Alan M. "Early Two-dimensional Reconstruction (CT Scanning) and Recent Topics Stemming from It." *Journal of Computed Tomography* 4, no. 5 (October 1980).

———. "My Connections with the Radon Transform." Paper presented at the conference "75 Years of the Radon Transform," Vienna, Austria, August 31-September 4, 1992.

———. "A Problem in Rotation Therapy with X-Rays." *International Journal of Radiation Oncology, Biology and Physics* 133 (1987).

Crease, Robert P. "Biomedicine in the Age of Imaging." *Science* 261 (July 1993).

Damasio, Antonio, and Hanna Damasio. "Brain and Language." *Scientific American* (September 1992).

Davis, Patricia C. "The Brain in Older Persons With and Without Dementia: Findings on MR, PET, and SPECT Images." *American Journal of Roentgenology* 162 (1994).

"Dementia: Treatable Causes." *Magnetic Resonance Update.* Squibb Diagnostics, 1993.

Donald, Ian. *Recent Advances in Ultrasound Diagnosis,* vol. 2. Amsterdam: Excerpta Medica, 1979.

Donaldson, S. W. "Roentgenogram as Evidence." *American Journal of Medical Jurisprudence* 1, no. 4 (December 1938).

"Echo-Planar MRI: Learning to Read Minds." *Science* 261 (July 1993).

Eleff, S., et al. "^{31}P NMR Study of Improvement in Oxidative Phosphorylation by Vitamins K_3 and C in a Patient with a Defect in Electron Transport at Complex III in Skeletal Muscle." *Proceedings of the National Academy of Science* 81 (June 1984).

Evans, K. T., and B. Knight. *Forensic Radiology.* Oxford: Blackwell Scientific Publications, 1981.

Fishman. Elliot K., et al. "Three-Dimensional Imaging." *Radiology* 1811 (1991).

Forsberg, David. "Quality Assurance in Teleradiology." *Telemedicine Journal* 1, no. 2 (1995).

Gershon, Diane. "Is There a Future for Clinical PET?" *Nature Medicine* 1, no. 6 (June 1995).

Gershon, Elliot, and Ronald Rieder. "Major Disorders of Mind and Brain." *Scientific American* (September 1992).

Ghosh, Pratik, David H. Laidlaw, Kurt W. Fleischer, Alan H. Barr and Russell E. Jacobs. "Pure Phase-Encoded MRI and Classification of Solids." *IEEE Trans. Med. Imag.* 14 (September 3, 1995).

Handley, Mark, et al. "The Infant Whiplash-Shake Injury Syndrome: A Clinical and Pathological Study." *Neurosurgery* 24, no. 4 (1989).

Harris, Julianna. "Illuminating Mysteries of the Brain." *UCLA Medicine* 11, no. 1 (spring 1990).

Harwood-Nash, Dreek. "Abuse to the Pediatric Central Nervous System." *American Journal of Neuroradiology* 13 (March/April 1992).

Helfer, Ray, and Ruth Kempe. *The Battered Child Syndrome.* Chicago: University of Chicago Press, 1969.

Herman G. T., and R. M. Lewitt. "Overview of Image Reconstruction from Projections." In *Image Construction from Projections,* ed. G. T. Herman. *Topics in Applied Physics* 32 (July 1979).

Hounsfield, Godfrey N. "Computed Medical Imaging." *Journal of Computed Assisted Tomography* 4, no. 5 (October 1980).

———. "Computerized Transverse Axial Scanning (Tomography): Part 1. Description of System." *British Journal of Radiology* 46 (1973).

Imaging Biological Function. Institute of Medicine. Washington, D.C.: National Academy Press, 1992.

"The Importance of X-ray in the Diagnosis and Treatment of Cancer." *Cancer News* (June 1947).

Isherwood, Ian. "Diagnostic Radiology." *International Journal of Radiation Biology* 51, no. 5 (1987).

Jack, Clifford R., Jr., Richard M. Thompson, R. Kim Butts, et al. "Sensory Motor Cortex: Correlation of Presurgical Mapping with Functional MR Imaging and Invasive Cortical Mapping." *Radiology* 190 (1984).

Jacob, Russell E., and Scott E. Fraser. "Magnetic Resonance Microscopy of Embryonic Cell Lineages and Movements." *Science* 263 (February 1994).

Jaffe, C. Carl. "Medical Imaging, Vision, and Visual Psychophysics." *Medical Radiography and Photography* 60, no. 1 (1984).

Jolesz, F. A. "MRI-Guided Interventions." In *The Coolidge Scientific Review* 2. Versailles, France: GE Medical Systems (November 1994).

Juades, Paula Kienberger. "Comparison of Radiography and Radionuclide Bone Scanning in the Detection of Child Abuse." *Pediatrics* 73, no. 2 (February 1984).

Kahn, Daniel, et al. "Diagnosis of Recurrent Brain Tumor." *American Journal of Roentgenology* 163 (1994).

Kanal, Emanuel, and Frank Shellock. "MR Imaging of Patients with Intracranial Aneurysm Clips." *Radiology* 187 (1993).

Kanal, Emanuel, Frank Shellock, and Lalith Talagala. "Safety Considerations in MR Imaging." *Radiology* 176 (September 1990).

Kanal, Emanuel, et al. "Survey of Reproductive Health among Female MR Workers." *Radiology* 187 (May 1993).

Kaufman, Leon. "Hardware Improvements Augment MRI's Utility." *Diagnostic Imaging* (January 1990).

Keyes, John W., Jr. "Perspectives on Tomography." *Journal of Nuclear Medicine* 23, no. 7 (1982).

Kienberger, Paula. "Comparison of Radiography and Radionuclide Bone Scanning in the Detection of Child Abuse." *Pediatrics* 73, no. 2 (February 1984).

Kim, Seong-Gi, et al. "Functional Imaging of Human Motor Cortex at High Magnetic Field." *Journal of Neurophysiology* 69, no. 1 (January 1993).

———. "Functional Magnetic Resonance Imaging of Motor Cortex: Hemispheric Asymmetry and Handedness." *Science* 261 (July 1993).

Kimme-Smith, Carolyn. "New and Future Developments in Screening-Film Mammography Equipment and Techniques." *Radiological Clinics of North America* 30, no. 1 (January 1992).

Kirschvink, Joseph L., et al. "Magnetite Biomaterialization in the Human Brain." *Proceedings of the National Academy of Science* 89 (August 1992).

Kleinman, Paul K., et al. "Investigations of Fatal Infant Abuse." *The New England Journal of Medicine* 320, no. 8 (February 1989).

Klucznik, Richard, et al. "Placement of a Ferromagnetic Intracranial Aneurysm Clip in a Magnetic Field with a Fatal Outcome." *Radiology* 187 (June 1993).

Kramer, Lynn D., et al. "Cerebral Cysticercosis: Documentation of Natural History with CT." *Radiology* 171 (1989).

Krels, Roland, et al. "Proton MRS in Children Resuscitated After Near-Drowning: A Possible Prognostic Indicator?" *Science of Magnetic Resonance in Medicine Book of Abstracts* 1 (1992).

Kwong, Kenneth, et al. "Dynamic Magnetic Resonance Imaging of Human Brain Activity During Primary Sensory Stimulation." *Proceedings of the National Academy of Science* 89 (June 1992).

Lassen, Niels, et al. "Brain Function and Blood Flow." *Scientific American* 239, no. 4 (October 1978).

Lauterbur, Paul C. "Cancer Detection by Nuclear Magnetic Resonance Zeumatography Imaging." *Cancer* 57, no. 10 (May 1986).

———. "Image Formation by Induced Local Interactions: Examples Emplying Nuclear Magnetic Resonance." *Nature* 242 (1973).

Ledley, R. S., G. Di Chiro and H. L. Twigg. "Computerized Transaxial X-ray Tomography of the Human Body." *Science* 186 (October 1974).

Leopold, George. "Seeing with Sound," *Radiology* 175 (April 1990).

Lindahl, Robert M. "Spiral Gives CTR Boost in Race Against MRI." *Diagnostic Imaging* (November 1993).

Mansfield, Peter, and P. K. Grannel. "NMR 'Diffraction' in Solids?" *Journal of Physics C: Solid State Physics* 6 (1973).

Mansfield, Peter, and P. R. Harvey. "Limits to Neural Stimulation in Echo-Planar Imaging." *Magnetic Resonance in Medicine* 29 (1993).

Mansfield, Peter, et al. "Volumar Imaging Using NMR Spin Echoes: EchoVolumar Imaging (EVI) at 0.1 T." *Journal of Physics E: Scientific Instrumentation* 22 (1989).

Mazziotta, John C. "Mapping Human Brain Activity In Vivo." *Western Journal of Medicine* 161 (1994).

Merten, David, et al. "The Abused Child: A Radiological Reappraisal." *Radiology* 146 (February 1983).

Meservy, Clifford, et al. "Radiographic Characteristics of Skull Fractures Resulting from Child Abuse." *American Journal of Roentgenology* 149 (July 1987).

Mettler, Fred A., Jr., and Robert D. Moseley, Jr. *Medical Effects of Ionizing Radiation.* Orlando, Fla.: Grune & Stratton, 1985.

"Multiple Sclerosis." *Magnetic Resonance Update.* Squibb Diagnostics, 1992.

Myers, William G., et al. "Use of Annihilation Radiation to Locate Positron Emitters." *The Journal of Nuclear Medicine* 7, no. 5 (May 1966).

"Nuclear Magnetic Resonance (NMR) Medical Diagnostic Device That Produces Pictures Based on Response of Atomic Nuclei to Magnetic Field Is Expected to Perform Significantly Better and More Safely than CAT Scanners." *New York Times* (November 28, 1982).

Ogawa, S., et al. "Functional Brain Mapping by Blood Oxygenation Level—Dependent Contrast Magnetic Resonance Imaging." *Biophysical Journal* 64 (March 1993).

Oldendorf, William. "Isolated Flying Spot Detection of Radiodensity Discontinuities—Displaying the Internal Structural Pattern of a Complex Object." *Biomedical Electronics* 8, no. 1 (January 1961).

———. "The Quest for an Image of Brain: A Brief Historical and Technical Review of Brain Imaging Techniques." *Neurology* 28, no. 6 (June 1978).

———. *The Quest for an Image of Brain: Computerized Tomography in the Perspective of Past and Future Imaging Methods.* New York: Raven Press, 1980.

———. "Some Possible Applications of Computerized Tomography in Pathology." *Journal of Computer Assisted Tomography* 4, no. 2 (April 1980).

Oldendorf, William, and William Oldendorf, Jr. *MRI Primer.* New York: Raven Press, 1991.

Oldendorf, William, Jr. "Spiral CT." *Decisions in Imaging Economics* 7, no. 2 (fall 1994).

———. "A Visionary Department: USC Radiologists Develop Advanced Technologies for Patient Care." *USC Medicine* (winter 1988).

Ordidge, R. J., Peter Mansfield, et al. "Real Time Movie Images by NMR." *British Journal of Radiology* 55, no. 658 (October 1982).

Pake, George E. "Nuclear Magnetic Resonance in Bulk Matter." *Physics Today* (October 1993).

Pennisi, E. "NMR Improvements Earn Chemistry Nobel." *Science News* 140 (October 1991).

Raichle, Marcus E. "Visualizing the Mind." *Scientific American* 270, no. 4 (April 1994).

Rao, S. M., et al. "Functional Magnetic Resonance Imaging of Complex Human Movements." *Neurology* 43 (November 1993).

Roberts, John D. "Useful Knowledge about the Application of Nuclear Magnetic Resonance to Medicine." *Proceedings of the American Philosophical Society* 133, no. 4 (1989).

Salzman, Edwin W. "Living with Parkinson's Disease." *The New England Journal of Medicine* (January 11, 1996).

Sato, Yutaka, et al. "Head Injury in Child Abuse: Evaluations with MR Imaging." *Radiology* 173 (1989).
Schapiro, Rolf L. "Opinions of an Editor." *Journal of Computed Axial Tomography* 1, no. 1 (1977).
Shatz, Carla. "The Developing Brain." *Scientific American* (September 1992).
Shellock, Frank. "Biological Effects and Safety Aspects of Magnetic Resonance Imaging." *Magnetic Resonance Quarterly* 5, no. 4 (1989).
———. "MR Imaging of Metallic Implants and Material: A Compilation of the Literature." *American Journal of Roentgenology* 151 (October 1988).
———. "The Safety of MRI." *JAMA* 261, no. 23 (June 1989).
Shellock, Frank, and John Crues. "Safety of MRI in Patients with Metallic Implants or Foreign Bodies." *Applied Radiology* (November 1992).
———. "Temperature Changes Caused by MR Imaging of the Brain with a Head Coil." *American Journal of Neuroradiology* 9 (March/April 1988).
Shellock, Frank, and Julie Swengros Curtis. "MR Imaging and Biomedical Implants, Materials, and Devices: An Updated Review." *Radiology* 180 (August 1991).
Shellock, Frank, and Emanuel Kanal. "Policies, Guidelines, and Recommendations for MR Imaging Safety and Patient Management." *Journal of Magnetic Resonance Imaging* 1, no. 1 (January/February 1991).
Shellock, Frank, et al. "Exposure to a 1.5-T Magnetic Field Does Not Alter Body and Skin Temperatures in Man." *Magnetic Resonance in Medicine* 11 (1989).
Shuman, William P. "The Poor Quality of Early Evaluations of MRI Imaging: A Reply." *American Journal of Roentgenology* 151 (November 1988).
Silverman, Frederic. "Unrecognized Trauma in Infants, the Battered Child Syndrome, and Syndrome of Ambroise Tardieu." *Radiology* 1004 (August 1972).
Skinner, Edward H. "Accidents in Radiology." *American Journal of Medical Jurisprudence* 1, no. 2 (October 1938).
Stark, David D. "Standards of Quality in Medical Research: Who Decides?" *American Journal of Roentgenology* 151 (November 1988).
Stark, David D., and William Bradley. "MRI of Hemorrhage and Iron in the Brain." In *Magnetic Resonance Imaging.* St. Louis: C. V. Mosby Co., 1988.
Stehling, Michael K., Robert Turner, and Peter Mansfield. "Echo-Planar Imaging: Magnetic Resonance Imaging in a Fraction of a Second." *Science* 254 (October 1991).
Stephens, Tim. "Manipulation of CT Data Brings Spiral Images Alive." *Supplement to Diagnostic Imaging* (November 1994).
Strauss, Ludwig, and Peter Conti. "The Application of PET in Clinical Oncology." *The Journal of Nuclear Medicine* 32 (1991).
Tancredi, Laurence, and Nora Volkow. "A Theory of the Mind/Brain Dichotomy with Special Reference to the Contribution of Positron Emission Tomography." *Perspectives in Biology and Medicine* 35, no. 4 (summer 1992).
Taveras, Juan M. "Nuclear Magnetic Resonance Imaging." *American Journal of Roentgenology* 139 (August 1982).
Torres, William. "Spiral CT Assists Liver, Kidney, Vascular Imaging." *Supplement to Diagnostic Imaging* (November 1994).
Volkow, Nora, and Laurence Tancredi. "Neural Substrate of Violent Behavior." *British Journal of Psychiatry* 151 (1987).
Wagner, Henry, and Peter Conti. "Advances in Medical Imaging for Cancer Diagnosis Treatment." Presented at the American Cancer Society National Conference on Advances in Cancer Imaging, New York, 1990. *Cancer* 67 (1991).
Wagner, Henry, et al. "Imaging Dopamine and Opiate Receptors in the Human Brain in Health and Disease." In *Biomedical Imaging,* ed. Osamo Hayaishi. Tokyo: Academic Press, 1986.
Walsh, David. "Deep Tissue Traumatism from Roentgen Ray Exposure." *British Medical Journal* (July 31, 1987), reprinted in *Health Physics* 38, no. 6 (June 1980).
Watkins, W. Warner. "Errors in X-ray Diagnosis of Industrial Injuries." *Radiology* 28 (1937).

Webb, Steve, ed. *The Physics of Medical Imaging.* Bristol and Philadelphia: Institute of Physics Publishing, 1988.

White, Robert I., Jr. "Interventional Radiology: Reflections and Expectations." *Radiology* 162 (1987).

Interviews

Interviews for this book were conducted with the following individuals, in person and by telephone. Taped interviews are designated by the letter T.

Herbert Abrams (T)
Richard Bing (T)
Douglas Boyd (T)
Ronald Bracewell (T)
William Bradley (T)
Thomas Brady (T)
Barbara Carter (T)
Peter Conti (T)
Alan Cormack (T)
Cynthia Corngold (T)
Raymond Damadian (T)
Agnes Denes (T)
David Ellenbogen (T)
Tori Ellison
Martin Harwitt
Sir Godfrey Hounsfield
Everett James, Jr.
John Jordan (T)
Emanuel Kanal
John Kassabian (T)
Leon Kaufman (T)
David Kramer (T)
Niels Lassen (T)
Paul Lauterbur (T)
Robert Ledley (T)
May Lesser
Sir Peter Mansfield (T)
John Mazziota
Steve Miller
Stella Oldendorf
William Oldendorf, Jr.
Michael Phelps (T)
Sheila Pinkel
Anne Roberts
John R. Roberts (T)
Bruce Rosen
Rolf Schild (T)
Joyce Cutler Shaw
Frank Shellock (T)
Fred Silverman (T)
Jay Singer (T)
Nina Sobell
Robert Stanley
Jay Stein (T)
Martin Weiss (T)
Samuel Williamson (T)

Index

(*Page numbers in italics refer to illustrations.*)

Aaron, Benjamin, 146
Acquired Immune Deficiency Syndrome (AIDS), 217, 258, 278
ACTA scanner, *see* Automatic Computerized Transverse Axial (ACTA) scanner
Acuson, 245
Adams, Jack, 118
AEC, *see* Atomic Energy Commission
agraphia, 103
agromeglia, 195
AIDS, *see* Acquired Immune Deficiency Syndrome
air as a contrast agent, 99, 100, 101, 104, 306
Akeley, Carl, 99
Albert Einstein Medical School, New York, 177–178
Allen, Woody, 172, 265, 317
Allman, John, 198
Altered States (film), 264, 315
Alzheimer's disease, 217; and MRI, 192, 194; and PET, 210, 216, *225*
Ambrose, James, 158–160, 161
American Academy of Railway Surgeons, 93
American Association for the Advancement of Science, 13
American Board of Radiology, 257
American Cancer Society, 253, 256, 317
American Civil Liberties Union, 265
American College of Obstetricians and Gynecologists, 243
American College of Radiology, 92, 161; accreditation program for mammography, 256, 317; establishment of, 85; and mammography, 253
American Genesis (Hughes), 4
American Institute of Electrical Engineers, 63
American Institute of Ultrasound in Medicine, 245
American Journal of Photography, 36
American Journal of Roentgenology, 57, 87
American Martyrs to Science through the Roentgen Rays, 48
American Medical Association (AMA), 59, 84; and mammography, 256; section Council on Radiology, 85, 307
American Missionary Institute, 58
American Radium Society, 92
American Registry of Diagnostic Medical Sonographers, 245

American Roentgen Ray Society (ARRS), 61, 87, 89, 92, 109; inaugural meeting, 84; membership, 85
American Sanatorium Association, 79
American Science and Engineering, 163, 185
American Women's Clubs, 121
amniocentesis, 228, 247, 313
Ampère, André, 16
Anatomy Lesson, The (Shaw), 292, *293*, 317
Anderson, Laurie, 295–296, 317
Anderson Hospital, Houston, 253
Andrews, E. R., 183
Andrews, Robert, 109
angiogram, 105–106
Antenatal and Postnatal Care, 243
Aragon, Louis, 131
Archaeology in Eden (Teplica), 283
Archives of Electrology and Radiology, 56
Archives of Radiology and Electrotherapy, 86
Archives of the Roentgen Ray, 86
Argonne National Laboratory, Ill., 211
Armstrong, Neil, 313
Army Medical Corps, 73
Arrowsmith (Lewis), 80, 307
ARRS, *see* American Roentgen Ray Society
art, and X-rays, 4, 6, 116–117, 141, 261–296. *See also* literature; motion pictures; paintings; photography; *individual titles of works*
Aschheim, Israel, 48
Atherton, Gertrude, 121, 307
Atkinson Morley's Hospital, Wimbleton, U.K., 156, *159,* 314
ATL, 245
Atomic Energy Commission (AEC): and availability of isotopes, 204, 205; and nuclear-related medicine, 141; and PET research, 211; and positron detector scanning, 208; and radiation protection, 254
AT&T Bell Laboratory, N.J., 198
attenuated rays, 20
Auden, W. H., 200
Autobiography (Rauschenberg), 271, 273
Automatic Computerized Transverse Axial (ACTA) scanner, 162, 165, 185, *314*
autoradiography, 206

back projections, 148
Bacon, Francis, 269–271, 270, 273, 313
Bacon, Roger, 14
Ballantine, Thomas, 234
barium, 70, 99
Barraud, Francis, 156
Battle of San Juan Hill, 69
Battle of the Marne, 72
Bauhaus School, 132
Bear, David, 169
Beatles, the, 156, 162, 300
Béclère, Antoine, 59, 67, 72, 79, 112
Becquerel, Antoine-Henri, 26, 27, 53, 305
Bell, Alexander Graham, 10, 17; and sound induction device, 11, 12, 13, 202, 305
Bell Laboratories, N.J., 163, 198
Bell Telephone Company, 10
Bellamy, Edward, 13
Bellevue Hospital, New York, 58
Berg, Hans, 111
Bergonie, Jean Alban, 52
Bethesda Naval Medical Center Hospital, 256
Bio-Medical Electronics, 151
Birth of Man with Homage to Michelangelo (Teplica), *282,* 283
Bismark, Otto, 89
bismuth, 67, 70, 99; subnitrate of, 51, 106
Black Oxen (Atherton), 121, 307
Bloch, Felix, 176, 177, 310, 311
Blood of the Poet, The (Cocteau), 140, 309
Blood Oxygenation Level Dependent (BOLD), 198, 316
Blue Cross, 92
Bocage, André Edmund Marie, 108, 109, 306
Boccioni, Umberto, 130
BOLD, *see* Blood Oxygenation Level Dependent
Bolt, Richard, 234
Booster (Rauschenberg), 271, 272, 273, 313
Boskirk, John Van, 69
Boston Dispensary, 111
Boston Medical and Surgical Journal, 51
Boston Tech, 63. *See also* Massachusetts Institute of Technology
Bouchard, Charles, 30, 67–68
Boyd, Douglas, 166, 316
Bracewell, Ronald, 163, 168, 169, 182, 312; and data strips, 158, 207; and mapping sunspots, 147–148
Brack, Viktor, 123
Brady, James S., 145, 146, 169, 315
Brady, Sarah, 146
brain, 225; and MRI, 193–197, 316; and PET, 216–221; and ultrasound, 233–234, 241, 310; using CT scanner on, 146, 149, 158–160, 161, *164;* X-rays, 36, 97–106, 122

"Brain Stealers of Mars, The" (Campbell), 118
Brainwave Drawing (Sobell), 315
Braque, Georges, 15, 124, 127
breast implants, 197
Breton, André, 131
Brinton, Christian, 129–130
British Journal of Radiology, 161
British Medical Journal, 53
Broadway, Len, 158, 162
Broken Column, The (Kahlo), 134, *135,* 311
bromide, 105
Brompton Hospital, U.K., 166
Brookhaven National Laboratory, N.Y., 208, 211
Brownell, Gordon, 208
Bruce, Ironside, 86
Buchsbaum, Monte, 215
Bucky, Gustav, 45, 64, 306
Bucky grid, 64–66, 306
Bucky-Potter grid, 108, 109; evolution of, 65–66, 306; variation of, 253
Budinger, Thomas, 208, 217
Buffet, Gabrielle, 126, 127
Bull, James, 158
Bull, William Tillinghast, 35, 36
Butler, Prescott Hall, 35, 36
Butler, Robert, 122

C tube, 74
Caffey, John, 193–194, 310
Caldwell, Eugene, 58
Califano, Joseph, 167, 171
California Institute of Technology (Caltech), Pasadena, 113; and cancer treatment, 141, 193, 198, 199; and MRI technology, 177
Call, Samantha A., 94
Call v. City of Burley, 309
Camp Greenleaf, Ga., 73
Campbell, John, 118
cancer, 52, 100; of the breast, 250–260, 306, 315; cure for, 80; detection of, 178, 184, *225;* and PET, 211–213, *214;* radiation-induced, 57, 89; treatment of, 70, 88, 141
Cannon, Walter Bradford, 70
Carbutt, John, 67
Carter, Jimmy, 167
Case Institute of Technology, Cleveland, 179
Cassandras, 124
Cassen, Benedict, 205, 310
CAT scanner, *see* computerized tomography (CT)
catheterization, 106, 308
cathode rays, 17, 24, 26, 55, 128
cathodography, 36
Cedars of Lebanon Hospital, Los Angeles, 102
Century of Progress Exhibition (Chicago, 1934), 111
certificate-of-need (CON) laws, 167, 189, 315
Cézanne, Paul, 208
Chamberlain, Edward, 112
Chamberlain, Mrs., *see* Green, Miss
CHAMPUS, *see* Civilian Health and Military Personnel
Chandler, Winthrop, 119
Chatte, La (ballet), 131
Chausse, M., 108, 306
chelates, 196
Chernobyl meltdown, 203
Chicotot, Georges, 250, *251*
child abuse, 193–194, 310
Children's Hospital of Michigan, Detroit, 219
Chronicle (London), 22
chronophotography, 15
Chugani, Harry, 217, 219, 220
cinemaradiology, 138
cinematography, *see* motion pictures
Civilian Health and Military Personnel (CHAMPUS), 221
Clark, Kathleen Clara, 269, 270, 271
Cleveland Clinic, 110, 163, 179
Cleveland University Hospital, 109
Clysson, William, 119
Cocteau, Jean, 131, 140, 141, 309
collimating, 64
Columbia University, New York, 25, 35, 47; and CT scanner design, 164. *See also* Presbyterian Hospital
Committee for the Study of Sex Variants, 122, 123, 309
Committee on Radiation Safety, 90
computerized tomography (CT), 38, 181, 184; compared to MRI, 173, 175, 183; cost of, 167–169; in court, 169–172, 315; as daughter technology, 1; evolution of, 2, 4, 5, 144, 145–155, 160–167, 208; and FONAR products, 186; health costs of exposure to, 193; leadership in, 185; market for, 155–160, 187, 210–211; and other daughter technologies, 221–227
computers, 3; development of, 5, 143, 147, 311; and X-rays, 4–5
Connell, Will, 137
Conti, Peter, 213
Coolidge, William David, 63, 64, 74, 306

Coolidge tubes, 99, 107; development of, 74–76; marketing of, 77, 79, 86; variation of, 113
Cormack, Alan, 157, 181, 182, 208; and CT development, 151–153, 245; EMI contact, 155, 165; and experimental scanner, 162, 168, 312; wins Nobel Prize, 169, 315
County General Hospital, Los Angeles, 226
Courbet, Gustave, 289
court system. *See* computerized tomography (CT): in court; positron emission tomography (PET): in court; X-rays: in court
Cox, John, 30
crime solving, *see* X-rays: in crime solving
Crookes, William, 16, 27, 119, 283, 304
Crookes tubes, 20, 24, 46, 118, 304; Edison's refinement in, 34; Lenard's refinement in, 17; and magnets, 26; popularity of, 16, 23
Crucifixion (Bacon), 270
cryptoscope, 35
CT, *see* computerized tomography
cubism, 124, 126, 130, 287
Culverhouse, Emily, 28
Cunnings, Tolman, 30, *31,* 305
Curie, Irène, *73,* 298; and artificial radioisotopes, 203, 309; and structure of the atom, 120–121; wins Nobel Prize, 72, 114, 309
Curie, Jacques, 298; and piezoelectricity, 27, 232, *304*
Curie, Marie Sklodowska, *73,* 232, 298; and cure for cancer, 80, 88; discovery of polonium and radium, 27, 70, 305; and handling of radioactive substances, 52–53; and mobile X-ray units, 72, 306; and structure of the atom, 120–121; wins Nobel Prize, 305
Curie, Pierre, 72, 298; discovery of polonium and radium, 27, 70, 305; effect of radium on, 52; and piezoelectricity, 27, 232, 305; wins Nobel Prize, 305
curie, 87, 308
Curie Institute, *see* Institute of Radium
Cushing, Harvey, 201–202, 308
Cushing's disease, 195
Cushman, C. R., *237*
cystic fibrosis, 247

Da Costa, James, 14, 83
dada, 132
Daguerre, Louis, 15
Dali, Salvador, 133
Dally, Clarence, 62; as Edison's assistant, 42; as "martyr to radiation," 47–48, 52, 305
Dally, Halls, 93
Damadian, Raymond: comparisons to, 184, 240; court suits of, 185–186; and NMR, 177–183, 187, 314; and superconducting magnet, 184, 189
Damasio, Antonio, 220
Damasio, Hanna, 220, 221
Dandy, Walter, 107, 149, 226; and use of air as contrast agent, 100–103, 306
Daniel, John, 47
Darrow, Karl, 213
Das ist das Heil, das sie bringen! (Heartfield), 139, *139*
Davis, David, 146, 161
Davis, Edward Parker, 62
Dean, Dizzy, 124
Degas, Edgar, 30, 124
Delacroix, Eugène, 136
DeLillo, Don, 266, 317
Delta scanner, 163, 165
Demoiselles d'Avignon, Les (Picasso), 125, *125,* 281, 305
Denes, Agnes, 278–281, 279, 315
Department of Health and Social Security (DHSS) (U.K.), 156, 158
Depression, 85, 91–92, 114
dermatitis, 49, *50,* 62, 89
Detroit Receiving Hospital, 255
Diaghilev, Sergei, 131
diagnosis and X-rays, 5
Diagnost-U, 253
diaphragm, 65
Diasonics, 185, 245
Diasonograph, *242*
Dieffenbach, Dr., 49
Dodd, Walter, 58
Donald, Ian, *242,* 243–244, 312
Donner Laboratory, Berkeley, 208, 211, 216
Doppler effect, 242, 243, 245, 312
Dow Chemical Company, 179
Down's syndrome, 247, 313
Downstate Medical School, New York, 177, 178
Dream, The (Kupka), 126–127
Du Pont, 110
Duchamp, Marcel, 126, 127, *128,* 132, 307
Duchamp-Villon, Raymond, 126, 127
Dudley, William L., 47, 51
Dufayel, M., 25
Dulcinea (Duchamp), 127
Dumit, Joseph, 216
Dürer, Albrecht, 278

Dussik, Friedreich, 233–234, 241, 310
Dussik, Karl, 233–234, 241, 310
Duncan, Isadora, 119

Eakins, Thomas, 136
Eastman Kodak, *see* Kodak
echoplanar MRI, 183, 197, 314
Edison, Thomas, 42, 62, 130, 179; attempts at brain X-rays, 99, 234; and cathode ray research, 17; and evidence of radiation, 47–48; marketing of fluoroscopes and X-ray units, 55; and phonograph, 13, 156, 305; and photography, 15; and portable X-ray units, 40; and X-ray machine construction, 33–38, 304
Edison Lamp Works, N.J., 47
Edler, Inge, 241, 312
Egan, Robert, 253, 312
Einstein, Albert, 65
Eisenhower, Dwight, 204
Eldridge, Dr., 49
Electrical and Musical Industries (EMI), 168, 183, 185; and CT development, 155–165, 181, 207, 208, 226, 300, 312, 314; and NMR research support, 184
Electrical Exhibition (New York, 1896), [illegible]
Electrical World, 22, 26
electricity, 16, 17
electron, 26
Electronic Numerical Integrator and Computer (ENIAC), 311
electrotherapeutics, 38, 49
XIth Surgical Congress (Paris, 1897), 70
Ellis, Havelock, 27
Ellison, Tori, 275–276, *276,* 278
Elvis Revisited with 3-D Spiral CT, 172
Emilia, queen of Portugal, 58
EMI, *see* Electrical and Musical Industries
emission, 204–205
encephalography, *101,* 306
ENIAC, *see* Electronic Numerical Integrator and Computer
Ernst, Richard, 182, 186, 314
Essay on the Shaking Palsy (Parkinson), 220
Ettinger, Alice, 111, 113, 114, 308
European Space Telescope, 163
Exner, Franz, 22
Experiments on Myself (Forssmann), 106
expressionism, 130

Family of Man (Nilsson), 286
Fantastic Voyage (film), 263, 313
Faraday, Michael, 16
Faraday House, London, 156
fast MRI (fMRI), 197–199; and BOLD contrast agents, 316; compared to other daughter technologies, 211, 223, 226, 227
Federal Health Planning Act of 1976, 167
Feld Ballet, 200, 261, 317
Feminine Mystique, The (Friedan), 229
Ferguson, Laura, *274,* 274–275, 278
film developments, 110–113
Firestone, Floyd, 233, 310
Fleischmann, Elizabeth: images compared to cubism, 125; as "martyr to radiation," 48, 52, 62, 305; X-ray facilities of, 40, 58, 84, 108, 113
Florensky, Pavel, 130
Fluorex, 112
fluoroscopy, 35, *37;* compared to daughter technologies, 225; examinations, *34,* 51, 139–140
FONAR Corporation, 179, 184, 185–186
Foot-O-Scope, 80
Ford, Betty, 256, 315
Forestier, Jacques, 103, 104, 306
Forssmann, Werner, 106–107, 308
Fourier transforms, 148, 158, 186, 312
Fowler, Joanna, 206, 314
Franklin, Dean, 243
French Academy of Sciences, 26
Freud, Sigmund, 27, 120, 122, 132
Friedan, Betty, 229
Friedlander, Robert, 55, 56, 57
From Beyond (film), 264
Fry, Francis, 235, 241
Fry, William, 235, 241, 310
Frye rule, 175, 215
Fuller, Loïe, 119
futurism, 130

Gabo, Naum, 131, 132, 273
gadolinium salts, 196
gamma radiation, 70
Garfield, James: assassination of, 9–10, 145, 298, 305; efforts to locate bullet in, 10–13, 42, 202
Garfield, Lucretia, 9
Garland, L. H., 94–95
Gaucher's disease, 276
Geiger, Hans Wilhelm, 87
Geiger-Muller counter, 87, 202, 205, 308
General Electric Company (GE), 187; and CT scanner, 148, 149, 164, 165, 245, 314
General Electric Company (GEC Ltd.), 57, 165
General Theory of Relativity, 120

George Washington Medical Center, Washington, 145, 161
George Washington University, Washington, 228
Georgetown University, Washington, 162
German Roentgen Society, 64
Gershon-Cohen, Jacob, 252, 310
Gershwin, George, 102, 103
Ghosh, Pratik, *190, 200*
Giacconi, Riccardo, 163
gigantism, 195
Girl Before a Mirror (Picasso), 133, *133,* 309
Glasgow Royal Infirmary, 138
Glasgow University, 23
Goodrum, Mamie, 81, 82, 83, 90
Goodspeed, Arthur, 24, 85
Gowing, Lawrence, 271
Gramophone Company, 156
Grant, W. W., 31, 32
Great Awakening, The (Merrill), 117
Green, Miss, 81–82
Grey, Alex, 283–284, *285*
Groote Schuur Hospital, Cape Town, 151, 157
Gros, Charles, 253, 310
Gross, Professor, 70

Haimes, Judith Richardson, 171
Haldane, J.B.S., 122
Halsted, William, 100, 250, 252
Hammersmith Hospital, U.K., 208
Hannah and Her Sisters (film), 172, 261, 265, 317
Harlem Hospital, New York, 97
Harper's Monthly, 13
Harris, W. S., 118
Hartley, Elizabeth Anne Hargreaves, 43, *305*
Harvard University, Cambridge, 49, 50, 51, 91, 178, 211, 249; and bismuth subnitrate experiments, 70; and cyclotron program, 152, 153; and NMR technology, 176
Hawks, Herbert, 25, 47, 58
Head Surrounded by Sides of Beef (Bacon), 269, *270,* 313
Health Care Finance Administration, 211
Health Insurance Plan of New York (HIP), 253
Hearst, William Randolph, 36, 118, 220, 233
heart X-rays, 106–107, 108
Heartfield, John, 137, *138, 139,* 309
hemispherectomy, 217, *218*
Henn, Christa, 289
Hennage, David, 152
Henry, George, 122
Henry, Joseph, 11, 16
Hertz, Helmuth, 241, 312
Herzfeld, John, *see* Heartfield, John
Heuter, Theodor, 234
Hevesy, George: and radioactive tracers, 71, 201–203, 207, 304; wins Nobel Prize, 311
Hickey, Preston, 87
Hide-and-Seek (Tchelitchew), 283, *284,* 311
Hinckley, John W., Jr., 145, 169–170, 315
Hirschfeld, Al, 257
Hitler, Adolf, 24, 111, 309; depiction in art, 137, *138*
Hitler Swallows Gold and Spouts Junk (Heartfield), 138, *138,* 309
Hoch, Hannah, 137
Hoffman, Edward, 209, 210, 219
Holder, George, 30
Holmes, Joseph, 236
Hôpital Edith Cavell, Paris, *73*
Hôpital Herald, Paris, 251
Hôpital Ténon, Paris, 68
Hospital of the Good Samaritan, Los Angeles, 161
Hounsfield, Godfrey Newbold, 184; and CT scanner, 155–163, 165, 166, 312; wins Nobel Prize, 168, 181, 209, 315
Howry, Douglas, 235–241, 243, 310
Hughes, Thomas, 4
Humphrey, Hubert, 240
Huntington Memorial Hospital, Pasadena, 165
Huntington's disease, 210, 216, 247
hydrocelphalus, 101, 102, 194
hyperphonogram, *233*

idiosyncrasy, 39, 46, 90, 307
impressionism, 30, 126
incandescent light bulb, 33–34
"Indomitable," 179, 184, 314
Industrial Revolution, 3, 24
influenza, 78
Inner Space (film), 263
Instinct Extinct? (Pinkel), *280,* 281
Institute of Electrical and Electronics Engineers (IEEE), 149
Institute of Radium, Paris, 72, 80, 88
Interactive Electroencephalographic Brainwave Drawing (Sobell), 294, *294*
International Commission on X-ray Units, 87
International Committee on X-ray and Radiation Protection, 88
International Conference on Radiology (London, 1925, Stockholm, 1928), 107, 306, 308

International Council of Scientific Unions, 86
International Protection Commission, 90
International Studio, The, 129
Internet, 293
Interscience Research Institute, Champaign, 235
Introspection III—Aesthetics (Denes), *279,* 280, 315
Invisible Man, The (Wells and films), 117, 141, 262, 305
iodine, 104–106

Jackson, Herbert, 61, 304
Jacobs, Russell, *190*
Jacobson, Cecil, 228–230, 248
Jamison, Kay Redfield, 267
Jarre, Hans, 140
Jefferson Medical College, Philadelphia, 62, 80, 250
John XXI, Pope, 105
Johns Hopkins Hospital, Baltimore, 100, 209, 228
Johnson & Johnson, 185
Johnston, George C., 61
Joliot, Frédèric, 114, 203, 309
Journal of Computed Axial Tomography, 169

Kachina Transform (Pinkel), *281*
Kahlo, Frida, 134, *135,* 273, 311
Kanal, Emanuel, 171
Karolinska Institute, Stockholm, 286
Kassabian, Mihran, *50,* 58–59, 62, 63; and heart X-rays, 106
Kaufman, Leon, 185, 186, 187
Kearney, Officer, 9
Kelley, Koett, 91
Kells, C. Edmund, 43, 48
Kelly, Elizabeth, 235, 241
Kelvin, Hughes, 245
Kelvin, William Thompson, Lord, 22
Kenerson, Vertner, 42
Kennedy, John F., 313
Kety, Seymour, 206
Kieffer, Jean, 109, 110, 308, 310
Kieffer laminagraph, 110, 310
kinetoscope, 16, 34
King, Rodney G., 175, 317
Kirlian, Semyon, 283
Kirlian, Valentina, 283
Kirlian photography, 283
Kirschvink, Joseph, 193
Kobrine, Arthur, 146
Kodak, 15, 55, 140; safety film, 110, 111, 308
Korean War, 179, 311, 312
Kuhl, David, 158, 168, 169, 184; and cross-sectional imaging, 153–155; invention of photoscan, 205–206, 207, 312; and PET scanning, 208, 209, 210, 314
Kundt, August, 17
Kupka, Frantizek, 126

laminagraphs, 110
Langevin, Pierre, 232, 306
Langmuir, Irving, 63
Larionov, Mikhail, 130
Lassen, Niels, 207, 314
Laue, Max von, 71, 307
Laurie Anderson MRI (Leibovitz), 295, *295,* 317
Lauritsen, Charles Christian, 113, 114, 308
Lauritsen, Sigrid, 113, 114
Lauterbur, Paul, 187, 240; and zeugmatography, 179–182, 183, 184, 186, 314
Lawrence, Ernest, 203, 308, 309
Lawrence, John, 203
Le Bon, Gustave, 119
Leborgne, Raul, 252–253, 310
Lechner, Ernst, 22
Ledley, Robert, 162, 185, 314
Le Fevre, Owen E., 31, 32, 95
Leibovitz, Annie, 295, *295,* 317
Leksell, Lars, 241, 312
Lenard, Philipp, 23, 186; and refinement of Crookes tube, 17, 18, 19; wins Nobel Prize, 24
Lenard-Roentgen rays, 23
Leonard, Chester, 47
Lesser, May, 290–292, *291*
leukemia, 62
Lewis, Sinclair, 80, 307
Life in a Thousand Worlds (Harris), 118
Life magazine, 247, 286, 313
Lima, Almeida, 105
Ling, Gilbert, 178
lipiodol, 103–104, 306
literature, 117–124
lobotomy, 105, 106
London, Jack, 118, 305
London School of Science, 117
Los Angeles Memorial Hospital, 113
Love, Susan, 254–255
Lovecraft, H. P., 264
Luckett, H. M., 97, 98, 99, 100, 306
Luddites, 124
Ludwig, Anna Bertha, *see* Roentgen, Anna Bertha

Ludwig, George, 234–235, 236
Lumière, Auguste, 15, 16, 25, 139, 305
Lumière, Louis, 15, 16, 25, 139, 305

McGill, A. G., 81
McGill University, Montreal, 30, 31
McKinley, William, 41–43, 145, 298, 305
Machlett, Robert H., 55, 57, 62
Machlett & Sons, 57
MacIntyre, John, 138–139
Magic Mountain, The (Mann), 79, 121, 307
Magie, Professor, 35
magnetic resonance imaging (MRI), 1, 2, 4, 5, 38, 118, 144, 173–175; and the brain, 193–197; developments in, 182–187; and fMRI, 197–200; magnets in, 189–193; marketing of, 188–189, 210–211; and nuclear magnetic resonance (NMR), 175–179; and other daughter technologies, 221–227; and surgery, 192; and zeugmatography, 179–182, 314
magnetic resonance spectroscopy (MRS), 199
magnetism, 16, 17, 189–193
magneto-encephalography (MEG), 301–302, 317
Malevich, Kazimir, 130
Mallard, John, 183, 184, 187
Mallinckrodt Institute of Radiology, St. Louis, 110, 161, 209, 310
mammography, 5, 225, 310, 312; accreditation program for, 317; development of, 250–260; magnification, 314
"Man Who Awoke, The" (Manning), 118
Man Who Fell to Earth, The (film), 264
Manhattan Project, 88, 204, 311
Mann, Matthew, 42
Mann, Thomas, 79, 121, 262, 307
Manning, Lawrence, 118
Mansfield, Peter, 182–184, 186, 197–199, 314
Mansurov, Pavel, 132
Marey, Étienne-Jules, 15, 127
Margulis, Alex, 185, 186, 187
Massachusetts General Hospital, Boston, 58, 153; and CT scanning, 160, 185; and MRI research, 198; and PET research, 208, 209, 211; and ultrasound research, 234
Massachusetts Institute of Technology, Cambridge, 50, 51, 63, 163, 208, 236; Acoustics Laboratory, 234; and ultrasound research, 235, 238, 310
Massiot, 109
mastectomy, 100
Mauguin, Jacques, 289
Mauguin, Veronique, 289
Maxwell, James Clerk, 16
Mayakovsky, Vladimir, 130
Mayer, Carol, 108
Mayo, Charles, 40, 240
Mayo, William, 40
Mayo Clinic, Rochester, Minn., 82, 240; and CT technology, 160, 161, 185; radiology course, 84
Mazziotta, John, 216
Mechanical Expression as seen through our own Mechanical Expression (Picabia), 127, *129,* 307
Mechanized Maternity (Rivera), 134
Medicaid, 188, 211, 221
medical applications, *see* X-rays: medical applications
Medical-Chirurgical College, Philadelphia, 58
medical imaging, 3, 5. *See also* X-rays
medical politics, 77–96
Medical Research Council (MRC), 156, 158, 165, 184
Medicare, 167, 211, 221; legislation, 188, 300, 315
Mellon Institute, Pittsburgh, 179
Memoirs of an Invisible Man (film), 263, 317
Memorial Sloan-Kettering Hospital, New York, 256
Merrill, A. A., 117
Metropolitan Home, 266
Metropolitan Museum of Art, New York, 278
Meyer, Ted, 276–277, *277,* 278
Michelangelo, 270, 283
Mies van der Rohe, Ludwig, 132
Miller, Lee, 137
Miller, Steve, *259,* 289, *290*
Millikan, Robert, 113, 114
Minnesota Foundation, 240
Mondrian, Piet, 269
Moniz, Egaz, 104–106, 308
Morton, William, 43
Moseley, H.G.J., 71, 307
motion pictures, 138–141, 262–265; first, 16, 25, 305
Mount Sinai Hospital, New York, 55
MRC, *see* Medical Research Council
MRI, *see* magnetic resonance imaging
MRI (dance), 200, 261, 317
MRI Film of an AIDS Patient (Lesser), 292
MRS, *see* magnetic resonance spectroscopy
Mudd, Seeley, 113
Muller, Herman, 308

Muller, Walter, 87, 90
multiple sclerosis, 194, 195, *196,* 298
Murphy Brown (TV series), 261, 265
Museum of Modern Art, New York, 283, 286
Mutscheller, Arthur, 89, 90, 306
Muybridge, Eadweard, 15, 16, 270
myelography, 104

Nafziger, Howard, 102
Napierkowska, Udnie, 127–128
National Academy of Sciences, 143
National Aeronautics and Space Administration (NASA), 147, 153, 168
National Breast Cancer Coalition (NBCC), 258
National Bureau of Standards, 88
National Cancer Institutes, 168; and CT research, 163; and mammograms, 253; and MRI technology, 178, 184; and ultrasound research, 239–240
National Committee on Radiation Protection and Measurement, 88
National Council on Radiation Protection and Measurements, 254
National Geographic, 217, 286, 287, 317
National Health Planning Act, 189
National Heart and Lung Institutes, 184
National Institute of Child Health and Human Development, 249
National Institute of General Medical Sciences, 240
National Institute of Mental Health, 206
National Institute of Neurological Diseases and Blindness, 206
National Institutes of Health (NIH), 156, 187, 206, 268; and CT technology, 146, 168; and MRI technology, 185; and PET technology, 211, 221; and ultrasound technology, 240–241
Nature, 181, 182, 287, 314
Naval Military Research Institute, Bethesda, 234, 235
Naval Observatory, 10
NBCC, *see* National Breast Cancer Coalition
Negro skin bleaching, 49
Nequa (Adams), 118
Neue Freie Presse (Vienna), 22
neurobiology, 103
Newcomb, Simon, 10, 11
New England Journal of Medicine, 169, 220
New England Medical Center, Boston, 111
New Museum of Contemporary Art, New York, 284
New York Academy of Sciences, 289
New York Newsday, 200
New York Sun, 22
New York through an X-ray (Picabia), 128, 307
New York Times, 22, 169, 187, 257, 265
Niarchos, Philip, 288
Nichols, K. D., 204
Niepce, Joseph, 15
Nile Campaign, 39
Nilsson, Lennart, 286, 313
Nimura, Yasuharu, 242
NMR Specialities, 178, 180, 181
Nobel, Alfred, 23
Nobel Prize, 24, 72, 86, 113, 114, 169; in chemistry, 202, 311; first, 23; in physics, 27, 176, 305, 311; in physiology or medicine, 105–106, 168, 315
noise, 21
nuclear medicine, 26, 207, 301; and daughter technologies, 225; and PET, 5; radium as major component of, 70, 71
Nude Descending a Staircase (Duchamp), 127, *128,* 307

Oak Ridge National Laboratory, Tenn., 211
O'Dell, Mark, *190*
Offenbach, Jacques, 275
Ogawa, Seiji, 198, 316
Ohio Nuclear, 163
Oldendorf, William, 205; comparisons to, 153, 244; and CT research, 148–151, 155, 162, 168, 169; and CT scanner, 312
Oppenheimer, Robert, 113
Origine du Monde, L' (Miller), 289, *290*
Orme, George A. C., 45–46, 49, 305
Osaka University, 242–243
Oxford Instruments, 184, 186
Oxford University, 156

paintings, 124–135, 269–284
Pall Mall Gazette, 116
pallidotomy, 220
Pan American Exhibition (Buffalo, 1901), 41–42
Pancoast, Henry K., 49
Pap test, 258
Parental Induced Trauma (PIT), 193
Parker, Barrington D., 170
Parker, Betty, 91
Parker, Carl H., 84, 85, 91
Parker, Donald, 91
Parkinson, James, 220
Parkinson's disease, 209, 210, 220, *225,* 298
Pasadena Hospital, 84
Pasche, Otto, 64

Pathé, 110
Pauli, Wolfgang, 175
Payne Whitney Clinic, New York, 122
Peacock, Warwick, 217, 219
Pennsylvania Hospital, Philadelphia, 41, 82, 83
Perthes, George, 52
PET, *see* positron emission tomography
Peter Bent Brigham Hospital, Boston, 201
Peterson, Ryan, 217
petit curie, 72
Pevsner, Anton, 131, 273
Pevsner, Naum, *see* Gabo, Naum
Pfizer Corporation, 162, 185
Phelps, Michael, 209–210, 219, 314
Philadelphia General Hospital, 104
Philadelphia Hospital, 59
Philip's Skull (CAT Scan) (Warhol), 288, *288,* 317
Philips Company, 91, 253
phonograph, 13, 34, 305
photography: beginnings of, 14–16; commercial, 305; use of, 27; and X-rays, 136–138, 283–289
photomontage, 137
photomultiplier tube, 205
photoscan, 205, 312
Physical Institute, Munich, 23
Physical Institute, Vienna, 22
Physical Review, 176
Physico-Medical Society of Würzburg, 20, 304
Picabia, Francis, 125, 127–129, *129,* 134, 135, 307
Picasso, Pablo, 15, 124, 125, *125, 133,* 133–134, 281, 305, 309
Picker, James, 55
Picker X-ray Corporation, 57, 91, 109; and CT scanner, 154, 165; and mammography units, 253; and production of Coolidge tubes, 74; and safety film, 110; and ultrasound technology, 245; and X-ray equipment, 114
pied forcé, 40
Pierson, J. W., 107
piezoelectricity, 27, 232, 304
Pinkel, Sheila, *280, 281,* 281–282, 283
Pinto, Dr., 69
PIT, *see* Parental Induced Trauma
pixels, 143, 205
planigraph, 108, 110
Planned Parenthood v. Casey, 249–250
pneumoencephalography, 101, 102, 107, 226, 305
Poincaré, Henri, 22, 26
poison gas, 78
Poland, 27, 182
Pollock, Jackson, 269
polonium, 27, 70, 305
Pomona College, Claremont, Calif., 84
Portes, F., 108, 306
Portrait of Veronique Maxe (Miller), *259*
Positioning in Radiology, 269
positron, 204, 308
positron emission tomography (PET), 4, 5; and brain scanning, 216–221; and cancer, 211–213, *214;* in court, 214–216; machine development, 205–207; market for, 210–211; and nuclear imaging and SPECT, 207–208; and other daughter technologies, 1, 2, 144, 204–205, 221–227; and research, 208–210
Potter, Hollis E., 65, 306
Potter, Tina, 289
Practical Radiography (Ward), 92, 304
Pratt, Joseph, 111
Pregnancy (Grey), 284, *285*
pregnancy monitoring, 5. *See also* ultrasound: use in pregnancies
Presbyterian Hospital, New York, 84, 163, 185
Presley, Elvis, 172
Proceedings (of the Physico-Medical Society), 20, 22
Project Nina, 257
Psychic Energy System, 284
Public Health Service, 253
pulse-echo technique, 238
Punzo, James, 45–46, 49
Pupin, Michael, 25, 35, 36, 47
Purcell, Edward, 168, 176, 310, 311
Puvis de Chavannes, Pierre, 30

Queen & Company, 55–56
Queen Mary College, London, 182

Rabi, I. I., 176, 310, 311
RADAR, 156
radiation, 70, 82, *225;* -induced diseases, 4, 5, 46–53, 62, 123, 309; measures of absorption of, 151, 308; safety standards for, 4, 33, 77, 85–88, 254–255, 306
radioactivity, 27, 70, 305. *See also* radiation
radiograph, 22, 35
Radiological Society of North America (RSNA), 85, 87, 92, 161, 222, 253
radiologists, 77–96; affiliation with medical professionals, 83–85, 103; fees, 58, 84
Radiology, 153
radiotherapy, 88

radium, 119; discovery of, 27, 305; as occupational hazard, 52, 53, 123; as a tracer, 70; for treating and curing cancer, 88
Rampage (film), 215–216, 224, 261, 265, 317
Rand, Carl, 102
Rauschenberg, Robert, 271–273, *272*, 313
Ravel, Maurice, 102–103
Ray, Man, 137, 140, 283
rayograms, 137
Rayonnists, 130
RCA, 156
Reagan, Ronald, 145, 315
Realist Manifesto (Gabo), 131, 307
Red Cross, 72, 86
Reed, Harvey R., 92
Rees, Martin, 297
Reflectoscope, 233, 310
Rembrandt, 278, 280, 281
Renoir, Pierre Auguste, 124
Reproductive Genetics Center, Vienna, Va., 228
retrospectography, 39
Rib Cage with Spine (Ferguson), 274, *274*
Riemannian mathematics, 120
Riis, Jacob, 136
Rivera, Diego, 134
Roberts, John D., 177
Rockefeller, Happy, 256, 315
Roe v. Wade, 247
Roentgen, Anna Bertha, 17, 19, 116; X-ray of hand, 20, *21*, 22, 35, 38, 141, 262, 286, 297, 302
Roentgen, Wilhelm, *18,* 71, 131, 169, 179, 186, 278; discovery of X-rays, 1–2, 3, 17–27, 30–31, 33, 34, 47, 51, 54–55, 61, 67, 70, 86, 130, 162, 197, 232, 244, 262, 298, 304; wins Nobel Prize, 22, 305
roentgen, 87, 88, 308
roentgen rays, 23
Roentgen Rays and Electro-Therapeutics (Kassabian), 59
Roentgen Rays in Medicine and Surgery, The (Williams), 51
Roentgen Ray Society, 85
roentgenographs, 23, 24
roentgenograms, 23, 282
roentgenologists, 23, 59
Rollins, William Herbert, 50, 51, 57, 67; "Notes on the X-light," 52, 262, 304
Roosevelt, Theodore, 42, 43, 69, 298, 307
Royal Air Force (RAF), 156
Royal Marsden Hospital, London, 158
Royal Society of London, 27
RSNA, *see* Radiological Society of North America
Ruhmkorff coil, 18
Rumford Award, 86
Runyan, Dr., 82, 83
Runyan, Kirby, and Sheppard, 81
Runyan v. Goodrum, 307
Rush Medical School, Chicago, 84
Russell, Ethel, 104
Rutgers University, New Brunswick, 166
Rutherford, Ernest, 71, 87, 119, 201, 298

Sacred Mirrors (Grey), 284
Sagittal Series 1/10 (Lesser), *291,* 292
St. Elizabeth's Hospital, Washington, 170
St. Louis Post-Dispatch, 22
St. Luke's Hospital, Little Rock, 81, 82, 83
Salomon, Albert, 252, 306
Salvioni, Professor, 35
Salzman, Edwin W., 220
San Francisco County Hospital, 94
Sanders, Roger, 228–229
Satomura, Shigeo, 242, 312
Schellhammer, Raymond, 171
Schuster, Arthur, 22, 43–44
sciatica, 103
Science, 22, 204, 287
Scientific American, 26
scintiscanner, 205, 310
Scott, Gilbert, 99, 100
Senograph, 253
Seurat, Georges, 30
sexual repression, 28–30, 122
shadow, 21
Shattuck, F. S., 93
Shaw, Joyce Cutler, 292–293, *293,* 317
Shepp, Larry, 163–164, 168, 185
Sicard, Jan Athanase, 103, 104, 105, 306
sickle cell anemia, 247
Siemens, 162; and CT technology, 165; and mammography units, 253; and MRI technology, 185; and PET technology, 211, 223; and production of Coolidge tubes, 74; and ultrasound technology, 234, 241, 245; and X-ray technology, 55, 57, 304
signal, 21
Singer, Jay, 177, 312
Single Photon Emission Computed Tomography (SPECT), 207–208, 211, 225, 312, 314
skiascope, 35
Sky Garden (Rauschenberg), 271, 273
Sling Shots (Rauschenberg), *273*

Smith, James, 31, 32, 92
Smith v. Grant, 305
Smith-Kline Corporation, 243, 245
Smithsonian Institution, 11
Sobell, Nina, 293–295, *294,* 315
Sochurek, Howard, 286–287, 317
Society for Clinical PET, 221
Society for Psychical Research, 27
Soiland, Albert, 85, 114
Sokoloff, Louis, 206, 312
Sokolov, S. Y., 233, 308
somascope, 235, 310
SONAR, *see* Sound Navigation and Ranging
Sorbonne, Paris, 126
Sound Navigation and Ranging (SONAR), 233, 234, 235
sound waves, 12, 74, 232, 241–243
Southern California Edison Company, 113
Southern Dental Association, 43
Southwest Museum, Los Angeles, 282
Spanish-American War, 58; X-rays used in hospitals, 40, 46, 69, 108, 305
SPECT, *see* Single Photon Emission Computed Tomography
Spectral Cow, The (Dali), 133
Sperry, 245
spiral CT, 166–167, 316
spiritualism, 27
spot-film device, 111–113
Sputnik, 313
SQUID, 302
Standard X-ray Company, 91
Stanford University, 147, 166, 168, 176, 177
Stanley, Robert, 161, 162
State Institute of Artistic Culture (U.S.S.R.), 132
State University of New York, Stony Brook, 180
State X-ray and Radiological Institute (U.S.S.R.), 131
Stava, Robert, 109
Stein, Jay, 163, 164, 185
stereopticon, 68–69
stereoradiology, 69
sterilization, 52, 89, 123, 311
steriography, 107–108
Sternberg, George M., 40, 46
stethoscope, 13
Stewart, Alice, 230, 245, 312
Stewart, William, 97, 99
stratigraphy, 108, 308
Street and Smith Publications, 124
Structural Abnormalities (Meyer), 276, *277*
Superman, 124, 264, 311
surrealism, 132–133
Swanson, Kenneth, 170–171
Swanson v. U.S. Government, 315
Sweet, William, 208
Swinton, A. A. Campbell, 58, 112
Swiss Avalanche Research Center, Neuchâtel, 153
Syncor International, 223

Tainter, Sumner, 10, 11
Talbot, Fox, 15
Tales of Hoffman (Offenbach), 275
Taylor, Lauriston, 88, 90, 254
Tay-Sachs disease, 247
Tchelitchew, Pavel, 283–284, *284,* 311
Technical Manifesto of Futurist Painting, 130, 305
Technicare, 163
telephone, 10, 13, 305
teleradiology, 299, 317
Teleradiology Center, N.C., 299
television, 3, 5, 143, 156, 311
Temple University Hospital, Philadelphia, 171
Teplica, David, *282,* 282–283, 289
Terman, Lewis, 123
Ter-Pogossian, Michel M., 208–210, 314
Thatcher, Margaret, 184
Them (film), 264, 313
They Whisper (Butler), 122
Thomson, Elihu, 49, 50, 55, 304
Thomson, J. J., 26
Thomson-Houston, 55
Thorotrast, 105
"Thousand Deaths, A" (London), 118, 305
Time magazine, 111
Times (London), 22
Titanic, 12, 232
tomographs, 108, 152
tomography, 110, 112, 205, 306, 308
Toshiba, 185
Total Recall (film), 264
Townsend, Smith, 9, 10, 12
Tribondeau, L., 52
tuberculosis, 78, 79, *225*
tubes, 61–63, 67, 75, 87, 88; in art, 127–128, 135. *See also* cathode rays; Coolidge tubes; Crookes tubes
Tufts University, Boston, 111, 152, 153
Tulane University, New Orleans, 81
Turner, Joseph, 93

ultrasonic therapy, 5
ultrasound, 1, 2, 4, 5, 144; development of, 228–241; and FONAR products, 186;

market for, 243–246; and other daughter technologies, *225;* as seeing with sound, 241–243; use in pregnancies, 246–250
Union College, Schenectady, 148
United Shoe Machinery Corporation, 80
U.S. Department of Defense, 168, 257, 258
U.S. Department of Energy (DOE), 211
U.S. Food and Drug Administration (FDA); MRI approval, 188, 189, 191, 312; PET approval, 215, 221, 317
U.S. Supreme Court, 249–250
University of Alabama, 161
University of California, 49, 166, 177, 185, 186; at Berkeley, 203, 209, 210, 211; at Irvine, 215, 216, 223; at Los Angeles, 205, 211, 216, 217, 219, 252, 254; at San Diego, 292
University of Chicago, 151, 211, 266
University of Colorado Medical Center, 235, 243
University of Illinois, 182, 235
University of Indiana, 89
University of Iowa College of Medicine, 220
University of Kiel, 87
University of Lund, 241
University of Michigan, 211, 233
University of Minnesota, 198, 236
University of Minnesota Hospitals, 148
University of Neuchâtel, 153
University of Nottingham, 182, 183
University of Pennsylvania, 24, 47, 49, 153, 205; PET research at, 208, 211
University of Pittsburgh, 171
University of Rochester, 211
University of Southern California, 113, 223
University of Washington, 243
University of Wisconsin, 177
University of Würzburg, 17

Vallebona, Alessandro, 108, 109, 308
Van der Naillen School of Engineering and Electricity, San Francisco, 40
Van Gogh, Vincent, 278, 281
Vanderbilt University, Nashville, 47
Varian Associates, 156, 177, 179, 180, 182
ventriculography, 100, 101, 102, 107, 306
Victorian era, 14, 28, 32
Vietnam War, 313, 315
Vlieger, Marinus de, 241

Wagner, Henry, 208–209, 213
Waite, Henry, 55
Waite & Bartlett, 55, 57
Wallace, Alfred Russel, 22
Ward, H. S., 92, 304
Warhol, Andy, 288, *288,* 289, 316
Warren, Stafford, 252
Washington University, St. Louis, 110, 161, 209, 211
Weisberg, Ruth, 275
Wells, H. G., 117, 141, 262, 305
Wernicke's area, 220
West Point, 63
Western Roentgen Ray Society, *see* Radiological Society of North America (RSNA)
Western Union Telegraph Company, 11
Westinghouse, 91, 112, 114
Whistler, James, 30
White Noise (DeLillo), 266, 317
whole-body: MRI, 183, 184, 186, 314; PET, 211, *212;* scanner, 162–167, 185, 314
Wild, John, 236, 238–241, 243, 253, 310
Wilhelm II, emperor of Germany, 58
Williams, Francis H., 59, 93, 95; and chest X-rays, 79; concerns about radiation, 67; use of air as contrast agent, 98; use of goggles, 68; use of X-rays and sound, 50–51, 57
Williams College, Williamstown, Mass., 9
Willow Grove Naval Air Station, Philadelphia, 153
Wold, Alfred, 206, 314
Wold-Chamberlin Air Station, Minnesota, 236
Wolfe, John, 255
Woman Walking on the Boulevard (Larionov), 130
Wonderful Century, The (Wallace), 22
World War I, 232, 283, 307; ambulance units in, 31; influence on art, 132, 137; use of X-rays in, 54, 71–76, 77–78, 120
World War II, 182, 234, 252, 254, 257, 261, 286, 311; and development of atomic bomb, 204; and development of SONAR, 233; technological advances of, 5, 112
Wright, Arthur, 64

X-Dress (Ellison), *276*
X-light, 67
xeroradiography, 255–256, 281–282, 314
Xerox Corporation, 255, 281
X-rays: and the arts, 4, 261–296; chest, 78–79; compared to daughter technologies, *225;* in court, 6, 30–32, 77, 92–96, 305; in crime solving, 6, 43–46, 92, 305; daughter technologies, 1, 5, 143–144 (*see also* computerized magnetic resonance imaging; positron emission technology; ultrasound);

X-rays *(continued)*
dental, 43; discovery of, 9–24; exposure to (*see* radiation); future of, 297–302; in the imagination, 116–135; impact on diagnosis, 5, 27, 39, 59; machine refinements, 59–60, 99; medical applications of, 33–43; military use of, 39–41, 305, 307; in motion pictures, 138–141; and private and public property, 265–267; process of, 64–66; the public and, 24–30; in see-through photography, 136–137; and sexual repression, 28–30; shielding devices, 55, 57; slot machines, 25, 80; societies, 84–85; in story, 117–118; technical innovation 1897–1918, 54–76; technical innovation 1918–1940, 97–115; women in the field, 113–114
X-ray's Boy's Clubs, 25

Yale University, New Haven, 64
Year Book of Radiology, 95
Young, Ian, 183
Yvonne and Madeleine Torn in Tatters (Duchamp), 127

Zangwill, Israel, 27
Zehnder, Ludwig, 17, 19, 22
zeugmatography, 179–182, 314
Ziedes des Plantes, Bernard, 108–109, 308
Zola, Emile, 136

About the Author

Bettyann Holtzmann Kevles is a journalist and author who has written a science column and book reviews for the *Los Angeles Times.* Her own books include *Females of the Species* (1986), an exploration of sexual behavior in animals, and *Watching the Wild Apes* (1976), which won the New York Academy of Sciences Award for best science book for young adults. She is on the faculty of the Art Center College of Design in Pasadena, California, where she explores science with art students. She was a recipient of a grant from the Alfred P. Sloan Foundation, which supported research for this book. She lives in Pasadena with her husband.